ABT

…FOR DUMMIES
BESTSELLING BOOK SERIES

Herbal Remed… ies®

Cheat Sheet

Herbs for Easing Common Symptoms and Conditions

Symptom or Condition	Herbal Remedy
Allergies (hay fever)	Nettle herb, eyebright, cayenne, garlic, horseradish
Arthritis pain	Meadowsweet, ginger, cayenne, black cohosh, yucca, devil's claw
Bladder infections (cystitis)	Cranberry juice, marshmallow root, pipsissewa, uva-ursi, echinacea, usnea
Burns, scrapes, rashes, bites	Calendula cream, chamomile cream, St. John's wort oil
Colds	Echinacea, cayenne, garlic, ginger, osha, sage, yerba mansa, elder flowers and berries
Congestion, sinus	Cayenne, horseradish, eyebright, eucalyptus, ma huang
Coughs	Sage leaf, loquat leaf, licorice root, wild cherry bark, marshmallow root
Fatigue	American ginseng, red ginseng, rosemary, rehmannia, licorice, gentian
Gas, intestinal	Peppermint, chamomile, cumin seed, caraway seed, fennel seed
Headaches	Feverfew, wood betony, willow bark, meadowsweet
Infections of the skin	Echinacea, tea tree oil
Insomnia	Valerian, California poppy, chamomile, linden flower, kava
Memory (poor)	Ginkgo, rosemary, gotu kola
Nervous tension	Eleuthero (Siberian ginseng), valerian, California poppy, passion flower, hops
Sore throat	Sage leaf, echinacea, licorice, marshmallow
Stomachache	Ginger, peppermint, chamomile, gentian, centaury
Stress	Eleuthero (Siberian ginseng), California poppy, ligustrum, ashwaganda, schisandra

Herbal Superstars

The following herbal superstars are consistently the top-selling, most advertised, and most-talked-about herbal supplements on the market today.

- Bilberry
- Cranberry
- Echinacea
- Evening primrose
- Garlic
- Ginkgo
- Ginseng
- Goldenseal
- Grapeseed
- Kava
- Milk thistle
- St. John's wort
- Saw Palmetto
- Valerian

Herbal Remedies For Dummies®

…FOR DUMMIES
BESTSELLING BOOK SERIES

Cheat Sheet

Substitutes for Rare and Endangered Herbs

Herb	How You Can Help
American ginseng	Buy cultivated or woods-grown roots or products, instead of wild American ginseng.
Black cohosh	Substitute red clover products if you're using black cohosh for its estrogenic effects. Substitute kava or cramp bark if using this herb for muscle spasms. Substitute meadowsweet for arthritis.
Blue cohosh	Substitute yarrow.
Echinacea	Buy products containing *Echinacea purpurea,* which are cultivated organically, instead of wild-harvested *E. angustifolia.* Both are equally effective, in my experience. *E. angustifolia* is increasingly available as a cultivated herb.
Goldenseal	Buy cultivated goldenseal or substitute Oregon grape root, barberry, or the Chinese herb coptis, all of which contain the same active ingredient, called berberine.
Pipsissewa	Use uva ursi and marshmallow root together to soothe and help reduce bacteria for urinary tract infections.
Slippery elm	Substitute marshmallow root, which has similar soothing properties to slippery elm and is a cultivated herb.
Wild yam	Wild yam doesn't have progesterone-like effects, according to studies and historical use. Use wild yam only for bowel cramps, spasms, colic, and nausea, or substitute chamomile flowers.

Medication Substitutes*

Medication	Herbal Alternative
Pain reliever	White willow, meadowsweet
Daytime cold medication	Echinacea, goldenseal
Nighttime cold medication	Loquat syrup
Stomachache/gas reliever	Black walnut, chamomile
Sleep aid	Kava, valerian
Anxiety reliever	California poppy, kava
Anti-depressant	St. John's wort
Antibiotic	Usnea, goldenseal

**See your doctor or herbalist about persistent, serious conditions.*

Dosage Guide

Product	Dose
Teas	1 cup, 3 to 4 times throughout the day
Powdered herbs	2 to 4 capsules, 2 to 3 times daily
Tinctures	2 to 5 droppersful, 2 to 3 times daily
Standardized extracts	1 tablet, 2 to 3 times daily

IDG BOOKS WORLDWIDE

Cheat Sheet $2.95 value. Item 5127-2.
For more information about IDG Books, call 1-800-762-2974.

…For Dummies®: Bestselling Book Series for Beginners

Praise fo… …mies

"Here's an informative, engaging, well-researched introduction to herbal medicine by one of the nation's leading scientific herbalists."

— Michael Castleman, Author, *The Healing Herbs* and *Nature's Cures*

"Christopher Hobbs provides us with a very useful, definitive, and accessible introductory guide to the world of herbal medicine. From echinacea to St. John's Wort, this book presents an array of our best natural remedies with information on the herbs and on how to use them safely and effectively."

— James A. Duke, Medical Botanist (USDA, ret.) and Author of *The Green Pharmacy*

"*Herbal Remedies For Dummies* is no less than I would expect from Christopher Hobbs — spend a chapter with him and you know you've found a friendly, caring guide through the world of herbal medicine. He anticipates questions and provides concise, interesting answers that are nevertheless laced with thoughtful attention to detail. His botanical knowledge, combined with his expertise in medical systems and a talented way with words, make this book invaluable to all who care about their good health."

— Jan Knight, Editor, *Herbs For Health* magazine

"This is a useful and easy-to-read book for beginners by one of the most renowned herbalists in the United States. Christopher Hobbs packs in a wealth of herb information from explanations of the herbal revolution in health care; to helpful advice about safe use; to details of how to grow herbs, make tinctures and creams, and much more. Highly recommended."

— Robert S. McCaleb, President, Herb Research Foundation

"Lucid and authoritative, written by an acknowledged master herbalist, this book removes much of the confusion many consumers have about the complex world of herbal medicines. I've been reading and writing about herbs for almost 30 years and even I found some new information that I didn't know!"

— Mark Blumenthal, Founder and Executive Director, American Botanical Council; Editor, *HerbalGram*

"As a fourth generation botanist, Christopher Hobbs combines over 30 years of personal experience with extensive scientific study and research to contribute some of the finest texts available in the herbal field today. A gifted writer, consummate herbalist, botanist, and doctor of Oriental medicine, Hobbs firmly preserves the age-old wisdom of herbalism while imparting a contemporary flavor. Wisely written, warm, and graced with simplicity, *Herbal Remedies For Dummies* holds appeal for anyone interested in health and healing — from the novice looking for a safe and sane approach to the skilled health care professional looking for reliable guidance into the world of medical herbalism."

— Rosemary Gladstar, author of *Herbal Healing for Women*, Founder of United Plant Savers

Other Books by Christopher Hobbs

Women's Herbs, Women's Health, Botanica/Interweave Press (1998)

Handmade Medicines, Botanica/Interweave Press (1998)

Stress and Natural Healing, Botanica/Interweave Press (1997)

Saint John's Wort, The Mood Enhancing Herb, Botanica/Interweave Press (1997)

Saw Palmetto and The Men's Herbs, Botanica/Interweave Press (1997)

Botanical Safety Handbook, CRC Press (1997) (with M. McGuffin et al.)

The Ginsengs, Botanica/Interweave Press (1996)

Medicinal Mushrooms, Botanica/Interweave Press (1995)

Kombucha, Manchurian Tea Mushroom, Botanica/Interweave Press (1995)

Handbook for Herbal Healing, Botanica/Interweave Press (1994)

Valerian, The Relaxing and Sleep Herb, Botanica/Interweave Press (1993)

Foundations of Health, Botanica/Interweave Press (1992)

Ginkgo, Elixir of Youth, Botanica/Interweave Press (1991)

Vitex, The Women's Herb, Botanica/Interweave Press (1990)

Echinacea, The Immune Herb, Botanica/Interweave Press (1990)

The Echinacea Handbook, Botanica/Interweave Press (1989)

Natural Liver Therapy, Botanica/Interweave Press (1986)

Milk Thistle, The Liver Herb, Botanica/Interweave Press (1984)

Peterson Field Guide to Medicinal Plants of the Western U.S. (Houghton-Mifflin, in progress, with Steven Foster)

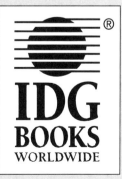

Herbal Remedies for Dummies®

HERBAL REMEDIES FOR DUMMIES®

by Christopher Hobbs, L.Ac.

IDG BOOKS WORLDWIDE

IDG Books Worldwide, Inc.
An International Data Group Company

Foster City, CA ♦ Chicago, IL ♦ Indianapolis, IN ♦ New York, NY

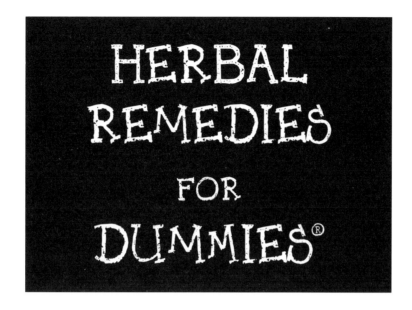

Herbal Remedies For Dummies®

Published by
IDG Books Worldwide, Inc.
An International Data Group Company
919 E. Hillsdale Blvd.
Suite 400
Foster City, CA 94404
www.idgbooks.com (IDG Books Worldwide Web site)
www.dummies.com (Dummies Press Web site)

Library of Congress Catalog Card No.: 98-88386

ISBN: 0-7645-5127-2

Printed in the United States of America

10 9 8 7 6 5 4 3 2

1B/QZ/QS/ZZ/IN

Distributed in the United States by IDG Books Worldwide, Inc.

Distributed by Macmillan Canada for Canada; by Transworld Publishers Limited in the United Kingdom; by IDG Norge Books for Norway; by IDG Sweden Books for Sweden; by Woodslane Pty. Ltd. for Australia; by Woodslane (NZ) Ltd. for New Zealand; by Addison Wesley Longman Singapore Pte Ltd. for Singapore, Malaysia, Thailand, and Indonesia; by Norma Comunicaciones S.A. for Colombia; by Intersoft for South Africa; by International Thomson Publishing for Germany, Austria and Switzerland; by Distribuidora Cuspide for Argentina; by Livraria Cultura for Brazil; by Ediciencia S.A. for Ecuador; by Ediciones ZETA S.C.R. Ltda. for Peru; by WS Computer Publishing Corporation, Inc., for the Philippines; by Contemporanea de Ediciones for Venezuela; by Express Computer Distributors for the Caribbean and West Indies; by Micronesia Media Distributor, Inc. for Micronesia; by Grupo Editorial Norma S.A. for Guatemala; by Chips Computadoras S.A. de C.V. for Mexico; by Editorial Norma de Panama S.A. for Panama; by Wouters Import for Belgium; by American Bookshops for Finland. Authorized Sales Agent: Anthony Rudkin Associates for the Middle East and North Africa.

For general information on IDG Books Worldwide's books in the U.S., please call our Consumer Customer Service department at 800-762-2974. For reseller information, including discounts and premium sales, please call our Reseller Customer Service department at 800-434-3422.

For information on where to purchase IDG Books Worldwide's books outside the U.S., please contact our International Sales department at 317-596-5530 or fax 317-596-5692.

For information on foreign language translations, please contact our Foreign & Subsidiary Rights department at 650-655-3021 or fax 650-655-3281.

For sales inquiries and special prices for bulk quantities, please contact our Sales department at 650-655-3200 or write to the address above.

For information on using IDG Books Worldwide's books in the classroom or for ordering examination copies, please contact our Educational Sales department at 800-434-2086 or fax 317-596-5499.

For press review copies, author interviews, or other publicity information, please contact our Public Relations department at 650-655-3000 or fax 650-655-3299.

About the Author

Christopher Hobbs, L.Ac., is a fourth-generation herbalist and botanist — his grandmother and great-grandmother were professional herbalists, and his father and great-uncle were professors of botany — with over thirty years experience with herbs. He studied acupuncture, Chinese herbs, and Chinese medicine at Michael and Lesley Tierra's East-West Acupuncture Program, Five Branches Institute of Traditional Medicine in Santa Cruz, and The Hangzhou School of Traditional Chinese Medicine in Hangzhou, China, earning his license in acupuncture in 1995. In 1989, he founded the American School of Herbalism in Santa Cruz, California (with Michael Tierra, O.M.D., L.Ac.) to educate professional and laypersons in the safe use of medicinal plants. He is currently the director of the Christopher Hobbs Clinic of Phytotherapy and Acupuncture, as a licensed primary health care provider in California.

In 1985, Christopher cofounded the American Herbalists Guild, the only national U.S. organization for professional herbalists, and along with David Winston and others, is a senior member on the admissions committee. As a consultant to the herb and natural foods industry, he was vice president and a board of trustee member of the American Herbal Products Association (AHPA) for seven years, has formulated many nationally-sold products as a consultant for a number of top companies. In 1984, he started a line of herbal products now known as Rainbow Light Herbal Systems. Christopher acts as director of herbal formulation for premium specialty brand Rainbow Light Nutritional Systems. He currently consults for the pharmaceutical and natural products industry and is a major contributor and herbal consultant to the successful herbal Web site, `www.AllHerb.com`. Christopher is a member of the Society for Medicinal Plants, the Society for Economic Botany, and the Society for Ethnobiology. He has lectured at Yale and Stanford Medical Schools; is a regular teacher at the University of California, Santa Cruz; and has taught at numerous schools, conventions, and symposia throughout the United States, Canada, Australia, and Europe. Christopher regularly contributes a clinic column in *Herbs for Health,* and his articles have appeared in *HerbalGram, Natural Health, Vegetarian Times, Let's Live*, and other national health magazines. Christopher is currently on the advisory boards of the American Botanical Council, United Plant Savers, *Let's Live* magazine, *Herbs for Health*, and other organizations and magazines. He owns one of the most extensive private libraries on medicinal plants, with over 6,000 volumes, including herb books that date from the 16th century. He is in the process of developing a 15-acre medicinal plant preserve and educational center called the *Living Farmacy* in Santa Cruz, California.

ABOUT IDG BOOKS WORLDWIDE

Welcome to the world of IDG Books Worldwide.

IDG Books Worldwide, Inc., is a subsidiary of International Data Group, the world's largest publisher of computer-related information and the leading global provider of information services on information technology. IDG was founded more than 30 years ago by Patrick J. McGovern and now employs more than 9,000 people worldwide. IDG publishes more than 290 computer publications in over 75 countries. More than 90 million people read one or more IDG publications each month.

Launched in 1990, IDG Books Worldwide is today the #1 publisher of best-selling computer books in the United States. We are proud to have received eight awards from the Computer Press Association in recognition of editorial excellence and three from Computer Currents' First Annual Readers' Choice Awards. Our best-selling *...For Dummies®* series has more than 50 million copies in print with translations in 31 languages. IDG Books Worldwide, through a joint venture with IDG's Hi-Tech Beijing, became the first U.S. publisher to publish a computer book in the People's Republic of China. In record time, IDG Books Worldwide has become the first choice for millions of readers around the world who want to learn how to better manage their businesses.

Our mission is simple: Every one of our books is designed to bring extra value and skill-building instructions to the reader. Our books are written by experts who understand and care about our readers. The knowledge base of our editorial staff comes from years of experience in publishing, education, and journalism — experience we use to produce books to carry us into the new millennium. In short, we care about books, so we attract the best people. We devote special attention to details such as audience, interior design, use of icons, and illustrations. And because we use an efficient process of authoring, editing, and desktop publishing our books electronically, we can spend more time ensuring superior content and less time on the technicalities of making books.

You can count on our commitment to deliver high-quality books at competitive prices on topics you want to read about. At IDG Books Worldwide, we continue in the IDG tradition of delivering quality for more than 30 years. You'll find no better book on a subject than one from IDG Books Worldwide.

IDG BOOKS WORLDWIDE

John Kilcullen
Chairman and CEO
IDG Books Worldwide, Inc.

Steven Berkowitz
President and Publisher
IDG Books Worldwide, Inc.

Eighth Annual Computer Press Awards 1992

Ninth Annual Computer Press Awards 1993

Tenth Annual Computer Press Awards 1994

Eleventh Annual Computer Press Awards 1995

IDG is the world's leading IT media, research and exposition company. Founded, in 1964, IDG had 1997 revenues of $2.05 billion and has more than 9,000 employees worldwide. IDG offers the widest range of media options that reach IT buyers in 75 countries representing 95% of worldwide IT spending. IDG's diverse product and services portfolio spans six key areas including print publishing, online publishing, expositions and conferences, market research, education and training, and global marketing services. More than 90 million people read one or more of IDG's 290 magazines and newspapers, including IDG's leading global brands — Computerworld, PC World, Network World, Macworld and the Channel World family of publications. IDG Books Worldwide is one of the fastest-growing computer book publishers in the world, with more than 700 titles in 36 languages. The "...For Dummies®" series alone has more than 50 million copies in print. IDG offers online users the largest network of technology-specific Web sites around the world through IDG.net (http://www.idg.net), which comprises more than 225 targeted Web sites in 55 countries worldwide. International Data Corporation (IDC) is the world's largest provider of information technology data, analysis and consulting, with research centers in over 41 countries and more than 400 research analysts worldwide. IDG World Expo is a leading producer of more than 168 globally branded conferences and expositions in 35 countries including E3 (Electronic Entertainment Expo), Macworld Expo, ComNet, Windows World Expo, ICE (Internet Commerce Expo), Agenda, DEMO, and Spotlight. IDG's training subsidiary, ExecuTrain, is the world's largest computer training company, with more than 230 locations worldwide and 785 training courses. IDG Marketing Services helps industry-leading IT companies build international brand recognition by developing global integrated marketing programs via IDG's print, online and exposition products worldwide. Further information about the company can be found at www.idg.com.

10/8/98

Dedication

I dedicate this book to my dad, Ken, who is very wise when it comes to knowing how to use herbs for staying healthy. He's 78 years young and still enjoys life thoroughly. A botanist and entymologist, he still likes to work and enjoys getting out in the field to collect plants and insects. Like so many other people over 60, my dad has had problems with his cardiovascular system. Fortunately, he's been taking hawthorn and ginkgo for years, and today his heart and cardiovascular system are in much better shape. My dad is the most steady and dedicated person I've ever seen when taking his herbs and the benefits are clear — his dedication more than anything else taught me how important it is to take herbs, regularly and for an extended time. I want to thank him for passing on his love of plants, insects, and the natural world; for his love of life; and, of course, for my life.

Author's Acknowledgments

I'd like to express my appreciation to my partner Beth for all her help with gathering and compiling information, editing, advice, good ideas, and emotional support. She's my grounding earth element and heart element.

I acknowledge the close members of my herbal family who have inspired me and helped carry the green wisdom for all these years. My deep love and respect go to Rosemary Gladstar, Michael Tierra, Cascade Anderson-Geller, Ed Smith, Sara Katz, David Winston, David Hoffmann, Kathi Keville, Steven Foster, Mark Blumenthal, Jim Duke, James Green, Roy Upton, Mindy Green, Rob McCaleb, and many more in our every-growing herbal family. I also acknowledge my teachers past and present, especially Paul Bragg, Carlos Castenada, Herman Hesse, Joanna Zhao, and Vivekananda.

Tere Drenth helped make writing *Herbal Remedies For Dummies* a pleasure and wonderful learning experience for style and clarity of writing. I want to express heartfelt appreciation to Tami Booth, our acquisitions editor, for her interest and excitement with herbs and natural healing. Thanks to Carol Roth for getting me together with IDG Books in the first place and for her valuable help in making the whole process more smooth. I am so fortunate to have D.D. Dowden provide the plant illustrations for this book. D.D. has a wonderful eye and feeling for plants and can express her vision magnificently on paper — she's a joy to work with. D.D., you're the best.

Darren Huckle, our farm manager, teacher of herbal cultivation, and gardener helped with the chapter on growing herbs at home. Thanks, Darren! A special thanks to David Hoffmann, one of the most dedicated, visionary, and influential herbalists in North America and other parts of the world. His keen eye for details, thorough knowledge of the scientific literature and of plant chemistry and pharmacology, coupled with his earth-centered and highly ethical and universal sense of herbalism and its importance for healing our Mother Earth, have been a valuable resource for this book.

Publisher's Acknowledgments

We're proud of this book; please register your comments through our IDG Books Worldwide Online Registration Form located at `http://my2cents.dummies.com`.

Some of the people who helped bring this book to market include the following:

Acquisitions and Editorial

Project Editor: Tere Drenth

Executive Editor: Tammerly Booth

Content Reviewer: David Hoffman

Editorial Manager: Mary C. Corder

Editorial Coordinator: Maureen Kelly

Illustrations: D. D. Dowden

Production

Project Coordinator: Regina Snyder

Layout and Graphics: Lou Boudreau, J. Tyler Connor, Angela F. Hunckler, Brent Savage, Rashell Smith, Kate Snell, Michael A. Sullivan

Proofreaders: Christine Berman, Kelli Botta, Rebecca Senninger, Ethel M. Winslow

Indexer: Sherry Massey

Special Help

Todd Fouty, Jonathan Malysiak, Heather Prince, Suzanne Thomas

General and Administrative

IDG Books Worldwide, Inc.: John Kilcullen, CEO; Steven Berkowitz, President and Publisher

IDG Books Technology Publishing: Brenda McLaughlin, Senior Vice President and Group Publisher

Dummies Technology Press and Dummies Editorial: Diane Graves Steele, Vice President and Associate Publisher; Mary Bednarek, Director of Acquisitions and Product Development; Kristin A. Cocks, Editorial Director

Dummies Trade Press: Kathleen A. Welton, Vice President and Publisher; Kevin Thornton, Acquisitions Manager

IDG Books Production for Dummies Press: Michael R. Britton, Vice President of Production and Creative Services; Cindy L. Phipps, Manager of Project Coordination, Production Proofreading, and Indexing; Kathie S. Schutte, Supervisor of Page Layout; Shelley Lea, Supervisor of Graphics and Design; Debbie J. Gates, Production Systems Specialist; Robert Springer, Supervisor of Proofreading; Debbie Stailey, Special Projects Coordinator; Tony Augsburger, Supervisor of Reprints and Bluelines

Dummies Packaging and Book Design: Patty Page, Manager, Promotions Marketing

♦

The publisher would like to give special thanks to Patrick J. McGovern, without whom this book would not have been possible.

♦

Contents at a Glance

Cartoons at a Glance

By Rich Tennant

"That should do it."

page 103

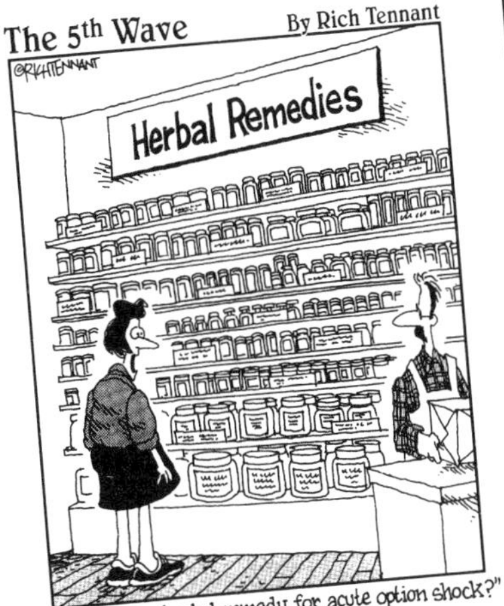

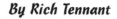

"Is there an herbal remedy for acute option shock?"

page 215

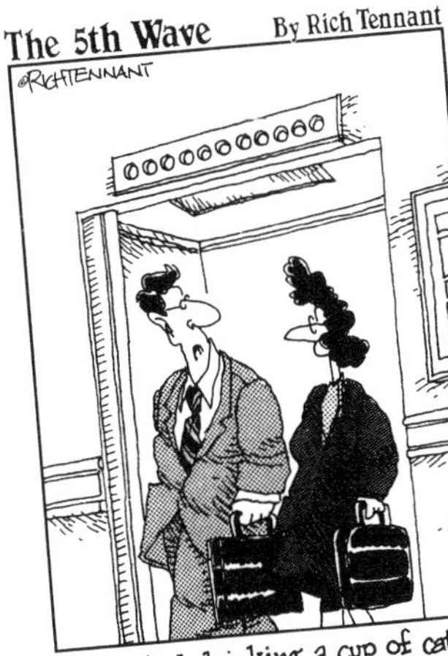

"I started drinking a cup of catnip tea to help me relax. It works fine, except I keep wanting to curl up on someones lap and take a nap."

page 191

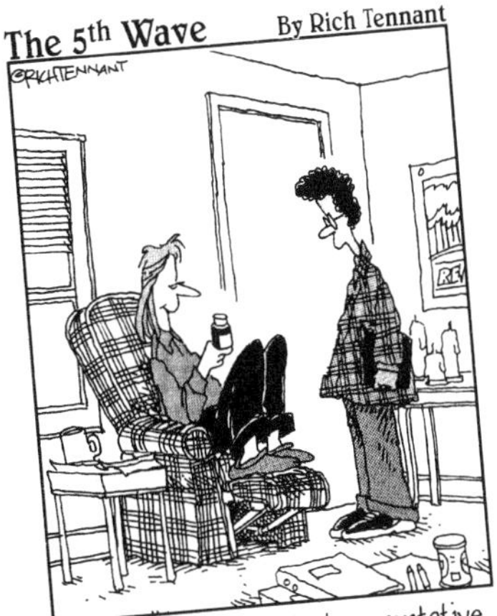

"Skunkweed has excellent preventative properties. It prevents guys from getting too close to me on first dates."

page 251

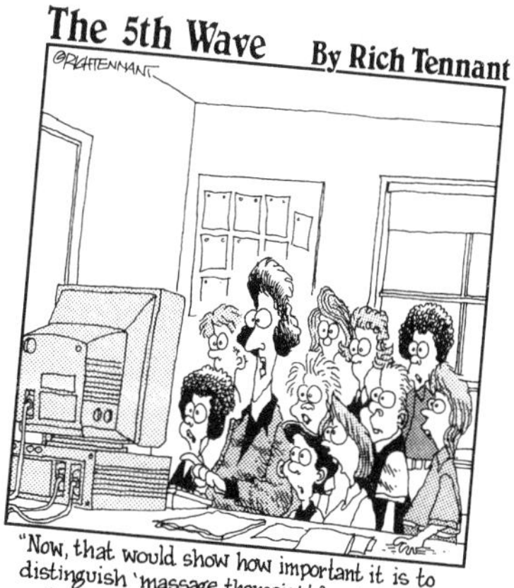

"Now, that would show how important it is to distinguish 'massage therapist' from 'massage parlors' when downloading a video file from the internet."

page 7

Fax: 978-546-7747 • E-mail: the5wave@tiac.net

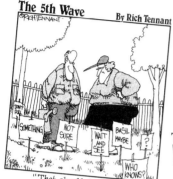

Recipes at a Glance

Products for External Use

Teas

More Products for Internal Use

Table of Contents

Introduction

If you're among the millions of people who don't seem to be getting well with traditional health care, have tried modern medical treatments unsuccessfully, or have experienced unpleasant (or even dangerous) effects from drug treatments, I invite you to try herbal remedies. This natural approach is a refreshing return to a healing art that was practiced long before the development of modern medicine and drugs. Using herbal remedies is a way of life — a celebration of the healing relationship with plants everywhere.

As a primary health care provider, I see many patients who aren't well-served by today's modern health care system — people who are often encouraged to depend on drugs and medical procedures to fix symptoms and conditions without any mention of the personal power they possess to create and maintain health. My experience shows me that people are likely to be healthier, happier, and more successful when they direct their own health care programs. This book gives you safe and effective herbal remedies and other natural means to ease your symptoms and prevent disease.

About This Book

The best way to experience the healing power of herbs is to actually use them, but reading about systems of herbal healing, how to take herbs, and what benefits herbs can bring is a good start. *Herbal Remedies For Dummies* helps you use herbs effectively and safely; discover the best herbal products for your own use; grow, harvest, dry, and store your own herbs; make herbal products at home — for yourself or for great gifts; and cook with common kitchen herbs.

In addition, along with this book, you get two bonus guides for quick reference. Flip to the *Symptom Guide* to look up any symptom or condition and obtain information on the best herbs to take. Then, check out the *Herb Guide* to get a full description (including an illustration) of each herb. Both are located in the green pages that are near the back of this book. The appendixes can help you, too, with a glossary, dosage table, and list of resources.

Be sure to read this!

The information in this reference is not intended to substitute for expert medical advice or treatment; it is designed to help you make informed choices. Because each individual is unique, a professional health care provider must diagnose conditions and supervise treatments for each individual health problem. If an individual is under a doctor's care and receives advice that is contrary to the information provided in this reference, the doctor's advice should be followed, because it is based on the unique characteristics of that individual.

How This Book Is Organized

Herbal Remedies For Dummies is an open door to the healing world of herbal remedies. My ultimate goal in this book is to help make herbal medicine accessible, clear, safe, and — most of all — useful. Whether you don't know a rose from rosemary or you've used herbs for years, this book gives you practical tips, recipes, and resources to help make your own natural health care serious fun, instead of just being serious.

Herbal medicine can be complicated and, without this book, you can easily get lost between the myriad of opinions and the bottles of tablets, syrups, and elixirs. *Herbal Remedies For Dummies* guides you each step of the way with practical advice and directions. And you don't have to start at the beginning — any page is a good place to start.

Here's how *Herbal Remedies For Dummies* is organized:

Part I: So, What Are Herbal Remedies, Anyway?

This part orients you to the fascinating world of herbs — the rich cultural flavor and the diverse systems of world healing. If you've explored every option that your doctor has and still find no relief from your symptoms, look in this part for an introduction to herbal products — a great way to experience the benefits of herbal remedies without having to grow, harvest, and make your own herbal medicines. From homeopathy to aromatherapy, herbal remedies come in many flavors. This part also leads you to the right remedy for kids, women, men, weekend warriors, and even pets.

Part II: Growing and Brewing Your Own Herbs

If you're eager to get your feet wet and your fingers into herbs, start with this part, where growing, processing, storing, cooking with herbs, and making your own products is much easier than you probably imagine.

This part helps you start a garden or window box so that you can grow your own immune-enhancing herbs, digestive aids, and energy-promoting herbs. From composting to sowing to harvesting, growing your own is easier than you may think. This part also helps you access the highest quality fresh and dried herbs for your needs. Find out how to harvest herbs, when to harvest them, and where to harvest the most potent plants. The drying, processing, and storing of herbs is a cinch with the information in this part, which also guides you through herbal medicine-making. Save money and get involved with your own health care in an entirely delightful process of smells and tastes. Make your own salves, tinctures, creams, teas, and extracts by consulting this part. Finally, this part is the place to look when you want to add the healing qualities of herbs to your favorite food recipes.

Part III: The Part of Tens

One of the most interesting, and certainly one of the most practical parts of *Herbal Remedies For Dummies* is the Part of Tens, where you get a series of "top-tens" about herbal remedies — ten reasons to take herbs, ten power herbs to take daily, and ten great teas to make.

Symptom Guide and Herb Guide

As an added bonus, this book contains two guidebooks, so you're getting three books for the price of one! The *Symptom Guide* is your compact sourcebook of natural healing programs for headaches, colds, flu, coughs, injuries, PMS, sore joints, and many other common symptoms. In this guide, you can find a description of each symptom and ailment described in terms that your doctor and herbalist may use, specific herbal remedies and simple herb formulas for each symptom that are time-tested for safety and effectiveness, and preparation and dosage guidelines. The *Herb Guide* gives you clear directions on how to use the top-selling and most-prescribed herbs for every health condition imaginable. This concise guide includes an A-to-Z listing of my favorite herbs, along with an illustration and description of each herb to aid you in identification, specific uses, the most effective kinds of extract or product to use, the exact dose instructions, and any possible side effects or problems to watch out for.

Appendixes

You can find three appendixes in this book.

Appendix A is a glossary of all of the herb talk you find in this book. Although all of the terms in Appendix A are defined somewhere in this book, you can use this glossary as a quick reference for tough terminology.

Appendix B gives you a dosage guide for the herbal remedies listed throughout this book. Simply look up an herb and Appendix B gives you the standard therapeutic dose.

Resources are especially important for the discovery and practical use of herbal remedies. In Appendix C, you can find information on purchasing herbs and equipment by telephone and online, journals and magazines for you to further your herbal education, and associations for more information or practitioner referrals.

Icons Used in This Book

Throughout the book, you can find icons that mark the vital information in your herbal education. Here's a listing of what they mean:

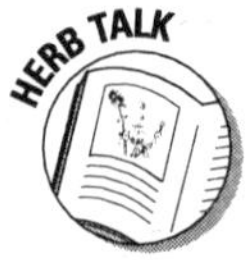

Although I try to keep jargon to a minimum, I use this icon to highlight special terms that herbalists use to describe certain aspects of the practice of herbal medicine. Using these terms will make you sound like an herbal guru in no time!

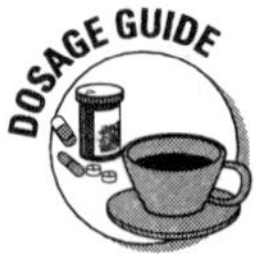

This icon helps you figure out how to take herbs, when to take them, and how often to take them.

Pay attention to these tips and ideas about how to use herbs safely and avoid rare, but unpleasant reactions. This icon also points out healthy habits (such as a balanced diet, exercise, and stress-relieving practices) to add to your herbal program for maximum effectiveness. Next to this icon, you can also find sources for herbal products.

This icon calls attention to the times that you want to talk to your doctor and get a complete diagnostic evaluation. Seeing your doctor helps you decide whether or not you're choosing the safest and most effective treatment program.

I use this icon to mark the times when you should visit an experienced herbalist. Whether you have doubts about taking herbs for any symptom or ailment, you feel you're experiencing side effects from herbs, or you have a chronic or acute condition that requires a strong or long-term course of herbal therapy, I always recommend seeking the advice of an herbalist.

I use this icon to point out tips and guidelines for using herbal medicines that you'll want to keep in mind long after you've finished this book!

A Word about Plant Names

Throughout this book, I use the common name of herbs to help identify each unique healing plant. Common names are sometimes confusing, though. For instance, depending on the state or region, three or four different herbs have the name *snake root.* To make sure of the identification and avoid confusion, herbalists often use the Latin name (also called a *binomial),* along with the common name. The Latin name always consists of two names — the *genus,* which is a group of related plants sharing many botanical and chemical characteristics, and the *species* name (also called specific *epithet),* which is the basic individual unit of the plant kingdom.

A genus consists of a group of closely-related species that share many features in common, but are often different enough so that when they cross-pollinate, a fertile seed isn't produced. Botanists and plant breeders use other names like *variety* and *sub-species* to describe small differences, such as flower color and leaf shape, between individual types of closely-related plants. When talking about herbs, herbalists don't pay too much attention to these subtle differences, but they do note the individual species, because certain species are more potent than others. A great example of an herbal genus that contains a few closely-related species that are still quite different is the genus *Mentha,* the mints. Though all mints help clear fever and ease stomach and digestive troubles, they all smell and taste quite different. Think of peppermint (*Mentha* x *piperita* L.), spearmint (*Mentha spicata* L.), and pennyroyal (*Mentha pelugium* L.). The capital letters or names at the end of the Latin name are an abbreviation of the botanist who first officially described the plant. In this case the Swedish botanist and physician Linneaus described all three mints, so you see the letter "L." The botanist or botanists names are known as the authority and help further clarify the exact and unique name for each plant.

Where to Go from Here

In this book, you can quickly and easily find every aspect of herbal healing, including how to use herbs correctly and safely — advice that's distilled from my thirty years of teaching, researching, experimenting, and practicing clinically with herbs. If the thought of making delicious *and* healing meals with kitchen spices appeals to you, turn to Chapter 6. How about choosing your own personal scent — for everyday use, for special occasions, or for filling your office with a relaxing or provocative smell that helps you focus and energize your mind? Flip to Chapter 3. Want more energy during your workouts, have a sick cat on your hands, or are tending to a child home from school with a fever? Browse through Chapter 4 and find fast herbal relief or flip to the *Symptom Guide,* in the green pages near the back of this book. In Appendix C, you can find suppliers of everything you may need (and a few things that you probably don't, but sound so interesting you may want to get them anyway!). So, dive in! Just pick a chapter and begin your herbal adventure.

For even more information about herbs, check out my Web site at `http://www.christopherhobbs.com`.

Part I
So, What Are Herbal Remedies, Anyway?

The 5th Wave By Rich Tennant

"Now, that would show how important it is to distinguish 'massage therapist' from 'massage parlors' when downloading a video file from the Internet."

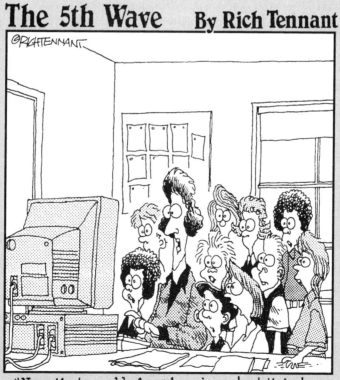

In this part . . .

Not long ago, many people thought of herbs as musty tea bags on the back shelves of health food stores or as brightly-colored roots and seeds in strange bottles lining the walls of dingy herb shops. Today, however, popular herbal medicines are advertised during prime time on national television — St. John's wort, echinacea, kava, and saw palmetto, just to name a few. Herbal medicine is big business in many countries, with sales in the billions of dollars, but it's also the medicine of the people. When you have trouble getting to sleep, you can grow valerian in your backyard, dig the aromatic roots, wash them, brew them, and drink a strong cup of tea before bedtime — all at a minimal cost, with no prescription or examination required.

If you don't choose to make your own herbal products, you can purchase all sorts of products to take internally from capsules and caplets to tinctures, syrups, and teas. For external use, choose from creams, salves, oils, and liniments. The only potential problem with all these interesting products is whether or not they are high-quality, and this part gives you guidelines for judging the quality of any herbal product.

This part also introduces you to herbal remedies, gives you suggested dosages, and describes the best herbs for women, men, kids, the elderly — even pets! And if you're interested in the aromatic side of herbs — aromatherapy — I've included a chapter for you.

So, what are you waiting for? If you want to know what herbal remedies are and how they can help you stay healthier, dive into Part I.

Chapter 1

Using (Not Abusing) Herbal Remedies

In This Chapter

- Choosing herbal remedies instead of pharmaceutical drugs
- Finding out how to use herbs for relieving symptoms and ailments
- Understanding dosage guidelines
- Finding a health care practitioner who is herb-friendly
- Discovering safe — and dangerous — herbs
- Understanding homeopathy

Unless you've been using herbs for years and feel comfortable dosing yourself with exotic tablets, capsules, and liquids, please read this chapter! Even if you feel comfortable with chamomile and friendly with feverfew, this chapter helps you gain a clearer understanding of how and when to use specific herbs for your personal needs.

In this chapter, I introduce you to herbal remedies and give you concise guidelines for using herbs every day. I also answer all of the burning questions that come up over and over again in classes and in my clinic — like which herbs to take for many common symptoms like fatigue and low back pain, how much of the herbs to take, when to take them, how long to take them, and what dosages to take. I also give you clear guidelines for determining the safety of the herbs you are using so that you can select the very safest herbs and teas.

How and Why Herbs Work

HERB TALK

Herbs work on many levels to help you maintain health or ease a troublesome or painful symptom. Modern science has expanded knowledge of herbs and their nature tremendously — people have begun to look deeply into these magic healers and discover the individual compounds that help make herbs work. Scientists can isolate and test some of these compounds in the laboratory and have discovered new ways to use herbs. Ginkgo nuts, for example, a traditional Chinese herb from the ancient tree from China (the maiden-hair fern tree called *Ginkgo biloba*), were an important cultural medicine for thousands of years. Today ginkgo has been rediscovered. German scientists have isolated compounds like *flavone glycosides* (from the leaves) that improve memory and brain function. Today, ginkgo leaf extracts are taken by millions, prescribed by doctors in Europe, North America, and even in China where it all began.

HERB TALK

Knowing the *active constituents* (active chemicals) in a plant helps scientists and manufacturers figure out exactly how to create the strongest herbal remedies, and herbalists how to use plant medicines effectively. An understanding of the toxic compounds in plants allows herbalists and doctors alike to help you avoid toxic reactions and side effects. The knowledge also helps farmers and manufacturers determine how best to grow plant medicines, when to harvest them, and how to extract them to maximize their potency. Knowing plant constituents also helps herbalists identify specific plants, check for authenticity of raw materials, and standardize herbal medicines to insure consistent activity.

The modern knowledge of medicinal plant constituents, pharmacology (the science that deals with the effects of herbs), and related sciences is revolutionizing herbal medicine today. Fortunately, you don't need to know that ginkgo contains flavone glycosides to use herbs effectively and safely. All the science, as well as all the wisdom of thousands of years of herbal use, are coming together now to give you access to the best natural herbal remedies in history.

Using Herbs as an Alternative to Drugs

Several years ago, doctors and medical researchers scoffed at herbal medicine as nothing more than quackery. When you disclosed, a little nervously, that you were using herbal remedies, the most enlightened docs said, "Well, it won't do anything, but at least it won't hurt you." The less enlightened believed that you were being swindled and might get sick or even die.

Herbs do more than heal your body

You can feel good about growing and using herbs for the benefit of all life on earth. Herbs deepen your appreciation of the natural world. By studying and maintaining your connection with healing plants, you gain a deep insight into the importance of caring for and protecting the wilderness. By going to an herb shop or drug store and buying a bottle of organically-cultivated echinacea tincture or capsules, you're voting with your dollars. You're saying, in essence, "I support natural medicine. I like that it's friendly to our earth; that it's sustainable; and that growing herbs, harvesting them, making medicines, and using them doesn't pollute the rivers and air I breathe. I appreciate that herbs don't pollute my bloodstream and internal environment. In fact, the herbs are a natural part of who I am. I'm continuing a long and honored relationship that has lasted for thousands of years."

Practitioners of modern medicine are savvy about what can go wrong in your body, and they attempt to mend problems with drugs, surgery, and other modern methods. However, in many countries, you don't go to your doctor when you get sick; instead, you go when you're well to get herbal remedies and advice on how to stay well. If you get sick, you stop paying!

Around the world, people use herbal remedies as an alternative to pharmaceutical drugs. While no medicine, natural or synthetic, is completely safe, herbal remedies are many times safer than pharmaceutical drugs. A recent study from the University of Toronto points out that pharmaceutical drugs are often not safe, even when used as directed. The study, which looked at the number of deaths from commonly prescribed medications in a hospital setting, reported shocking figures. The researchers who conducted the study concluded that even when prescribed properly, prescription drugs are between the fourth and sixth leading cause of death in the United States.

Drugs aren't inherently bad; in fact, they save lives. When my child has meningitis, give me the penicillin! (Even this life-saving drug comes directly from plants — it's purified and packaged from a fungus.) But using antibiotics repeatedly can cause harm. Any new drugs must now be developed to kill bacteria resistant to older antibiotics, because people overuse them, often for any minor infection, including viral infections like colds and flu that aren't helped by antibiotics. Herbs, on the other hand, have immune-supporting substances that help bolster the body's own natural resistance — the ultimate answer to antibiotic-resistant infections.

Ways that herbal medicine brings you total health

- Herb cultivation, processing, and product manufacture are sustainable processes that support the health of the natural environment.
- Growing medicinal herbs, shrubs, and trees adds oxygen to the air and removes waste products from the environment (by breaking them down).
- Herbal medicine is life-affirming and seeks to understand the causes of disease and how to maintain health of mind, body, and spirit.
- Herbs often smell good and taste good — the flavors and aromas enhance the enjoyment and digestion of your food.
- When used properly, herbs have few side effects.
- All things being equal, herbal medicine saves you money, especially if you grow and make some of your own herbal medicines.

Using Herbs for Acute Symptoms That Come and Go Quickly

Many symptoms and ailments are mostly *self-limiting* — that is, they eventually go away by themselves if the body is just given half a chance to heal itself. Good nutritious food, herbs, and plenty of rest and relaxation are the key ingredients of a successful health program.

If you've consulted with your doctor about on-going symptoms and either get no results or actually feel worse after taking drugs, herbs are worth a try. Do the following:

1. **Begin by choosing one or two herbs or one formula.** Match the symptoms you feel with individual herbs or a formula that sounds close to what you are experiencing. Refer to the *Symptom Guide* in the green-colored pages near the back of this book.

2. **Pay close attention to how you actually feel, as opposed to *how you think you feel* or what someone else says about your condition.**

   Be aware, too, that a diagnosis from a doctor is not conclusive or set in concrete — a diagnosis is only one piece of interesting information to start your healing journey. Notice actual symptoms without interpreting them. If you feel a headache, note where the pain is located and where it's coming from. If you feel an upset stomach, press on the area of the discomfort and feel it closely. Then proceed with the herbs.

3. **Start with a low dose — usually one-half of the recommended therapeutic dose that's listed in Appendix B.**

   Take this gentle dose for several days and then increase to a full dose if you experience no additional symptoms. You can go right to a full dose if you are using one of the extremely safe herbs listed in the "Choosing the safest herbs — safe-teas first" section (later in this chapter), or if you've used the herb before with no special reactions.

4. **Take the herbs regularly.**

   I can't stress often enough the importance of taking herbs regularly, especially for stubborn symptoms. How regularly depends on the condition. For symptoms that demand immediate attention, like a sudden case of nausea or pounding headache, take the herbs hourly or at least every few hours for most of the day, and before bed to try and ease the symptoms. If the condition is acute, but has been going on for up to ten days (like a cold or bronchitis), take the herbs every few hours for a week to ten days.

5. **Continue for a few days after symptoms are gone.**

   This helps ensure that they won't return.

Discovering Herbal Tonics for Chronic Ailments

For chronic symptoms that drag on and on or come and go, a different set of herbs are appropriate — the tonics. *Tonics* are herbs (and foods) that support and nourish the body's cells, tissues, and organs. They contain nutrients that the body needs like vitamins, minerals, and special large sugars and proteins called *polysaccharides* and *protein-bound polysaccharides* that help support proper immune function. Tonics are best taken as teas, dried teas, dried plant juices, or whole herb powders.

Many of the healing tonic properties of plants aren't compatible with alcohol or are destroyed by alcohol, so the popular concentrated alcoholic herbal extracts available in herb shops and natural food stores (called *tinctures*) aren't the best way to take tonic herbs. Most herb tonics need to be taken for at least one month and up to nine months to be fully effective — too long for many people to consume alcohol daily. The exception to this rule is *bitter tonics,* specific bitter-tasting herbs and herb blends that stimulate and invigorate the digestion, leading to more complete and pain-free absorption of nutrients and elimination of wastes.

Understanding ancient healing systems

Herbs have been used as medicine for thousands of years. Here are some examples of traditional, medicinal uses of herbs from around the world:

- *Traditional Chinese Medicine (TCM)* is a holistic system in every sense of the word. Unlike modern medicine, which looks at individual processes related to disease and how to use drugs to alter those processes to eliminate symptoms, TCM looks at the big picture — the TCM body organs are seen more as functional systems than anatomical ones. Looking at the body as an integrated whole with functioning organ systems allows subtle diagnosis and treatment of disease. A TCM practitioner can easily detect a budding anemia, where the blood is deficient and not doing all of its jobs, even before major symptoms occur. At this early stage, you can use herbs and diet to strengthen the blood before any damage to the body occurs.
- *Ayurveda* is an ancient East Indian system of healing. The system integrates diet therapy and herbal therapy with an active spiritual life, to create health and balance.
- The *Native American Indian* way of life honors plants and animals as important and necessary to the health of the entire planet. The health of the individual is dependent on living in harmony with nature, the seasons, plants, and animals.
- Modern *phytotherapy* is a synthesis of ancient principles of healing with the modern scientific knowledge of medicine, botany, chemistry, toxicology, and pharmacology. The system is oriented toward the modern practice of medicine, with its emphasis on disease, symptoms, and modern tests and procedures, but still manages to keep its healing roots, embracing traditional aspects of healing.

Take enough of the tonic to do some good. One cup of a strong herb decoction, morning and evening made with at least 2 ounces of herbs per day is the right amount. Concentrated extracts in tablet and capsule form are more convenient, but cost more. Take about 3 or 4 pills with meals, 2 times daily. If you are making a tea, buy your herbs by the pound from one of the high-quality suppliers listed in Appendix C. Except for growing your own (covered in Chapter 5), buying by the pound is the most cost-effective way to use tonic herbs long-term. Plan on spending about $25 to $40 per month on bulk herbs and about $40 to $60 on ready-made extracts.

Tonics are especially indicated for chronic conditions and symptoms, especially when they've been present for a month or more — even for years. The following list gives information on tonics for various symptoms. Note that I call a one to nine month period of taking tonics one *course*.

- **Fatigue:** If you feel tired and run down much of the time, you may benefit from a course of tonics. I recommend ginseng (GIN-seng), codonopsis (coh-doh-NOP-sis), ligustrum (lih-GOOSE-trum), and bitter tonics.
- **Coldness:** If you avoid cold, rain, and damp, or even have a fear of coldness, you can benefit from a course of warming tonics, such as ginger, cinnamon, American calamus (CAL-uh-muss) root, the Chinese herbs atractylodes (uh-track-tuh-LOW-dess) or cordyceps (CORE-dih-seps), cayenne pepper as a circulatory stimulant, the Chinese ready-made formula *Liu Jun Zi* (loo-JEN-zuh), or 8-flavor tea pills (also called Rehmannia 8 [ruh-MAH-nee-uh] or Sexoton [SEX-oh-tahn] pills). Take 6 to 8 of the small pills, 3 times daily, preferably before meals.
- **Paleness of the cheeks and tongue:** If your friends say you look like a ghost, or that you've just seen one, you probably need blood tonics. When a woman's menstrual blood is pale, begins to flow for fewer days, or stops altogether, she is often experiencing *blood deficiency* or *weak blood,* which is similar to anemia, but can be in the beginning stages. *Weak blood* is a common condition in which your blood is not completely balanced and healthy. Your blood can have fewer red blood cells, immune cells, proteins, hormones, and enzymes than is optimum for your needs. If you have weak blood, you may not be getting the proper oxygen and nutrients that your organs and tissues need for ideal health.

  Effective blood tonics include nettles tea, yellow dock tincture, edible seaweeds (also called sea vegetables) like nori (NORE-ee) or wakame (WAH-kuh-may), and foods like almonds, dried figs, and molasses. Red meat is one of the strongest blood tonics, but I discourage its use more than once or twice a week. Red meats are too warming and stimulating for many people and can increase your risk of developing heart disease.
- **Don't like being with people:** If parties, big gatherings, and lots of loud conversation and other noise intimidate you, or if you feel withdrawn for periods of time for no apparent reason, you can often benefit from a course of warming tonics. Use the same tonics I recommend under "Coldness," earlier in this list.
- **No interest in sex:** If even the girl or guy of your dreams doesn't pique your interest, then you may need a round of warming hormone tonics. Take one or more of the Chinese herbs ginseng, ligustrum, dendrobium (den-DRO-bee-um), or the Chinese ready-made product, 8-flavor tea pills (also called Rehmannia 8 or Sexoton pills).
- **Abnormal interest in sex:** A person who thinks about sex all the time and has on-going fantasies is usually suffering from a severe hormone deficiency. It can be from the body feeling threatened by the continued and fundamental weakness and wanting to reproduce before time runs out. This condition clears up when the deficiency is removed. Use hormone tonics like ligustrum, rehmannia, and the formula Rehmannia 6.

- **No strength:** If you can't lift a finger without feeling worn out, and your muscles get sore and weak with only a little physical effort, digestive tonics may be important remedies for you. Take a course of herbs like ginger, ginseng, atractylodes, or a good bitters formula for at least three months.
- **Chronic low back or knee pain, weak low back or knees:** These are classic signs that your hormones are out of balance and need support from a long course of herbal tonics. Take hormone tonics like the Chinese herbs rehmannia or dipsacus (DIP-suh-cuss) root, or one of the ready-made formulas Polygonum Juice (Shou Wu Zhi [SHOW-woo-zhuh]), Anti-Lumbago pills (Yao Tong Pian [yeow-tong-pe-AN]), 8-flavor tea pills (also called Rehmannia 8 or Sexoton pills), or American ginseng. Strengthening Western herbs for your bones include nettles herb and horsetail extract (available as a standardized extract to organic silica).
- **Shortness of breath:** When you find yourself laboring to take that next breath, even when you aren't exerting yourself much, you need lung and digestive tonics. Try the herbs codonopsis, reishi (REE-she), and a little red ginseng.
- **Frequent colds or infections:** These often indicate immune weakness. Take a course of immune tonics like the Chinese herbs astragalus, ligustrum, shiitake (she-uh-TAH-key), or reishi. Just before, during, and after the acute phase of a cold or infection, stop taking the tonics and use immune stimulants like echinacea.
- **Dizziness, spaciness, poor memory:** These mental symptoms often accompany weakness of the hormonal and nervous systems. Try the hormone tonics rehmannia or American ginseng roots. The premier nervous system and brain tonic is a combination of ginkgo and gotu kola (GO-tah CO-lah) leaf extracts. These can be used in extract form in tablet or capsules or in liquid extract form for periods of up to three weeks or longer as needed.

SEE YOUR HERBALIST

I can't stress enough the importance of taking your tonics regularly and daily for at least one month. After one month, try to take an unbiased assessement of how much you have improved. Ask your friends if you look better or act more energetically or positively. If you do feel some difference, continue with the herb. If you don't, or you feel worse, I recommend consulting a qualified herbalist for a complete program. Remember that you can heal almost any symptom or ailment given time, patience, herbs, and the practice of healthy habits.

TIP

Stop taking tonics during the acute phase of an infection or flare-up of an inflammatory condition like arthritis. They can feed the infection or aggravate inflammation. Begin taking them again as soon as the acute phase is over.

Ineffective or Active Herbal Therapy — It's All in the Dose

Take the same herb like echinacea (eck-in-AY-sha) in a small dose and a large dose, and you get a completely different response. Studies show that a small dose often provides little or no benefit. When a certain threshold is reached, for instance 40 drops of the liquid tincture four times daily, an immune response happens that can help relieve symptoms like sore throat or a stuffy nose that go along with a common cold.

Factors such as your body size and weight, strength, health history, and sensitivity to herbs and drugs in general are all important factors when determining the proper dose for you.

- **Adjust the dose according to your size, weight, and strength.** I can't give you a hard and fast rule, because every individual is different. My experience tells me that proper dose is important in determining how effective and safe an herb or formula is for your needs. Fortunately most, if not all, of the herbs in this book have a wide range of safety. Even if you take double or triple the amount, you rarely experience major side effects. At most, you may irritate your stomach and feel a slight abdominal discomfort. Take a look at the "Are They Safe? After All, They're Natural!" section, later in this chapter.
- **Start low, increase the dose, and taper off.** With this process, your body doesn't experience too dramatic a change. As with any kind of medicine, your body doesn't like abrupt changes and often uses up additional vital energy to deal with them.
- **Make sure to take enough of the herbs.** Over the years, after tasting and brewing many doses of herbs, roots, and other plant parts, I'm certain that most herbs are safe. In my clinic, I've increased the dose I prescribe to patients and have seen good results with few side effects. My bottom line is to make sure to start with a low dose to check for individual sensitivity, but don't be afraid to take a full therapeutic dose when needed.

Timelines

For acute ailments, take herbs at the first sign of symptoms, stepping up the dose and frequency during acute symptoms, and take them for at least a day or two after the symptoms disappear.

TIP

Finding an herb-friendly health care practitioner

Doctors are trained thoroughly in how the body works, what symptoms mean, and how to use drugs. However, they often receive little or no training in how to create wellness and prevent illness in the first place, especially with herbal remedies. Several different kinds of other practitioners receive just as much training in health and how to maintain it with herbs and natural remedies (what can go right with the body) as a doctor does in disease (what can go wrong with the body).

- **Naturopathic physicians.** These doctors are well-trained in medicine *and* nature cure, the use of hot and cold water, diet, supplements, herbs, and manipulation of the body to create health and treat disease. They're the general practitioners (GPs) of natural healing.
- **Lay herbalists.** Herbalists, both modern and ancient, are traditionally outlaws by nature. For this reason, many fine herbalists with years of extensive training have no license at all. They passionately care about health and helping their clients or patients discover the healing powers of their own bodies. Many teach classes in the art of herbal medicine, including *herb walks,* in which teachers take the students through botanical gardens or to wilderness areas to teach them how to identify the medicinal plants. The downside of the unregulated nature of herbal practice today is that the quality of herbalists varies widely, so the word "herbalist" has no meaning in a modern regulatory sense — no educational standards exist. Call the American Herbalists Guild (435-722-8434) for a list of professional practitioners.
- **Licensed acupuncturists and Oriental medical doctors.** To receive a license from individual states, acupuncturists and Oriental doctors must receive up to 6 years of education and training as well as pass a rigorous exam. Many practitioners of TCM work exclusively with Chinese herbs, though increasingly, those trained in the United States are also familiar with traditional North American herbs and modern European herbal medicines.
- **Chiropractors.** Trained in how the body works structurally, chiropractors are able to manipulate the bones, joints, and muscles to restore proper energy flow and relieve symptoms. Chiropractors are especially helpful for injuries and chronic pain. They're often poorly trained in herbal medicine, but some chiropractors take extra classes in herbs and have a basic understanding.
- **Licensed massage therapists.** These hands-on body workers are trained to help you relax, release tension, and get more in touch with your body. I encourage my patients to receive the healing gift of touch at least once a month — it's an investment in yourself. Some massage therapists and body workers are familiar with herbal medicines, but they aren't required to receive this training.
- **Medical doctors.** Although they're unlikely to receive any training in natural medicine or herbalism, an increasing number are studying herbs. The reason for this is often simple — their patients ask about herbs and natural medicine, and many want to be able to give answers.

Take your herbs for two additional days after symptoms of an acute illness such as a cold or flu disappear, for each week that the symptoms occur. If the symptoms of an acute ailment like a cold or flu last ten days, take your herbs for about three extra days.

If you have been getting repeated colds on and off for a month, take your herbs steadily for at least a month — even if the symptoms disappear. Chronic ailments like immune weakness take time to develop — often years. Remeber to be patient with your body. The herbs and other healthy habits that you practice during your time of healing are working behind the scenes to repair unhealthy tissues and cells, assist in removing toxic waste products, and help restore vital health. I've seen cures of chronic diseases that many would call miraculous — when patients have persisted with the herbs and health program. Your body can heal itself of seemingly serious ailments when given the support, love, and care it needs.

Mixing herbs for even better results

The use of single herbs for health and healing is called *simpling*. This is indeed a simple approach, and one that works well for the beginning herb user. This way, if you experience unpleasant symptoms, you know which herb to reduce or discontinue. If you get great results, you have one herb you can count on if symptoms return.

Many herbalists feel, though, that better results can often be achieved with several herbs in one formula. Here are a few good reasons to try your hand at blending two or three herbs together to start with as you become more familiar and confident with your herbalism. (Try some of the time-tested blends throughout this book to get a feel for formulas.)

- **Several body systems can be affected at one time.** If you have a cold with a runny nose and sore throat, you can use respiratory herbs to decongest and soothing herbs like licorice for your throat. In addition, an immune-stimulating herb, such as echinacea, can help discourage the cold virus from settling in for an extended visit.

- **Side-step the side effects of active herbs.** A spicy, hot herb like ginger can help settle the stomach and get your digestion moving, but if your stomach is a little hot already from a flu bug or that extra dash of salsa on the Mexican food you ate last night, be friendly to your body and add a cooling and soothing herb, such as marshmallow root, to the ginger.
- **Herbs work synergistically.** If you can't sleep because of a party down the street or things that go bump in the night, consider taking a calming and sleep-promoting herb like kava (KAH-va). You can often get a better night's sleep with this one herb, but I find that by blending three or four calming herbs together, the effects are greater. Kava plus chamomile (KAM-oh-meal), hops, and hawthorn can help relax your body, mind, heart, and digestion, promoting a more refreshing night's sleep.
- **It has to taste good.** After years of formulating for herbal and health companies, I've developed three important guidelines for successful products.
  - It has to taste good.
  - It has to taste good.
  - It has to taste good.

  You get the idea. No matter how powerful and effective an herbal formula is, if you don't take it, *it won't work*. Simple idea, but it's true. So, if you mix in herbs to make your formulas and concoctions pleasant and enjoyable to use, you'll use more of them.

  - A few herbs that I can always count on for good flavor are ginger, peppermint, wintergreen, stevia (the sweet herb, pronounced STEE-vee-uh), licorice, and orange peel.
  - Essential oils of aromatic and flavorful herbs are useful and convenient additions to flavor your formulas and teas. Many tongue-teasing oils are available — I like cinnamon, orange, grapefruit, lavender, rosemary, and peppermint. Add 1 to 3 drops of an essential oil for 1 cup of tea or 1 ounce of tincture. (See Chapter 3 for more on essential oils.)

Are They Safe? After All, They're Natural!

No responsible herbalist will tell you that herbs are always safe. Consider the common garden herb foxglove — a powerful heart stimulant that can kill if used incorrectly (don't use it at home without the guidance of a naturopathic doctor or physician). This herb grows wild in parts of North America and Europe, and every few years someone dies after mistakenly eating it as a pot-herb. This is not an herb to use at home. However, after 30 years of experience and after comparing notes with many other herbalists, I know that most herbs are quite safe under most circumstances — that's one reason that they're so popular. Across the board, I believe that herbs are far safer and have much fewer side effects than pharmaceutical drugs and over-the-counter (OTC) drugs such as aspirin and sleeping pills.

Rob McCaleb of the national Herb Research Foundation examined the reports of the American Association of Poison Control Centers, which collects data on all reports of human poisoning, and found that nearly all reports of adverse effects from plants were from accidental consumption of common toxic houseplants and ornamental shrubs like diffenbachia and oleander, and poisonous weeds.

Choosing the safest herbs — safe-teas first

Some herbs are exceptionally safe. Under nearly every situation they can be depended on to provide helpful benefits with virtually no risk — even if you are currently taking pharmaceutical or OTC drugs.

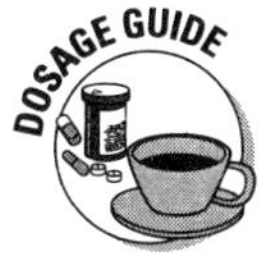

If you hold the common notion that if a little is good, more is better, these especially safe herbs are a good place to start or to return to if you're feeling uncertain about using herbs.

- **Peppermint leaf.** A fragrant cup of peppermint tea is one of nature's finest remedies for settling the stomach, reducing pain from gas, and easing intestinal cramps. Steep 1 teaspoon of the herb in one cup of boiled water for 15 minutes.
- **Ginger root.** Spicy ginger is an herb that you can always keep on hand — in your spice rack or in your refrigerator as a fresh root for cooking. A cup or two of the spicy brew helps alleviate nausea and vomiting, as well as encourage complete digestion. Lightly simmer 1 teaspoon of the herb in 1 cup of water for 15 minutes.

- **Chamomile flowers.** An aromatic, pineapple-like scent accompanies this pleasant-tasting, relaxing tea. Steep 1 teaspoon of the herb in 1 cup of boiled water for 15 minutes.
- **Cinnamon bark.** Increasingly popular in recent years, this warming bark tea is available both in bulk form and in tea bags (with or without caffeinated black tea). Besides tasting great, the herb can help prevent a cold from settling in the bronchial or lung area and can speed healing. Lightly simmer 1 teaspoon of the herb in 1 cup of water for 15 minutes.
- **Mullein leaf.** This common garden and wild herb is one of the best all-around respiratory tonics available. The tea is mild and soothing. Steep 1 teaspoon of the herb in 1 cup of water for 15 minutes.
- **Red raspberry leaf.** Red raspberry leaf is an important and widely-respected female reproductive organ tonic, but it's useful for men to relax the stomach and bowels. Steep 5 or 6 leaves in a cup of boiled water for 15 minutes to make a refreshing and mildly astringent tea that is reminiscent of green tea.

Those problem herbs — the infamous three

Over the last few years, as the use of herbs has exploded into the mainstream, and millions more are using them regularly, only a few problem herbs have come to light. These are somewhat infamous among herb users.

- **Comfrey.** This garden herb, shown in Figure 1-1, is a bristly perennial used for centuries to help heal wounds, burns, and broken bones. Modern science, however, has identified alkaloids in this plant that stress the liver. Children, pregnant women, and people with pre-existing liver conditions should avoid this herb altogether. Otherwise, it can safely be applied externally in creams, salves, and poultices. Restrict internal use to two one-week periods per year.
- **Chaparral** (shap-ah-RAL). This desert shrub (see Figure 1-2) was a favorite cold and flu remedy of native American Indians of the southwestern United States. Capsules of the powdered herb were widely sold to fight cancer in the 1970s and early 1980s. Recent reports, however, link the herb with liver stress in susceptible people. Moderate use for three or four two-week periods a year is not a problem for most people.
- **Ephedra** (eh-FED-ruh) **or ma huang** (ma-HWANG). This popular and ancient Chinese herb is one of the most controversial herbs available. Used for thousands of years for its ability to decongest sinus passages and help give cold sufferers a good night's sleep, it contains a potent plant constituent, the stimulant alkaloid, called *ephedrine*. *Alkaloids* are natural plant active chemicals that contain nitrogen as part of their

structure. Many strongly affect the nervous system — caffeine and nicotine are common examples. Because of its ability to give many users an extra jolt of energy and possibly melt away unwanted fat, the herb has seen sales increases of millions of dollars over the last ten years. Easy-to-purchase products have sprouted up in gas stations, convenience stores, and markets everywhere.

REMEMBER

For sensitive individuals, side effects include disturbed sleep, nervousness, anxiety, heart palpitations, and in a few cases, death. The Food and Drug Administration and the attorneys-general of several states in the U.S. have responded by calling for stricter regulations.

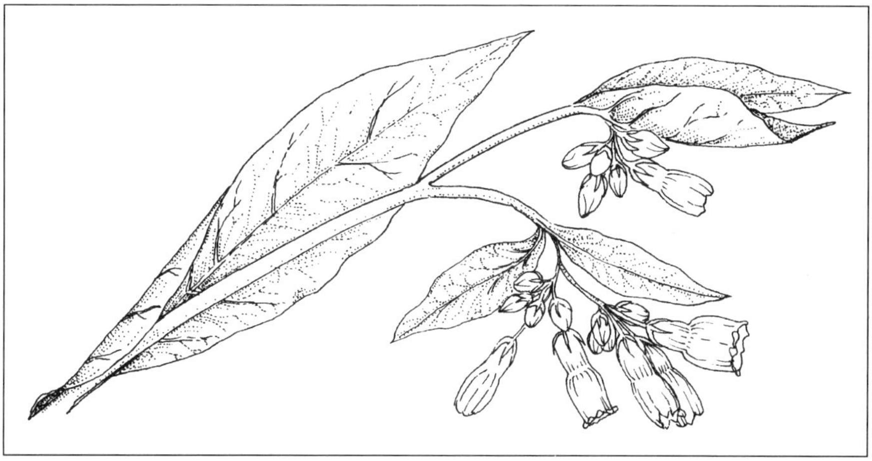

Figure 1-1: Comfrey is also known as knitbone for its ability to heal broken bones. It is one of three problem herbs.

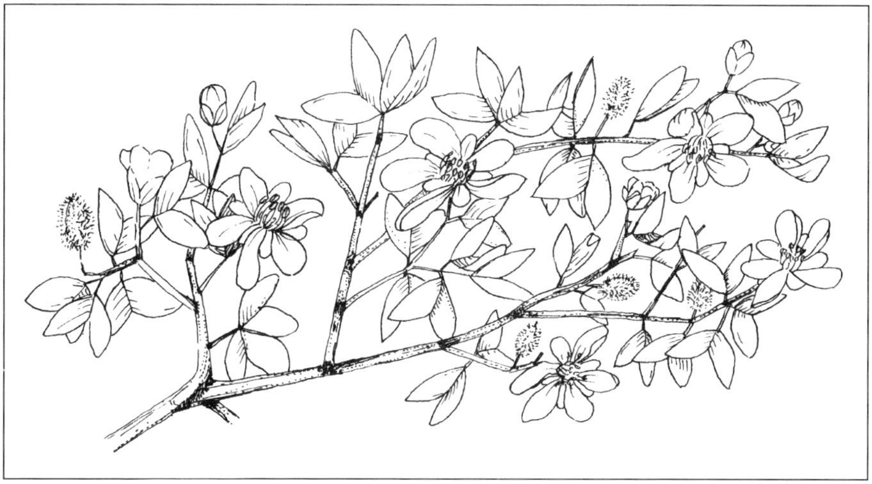

Figure 1-2: The pleasant scent of chaparral is in the air in many open deserts. It's another problem herb.

Can herbs be regulated?

Are herbs really medicines (with properties that affect your body's internal functions) that should be regulated like drugs? Or are they benign dietary supplements that pose little safety risk? The United States government agency called the *Food and Drug Administration* (FDA) is charged with regulating many of the substances that people eat, drink, or otherwise consume every day. The question, "Are herbs foods or are they drugs?" has haunted the agency since it was first created, partly to control the wild promotion and sale of quack medicines in the early 1900s. Most of these remedies contained herbs like sarsaparilla and cascara, for which unbelievably extravagant claims of miraculous cures were made.

Today, the regulatory climate in the United States is favorable to the exploration and use of herbs and other health supplements, because massive popular support and a proactive herbal and dietary supplement industry worked hard to convince congress to pass the Dietary Supplement Health and Education Act (DSHEA) in 1994. Few, if any, herbs in the United States are forbidden for sale and no specific guidelines exist regarding what form and manufacturing process must be used to produce a product. In Germany, many more pre-approved health claims can be made for herbs than in the United States. But some herbs that have no scientific testing to prove effectiveness and safety aren't allowed in products.

Other herbs to watch out for

Many of the common drugs prescribed by doctors today are derived from plants. So it's not surprising that some plants are extremely potent and have a small therapeutic-to-toxic window of action — that is, when the dose is low and the user is not abnormally sensitive or allergic to the herb, the herb can be highly effective. If the dose is just a little too high, unpleasant symptoms such as digestive upset, nausea, or a feeling of heaviness of the legs and arms can occur. Higher doses can be dangerous or even fatal.

REMEMBER

These types of potentially toxic herbs are known as *heroic medicines.* Digitalis (didge-ih-TAL-iss) or foxglove, belladonna, nux vomica (nux VOM-ih-cah), aconite (AAH-co-nite), rauwolfia (rau-WOOL-fee-uh), and mandrake (MAN-drake) are common examples. Fortunately, they aren't sold in stores except in highly dilute homeopathic preparations, which I talk about in the "Homeopathic Remedies — Less Is More" section of this chapter.

TIP

A few herbs fall somewhere in-between toxic and non-toxic — you can use them, but you must be very cautious. Knowing about these herbs can help you avoid an unpleasant experience. Though in some cases they are effective remedies, you need a lot of experience to get to know the nature of these potent herbs in order to use them safely. Although sometimes sold in stores, take these potent herbs only as directed by a professional herbalist skilled in their use. However, they're rarely, if ever, fatal.

- **Poke root.** Also known as *poke salat* (poke SAL-it), these fresh spring greens are traditionally boiled as a vegetable in the southeastern United States. You may have heard of poke salat Annie, the heroine of a popular song who went out into the woods and picked greens. The root is a powerful immune stimulant and is used by herbalists to treat tumors, cysts, and swollen lymph nodes. The tincture or tea of the root or berries (see Figure 1-3) acts as a strong purgative. Vomiting usually occurs 20 to 30 minutes after ingestion.
- **Lobelia** (low-BEE-lee-uh). *Indian tobacco,* as it was formerly called, contains a potentially toxic alkaloid called *lobeline* (LOW-bell-een) that has a similar nerve-suppressing effect on the spinal cord as nicotine in tobacco. For this reason, the herb is often used in herbal stop-smoking formulas. Lobelia is also a famous remedy for asthma, helping to relax the bronchial airways. Taking too much lobelia, shown in Figure 1-4, can lead to nausea and vomiting.

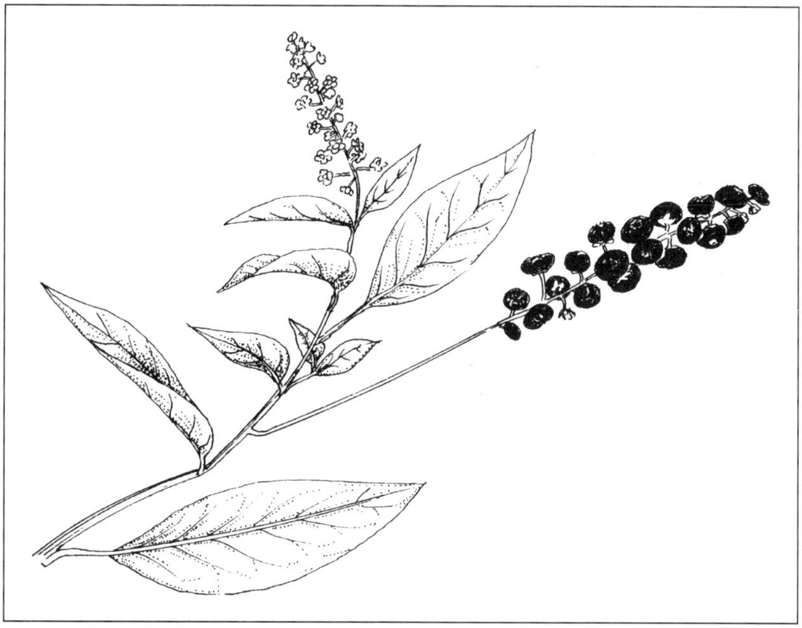

Figure 1-3: The big, stout poke plant is a common sight in the eastern United States with its bright red stems and purple berries.

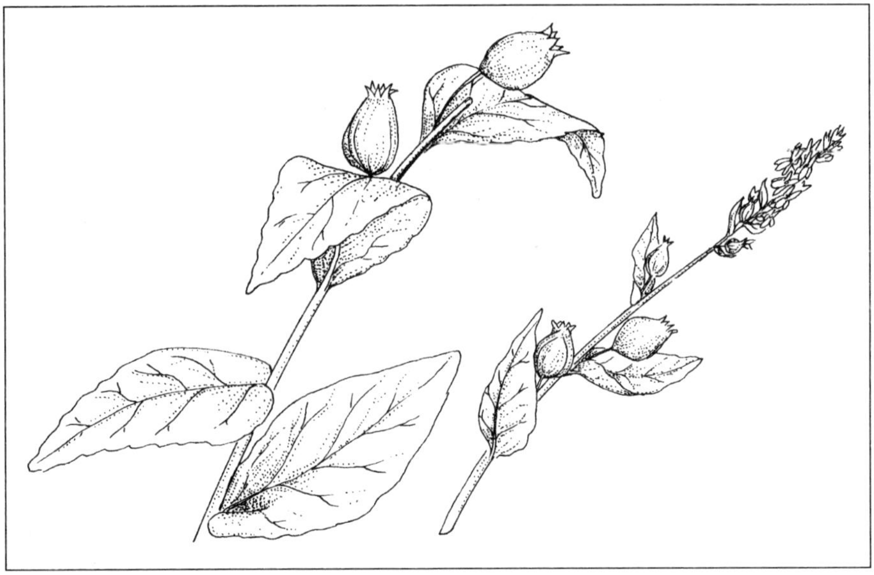

Figure 1-4: Lobelia was called Indian tobacco by the early Europeans who came to North America because people smoked it to relieve asthma symptoms.

- **Mistletoe.** Wild American and European mistletoe are the familiar kissing herbs hung up in doorways at Christmas time. The origins of this ritual came from the Druids who valued the plant in rituals to promote fertility. Leaves and stems of the European mistletoe, *Viscum album,* are used by doctors and herbalists alike to treat cancer and high blood pressure. American mistletoe, shown in Figure 1-5, is considered toxic, leading to symptoms such as heart palpitations. The berries can potentially kill children who eat them.

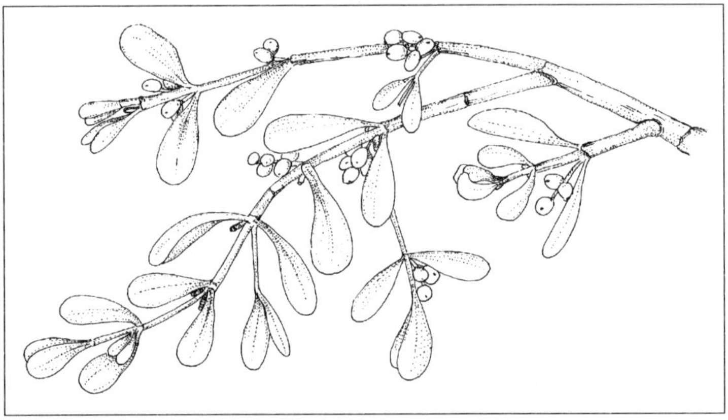

Figure 1-5: Mistletoe is the traditional Christmas kissing herb.

- **Chinese aconite.** Plants from the genus *Aconitum,* or the aconites, grow worldwide and are among the most toxic of all plants. Because only a small amount of the fresh or dried plant, shown in Figure 1-6, can be lethal, the Chinese use vinegar to remove the toxic alkaloids. The processed herb is considered the remedy of choice for stimulating and warming up the metabolism for people who are cold and have a low sex-drive. Sometimes even the processed herb produces toxic symptoms such as nausea and dizziness. The herb can be found in commercial prepared Chinese pills available in herb shops and natural food stores. I recommend consulting a licensed practitioner of Traditional Chinese Medicine before using these products.
- **Bloodroot.** This native American plant (shown in Figure 1-7) can be found growing in the lush hardwood forests of the eastern United States and southern Canada. As its fiery red roots suggest, the root is extremely bitter and harsh and can burn your mouth and stomach if used undiluted. Small amounts of a liquid extract (called *tincture* — see Chapter 2) of bloodroot are used in commercial mouthwashes and toothpastes to kill the bacteria associated with gum disease and tooth decay on contact.

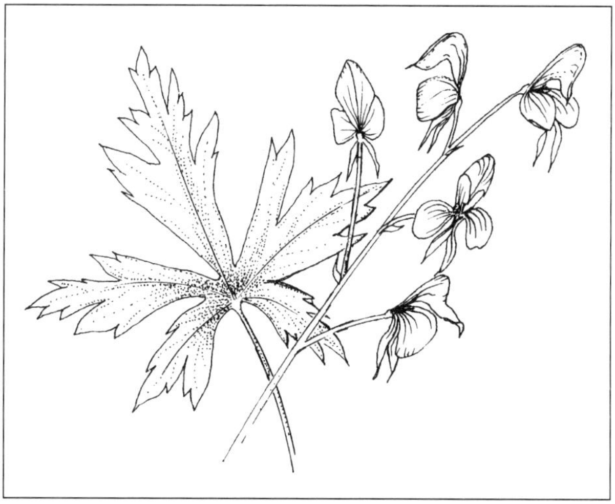

Figure 1-6: Aconite is a beautiful plant of the mountains that is related to the familiar garden larkspur.

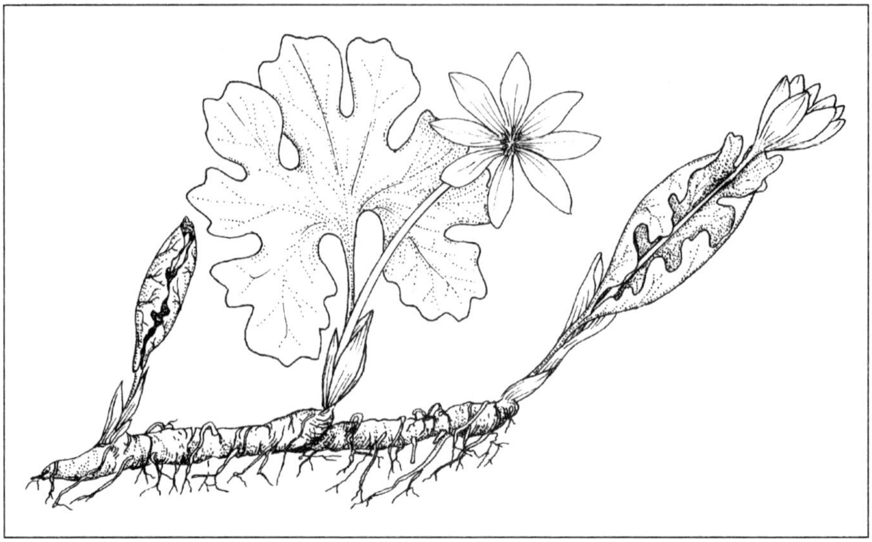

Figure 1-7: The single, white flower of the bloodroot is one of the first to bloom in the early spring.

- **Arnica.** This is a yellow, daisy-like plant (shown in Figure 1-8) that grows in the high mountains of Europe and North America. Externally, oils and creams made from arnica (ARE-nih-cah) can speed healing of strains, sprains, and inflammation. Internally it can produce nausea, dizziness, and even death.

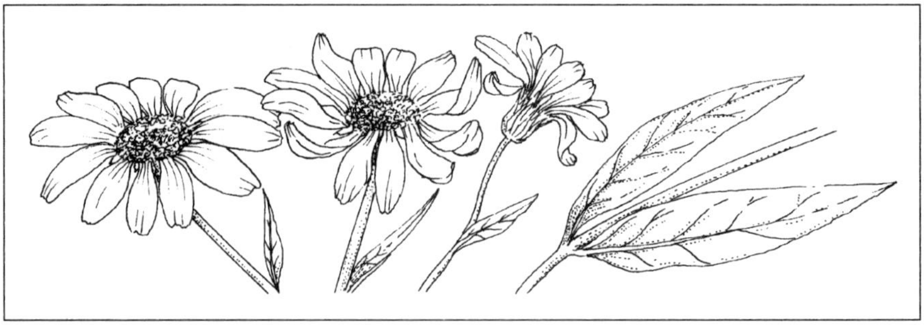

Figure 1-8: The cheerful, yellow, daisy-like flower of arnica graces high mountain meadows throughout the world.

- **Pennyroyal oil or tincture.** The common garden pennyroyal is a wonderfully fragrant member of the mint family. A tea of the dried herb is safe to use for settling the digestion, relieving gas, and to promote timely menstruation. The tincture (see Chapter 2) and essential oil (discussed in Chapter 3) are known to cause deaths in women trying to use the products to abort a fetus. Never use these products internally.
- **Apricot or bitter almond kernels.** The seeds of the apricot or bitter almond trees are effective ingredients in Chinese products for relieving coughs. Both herbs contain cyanide-like compounds that have led to dizziness and nausea in sensitive individuals. Children are especially sensitive — deaths with as little as eight kernels are reported.
- **Germander.** A common garden plant from the mint family (shown in Figure 1-9) that you should avoid for internal use because of reports that it can cause liver damage. Fortunately germander is rarely included in herbal products.

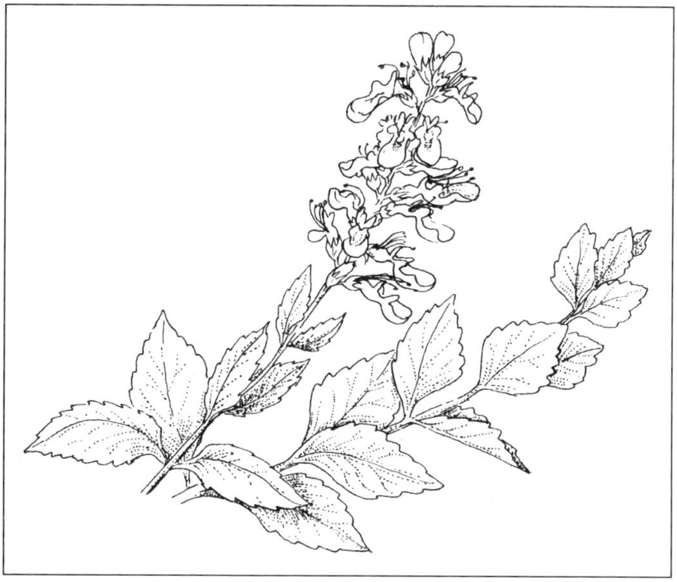

Figure 1-9: The germander has delicate two-lipped flowers that are characteristic of the mint family.

Maximizing the safety of herbs

Although the vast majority of herbs are safe to use under many circumstances, here are a few easy tips to help make them even safer.

- **Start with one herb or formula at a time.** If you find yourself thinking, "Gee, many of the herbs sound good, and I want to try them all" or "I'm a wreck, I need *all* of them," remember that patience is a big virtue when it comes to natural healing. Jumping in with both feet and taking several formulas or products at once can really confuse your body. I see patients get the best results with the least problems when they start with one new formula or two new herbs at a time. Take them for two weeks and then add another formula or two more herbs if you feel adventurous.
- **Begin with a low dose and work your way up.** You can check your sensitivity to an herb or formula by starting with half the dose recommended on the package, bottle, or in this book. Take this low dose for three days. If you notice a positive effect, or none at all, try increasing to a full therapeutic dose. If you believe that you feel mild side effects, such as a headache, continue taking the herb for another five days and reevaluate. If you continue to experience these symptoms or if you feel strong side effects at any time, discontinue them and consult with your herbalist or other practitioner trained in the use of herbs.
- **Pay attention to quality.** Herbs are grown in countries around the world, and some of these countries allow pesticides and herbicides to be used during the growing season. In addition, fumigants and preservatives are sometimes added during processing and storage to control insects, bacterial or fungal growth, and to maintain their color. A number of plants can absorb heavy metals from synthetic fertilizers or when grown next to industrial areas. Some people can react to these substances, even if they only occur as residues in a finished herbal product.

  In order to use herbs and herbal products that are as free as possible of these chemicals, choose organic products. If you're not sure about which herbs or products you want to use, ask the herbal or supplement specialist in a natural food store or herb shop. If they don't know, feel free to call the supplier or manufacturer and ask the hard questions — where do your herbs come from? Are they *certified organic* (grown without synthetic pesticides, herbicides, or fertilizers) and if so, by what organization are they certified? Call the certifying agency to follow up if you want to be absolutely certain.

  Asking for organic herbs and foods, even when a store doesn't have them, may encourage the store to begin carrying organic products. Thousands of tons of unneeded toxic chemicals are dumped on your foods and herbal medicines every year. Many of these chemicals end up in your water, food, and air — one way or another. Herbalists universally feel that plants that are picked from a healthy wild environment or grown in natural soil, full of rich natural humus and organic matter, create the most effective herbal medicines. After all — when you're trying to heal yourself, do you really want to stress your bodies with even small amounts of unneccessary toxic chemicals?

- **If you have a serious health condition, consult your health care provider first.** Use only mild herbs in light to moderate doses if you can't consult with a herb-savvy physician or trained herbalist.
- **Understand the healing crisis — when feeling bad is not necessarily bad.** A *healing crisis* is a short period of discomfort resulting from your body's own attempts to throw off toxic wastes to help heal itself. This common response to a new herb or herb formula is sometimes necessary in order to get well. Years of accumulated waste products can be stored in your fat tissues, liver, and other organs. Cleansing herbs and herbs that specifically work on the liver are notorious for initiating a *cleansing response,* in which toxins are thrown off into the bloodstream. With increased vital energy to work with, the body in its wisdom attempts to throw these unhealthy substances off through the urine and bowels. As they circulate through the body they can produce symptoms such as nausea, dizziness, headaches, rashes, fatigue, and heightened emotional responses (irritability and anger). If you experience some of these symptoms, I recommend sticking with the herbs at half the dose for one to two weeks. Drink a few cups of warm elderflower tea (see Chapter 6) or pure water with half of a fresh-squeezed lemon throughout the day. If the symptoms clear, you can be fairly certain that you're on the right track.

  If your symptoms continue to get worse or don't clear up, then you may be taking the wrong herbs for your personal constitution or present condition. Consult your health care provider, or try another formula that sounds right for you.

Watching out for potential side effects

Because common foods like bread, milk, and cheese cause allergic reactions in millions, you probably won't be surprised to find out that herbs can lead to unwanted effects at times, too. These effects fall into several categories.

Some side effects can be caused by a healing crisis.

- **Allergic reactions.** Although uncommon, some individuals can immediately react to an herb with symptoms including scratchy throat, headaches, mild insomnia, and digestive upsets. This is often due to a specific immune response to natural chemical compounds in a plant. Try discontinuing the herb for a few days. When the symptoms clear up, take a half dose of the herb and see if the same symptoms return. If they do, discontinue the herb — you may be allergic. Keep in mind that some allergies develop only after several weeks or months of use.

- **Throat irritation.** Some harsh, bitter herbs can irritate your throat, giving you an unpleasant prickly feeling. Watch out for herbs like bloodroot, *Echinacea angustifolia* root, prickly ash bark, celandine (SELL-un-deen), skunk cabbage, ipecac syrup, and lobelia herb. This irritation usually persists for only a short while. Try drinking several cups of a mild decoction of marshmallow root and/or plantain leaf and licorice root. Or suck on a small piece of licorice or licorice candy.
- **Stomach irritation, upset stomach.** A few herbs are well-known to upset even the most robust stomachs. Some of these herbs are known as *emetics*. The most likely are lobelia herb, poke root, bloodroot, and sometimes, spicy, hot herbs like garlic and cayenne pepper.
- **Loose bowels.** Laxative or *purgative* herbs can create a need for sudden unscheduled stops to the toilet — at times in the most awkward situations. The famous examples include cascara sagrada (cass-CARE-uh sah-GRAH-duh) bark, buckthorn bark, aloe resin, rhubarb root, and senna (SEN-nuh). Cascara is the mildest, but the other herbs can be dramatic in their action.

  Herbalists also say that cold bitter herbs, such as goldenseal, can shut down the digestion, leading to loose stools when used for more than a week or two in amounts that are higher than the standard therapeutic dose.
- **Headaches.** A few herbs can lead to a dull headache, mostly when used in amounts that are higher than recommended or when they stimulate the liver too much. Valerian (va-LEHR-ee-en), the calming herb, is famous for creating headaches in some sensitive people, especially when used excessively.

When I talk about herbs being used in "higher than recommended amounts" or "increased amounts," or "a high dose," I mean taking more of an herb or herb product than is recommended in the dosage guide in Appendix B.

Avoiding cross-reactions with herbs and food or drugs

Science has actively and intensively studied how drugs interact with other drugs and how foods and beverages can increase the risks or decrease the benefits of drugs. Not much testing has been done with herb and drug interactions, however. Why? Because little patent protection is offered to companies who *do* spend millions on testing herb combinations.

Few studies look at the interaction of herbs and drugs and the side effects these interactions may produce. Even so, you are much more likely to have an unpleasant or dangerous reaction with a drug-drug interaction than an herb-drug interaction — some people take three or four drugs at a time and as people get older, doctors often add even more to the cocktail, including up to *ten drugs* at once.

Fortunately, most herbs are gentle medicines with hardly any side effects. If you use the herbs covered in this book, you will have few potential problems with interactions because I only include herbs with a long, safe human use — herbs are widely known and used by millions around the world. Many have scientific testing to help support their safe use. The exceptions are herbs that I label as toxic or problematic.

Meanwhile, here are a few general guidelines to help you minimize drug-herb or food-herb interactions and maximize your healing experience.

- Before you take a pharmaceutical drug, don't take herbs that have a high mucilage content like marshmallow root, flax, or psyllium seed — they can inhibit the absorption of many drugs. Take these soothing and bowel-tonic herbs at least an hour *after* you take your drugs. Herbs with a high mucilage content can also cause a change in your blood sugar, so be careful with them if you're a diabetic.
- Stay away from very spicy herbs like ginger and cayenne when you take drugs — these are known to enhance absorption of some chemicals. Eat spicy foods at least an hour *after* taking a drug.
- Avoid heart tonic herbs such as hawthorn or cactus if you're taking digoxin or other heart medications, unless you're under the care of a doctor and herbalist.
- When taking heart medications or mood-altering drugs like Prozac, Zoloft, or Paxil, be careful with caffeine-containing herbs like guarana, green tea, yerba maté tea, kola nut, and chocolate, or other herbal stimulants like ephedra (ma huang). Stimulant herbs can make your nervous system more responsive to many kinds of drugs that affect your nervous system or cardiovascular system.
- Many Chinese ready-made pills and tablets, as well as herbal tea formulas that you make, contain licorice. Don't use licorice or formulas that contain it when taking diuretics like furosemide (Lasix) because licorice can cause potassium depletion in your body, especially when you use the herb for more than ten days or so.
- If you're taking any pharmaceutical drug called a MAO inhibitor for depression, don't take the African aphrodisiac herb yohimbe.

TIP

Be careful during pregnancy or nursing

Pregnancy is a special time when the mother makes a safe and nurturing environment inside of her body for the growing fetus. Herbs can be an important part of this process. Some have been used for over 2,000 years to help prevent miscarriages, ease unpleasant symptoms like morning sickness, and help prepare the womb for birth.

Many herbs are too strong to use during pregnancy because they contain compounds that may stimulate the uterus or affect the fetus.

Numerous chemicals can go through mother's milk right to a nursing baby. Some of these can be beneficial, while some are undesirable.

Avoid strong or potentially toxic herbs and any laxatives altogether during pregnancy and nursing, except under the direct guidance of a practitioner specifically trained in their use, preferably with years of practical experience. See Chapter 4 for a list of herbs to avoid during pregnancy or nursing.

Homeopathic Remedies — Less Is More

HERB TALK

Homeopathy is a system of medicine that was created by a German physician, Sameul Hahnemann, in the early 19th century. He developed the idea that tiny amounts of an herb can eliminate the symptoms that large amounts of the same herb created. For instance, when a researcher takes a substantial dose of belladonna tincture (see Chapter 2 for more on tinctures) on several occasions, it produces symptoms like headache and fever. This is called a *proving.* After the herb tincture is highly diluted and taken, the symptoms are relieved. This effect is known as *like cures like.*

Homeopathic remedies are found as liquids (in dropper bottles) and as small tablets (in vials or bottles). The products have become increasingly popular over the last few years because of the claims that manufacturers can make on their packaging, alerting the customer about their intended use. See Table 1-1 for ideas on homeopathic products that may work for your symptoms.

Table 1-1 Finding a Homeopathic Remedy

Symptom or Condition	*Homeopathic Remedy*
Anger	Chamomilla
Anxiety	Phosphorus, Arsenicum
Asthma	Ipecac, Arsenicum

Symptom or Condition	***Homeopathic Remedy***
Backache	Ruta Graveolens
Bee sting, insect bite	Apis Mellifica
Bleeding	Phosphorus
Bone break and fracture	Ruta Graveolens
Breast-feeding	Pulsatilla
Bruise	Arnica
Cold sore	Rhus Tox.
Cold	Gelsemium, Bryonia Alba, Arsenicum
Conjunctivitis	Sulphur, Arsenicum
Constipation	Nux Vomica, Bryonia Alba
Coughs	Pulsatilla, Nux vomica, Ferrum Phos., Bryonia Alba
Cramp	Magnesia Phosphorica (all kinds)
Dental problem	Ruta Graveolens, Arnica
Dizziness	Gelsemium
Earache	Ferrum Phos., Chamomilla, Belladonna
Eyestrain	Ruta Graveolens
Facial pain	Gelsemium
Fear	Gelsemium
Fever	Chamomilla, Ferrum Phos., Bryonia Alba, Belladonna, Aconitum
Flatulence	Pulsatilla
Flu	Nux vomica, Gelsemium, Bryonia Alba, Arsenicum
Food poisoning	Arsenicum
Fright	Gelsemium
Hangover	Nux Vomica
Headaches	Gelsemium, Ferrum Phos., Bryonia Alba, Belladonna
Heartburn	Pulsatilla
Hemorrhoid	Nux vomica

(continued)

Table 1-1 *(continued)*

Symptom or Condition	***Homeopathic Remedy***
Impatience	Chamomilla
Indigestion	Pulsatilla, Nux Vomica
Injury	Arnica
Irritability	Bryonia Alba
Itching	Sulphur
Menstrual flow irregularity	Pulsatilla
Moodiness	Pulsatilla
Morning sickness	Nux Vomica
Nausea	Ipecac
Pain	Chamomilla, Belladonna, Aconitum
Rashes	Rhus Tox.
Rheumatism	Rhus Tox., Bryonia Alba
Sciatica	Ruta Graveolens, Rhus Tox.
Shock	Arnica
Shortness of breath	Sulphur
Skin problem (acne, eczema), poor health	Sulphur
Sleeping problem	Nux Vomica, Gelsemium
Sore muscle	Rhus Tox.
Sore throat	Gelsemium, Belladonna, Arsenicum
Stomachache	Bryonia Alba
Strains	Ruta Graveolens, Rhus Tox.
Stye	Sulphur, Pulsatilla
Throat strain (hoarseness, also laryngitis)	Phosphorus, Ipecac
Vomiting	Ipecac, Chamomilla, Arsenicum

REMEMBER

Government regulatory agencies are often uneasy about the sale of homeopathic remedies because of the lack of solid studies that are up to modern scientific standards that can prove conclusively that they work. Safety is not often an issue because the remedies are so highly diluted they pose no real health risk.

Homeopathic dilutions — strength in numbers

If you're a label-reader, you may notice herbs listed on a homeopathic product that you know are toxic — for example, belladonna — and wonder why they're included. In the system of homeopathic medicine, highly diluted toxic herbs are often used to make healing adjustments in the body's internal workings without the danger.

Soaking (or *macerating*) an herb in a specified amount of solvent (or *menstruum*) for two weeks or so is the first step in the making of homeopathic remedies. The most common *extraction ratio* — how much of an herb is placed in a given amount of liquid — is one part herb to ten parts of menstruum. This yields a weak tincture, known as a *mother tincture.* Ten milliliters (about 350 drops) is then placed in 100 milliliters of alcohol and/ or an alcohol-water blend, and the resulting mixture is then vigorously shaken (called *succussion*). This dilution is called *1x.* The process is repeated again and again, up to 6x, and beyond to 80x, 100x (which is also called *1C*), and even 1000x (called *1M*).

According to true believers of homeopathy, the vigorous shaking of the plant extract in water and alcohol sets up a vibrational pattern unique to each plant in the molecules of the new batch of liquid. This transfers the healing energy of the plant to each succeeding dilution. Traditional physical science holds that fewer and fewer molecules from the original plant exist in each succeeding dilution. In fact, by the time a remedy reaches 12x, no actual physical molecules from the plant are left in the solution. This is great from the safety standpoint, because scientists and government agencies don't believe that you can become sick from pure, unseen (and therefore, unmeasurable) energy. By the same standard, they have difficulty believing that higher dilutions can have any effect at all in the human body, let alone get rid of headaches and stomachaches.

But does it work?

A number of scientific studies have attempted to prove that homeopathy works. While interesting, none of them have proven to the satisfaction of most modern scientific and medical investigators that the reported successes with homeopathic medicines are anything more than just in the belief of the users — in other words, all in their heads.

Although most scientists, physicians, medical researchers, and regulators are skeptical about the effectiveness of homeopathic remedies, the companies that are selling them are mostly left alone for the present. A likely reason for this is the safe track record they have. For this reason, homeopathic remedies are popular for children's ailments such as teething, headaches, nervousness, and fevers.

Ironically, homeopathic practitioners feel that remedies of extremely high dilutions, say over 80x, can be dangerous when used improperly. This is because the more a remedy is diluted, the more potent it is said to become. Dilutions over 30x are considered quite potent, and higher dilutions are increasingly powerful. These high dilutions are often not sold in stores and must be prescribed by a practitioner.

HERB TALK

Although I'm not a homeopath, I don't necessarily disbelieve in the basic concepts of homeopathy. Most herbalists feel that plants have healing powers that are unseen and difficult to measure. According to Rupert Sheldrake, a well-known biochemist, every physical object, whether alive or inert, has an energy field that defines its unique identity, which he calls *morphic resonance.* If he's right, this field may be transferred to water and alcohol solutions. Further studies are underway that may eventually prove their effectiveness to the satisfaction of science. At present, the whole concept is foreign to many, but stranger things have happened throughout human history.

Top homeopathic remedies for babies and kids

Homeopathic remedies are perfect for babies and children, because they come in tiny, sweet-tasting tablets that dissolve quickly in the mouth and are extremely safe.

- Bedwetting: Pulsatilla
- Chickenpox: Pulsatilla
- Colds: Aconite, Belladonna
- Colic: Bryonia, Chamomilla
- Coughs: Pulsatilla
- Diarrhea: Chamomilla, Nux Vomica
- Earaches: Belladonna, Chamomilla, Pulsatilla
- Fevers: Belladonna
- Grumpiness: Byronia
- Influenza: Belladonna
- Nervousness: Chamomilla
- Stomachache: Aconite, Nux Vomica
- Sleeping problems: Chamomilla
- Teething: Belladonna, Calcarea Phosphorica, Chamomilla
- Temper tantrums: Chamomilla
- Toothaches: Chamomilla
- Vomiting: Aconite, Byronia

Chapter 2

Choosing the Best Herbal Products

In This Chapter

- Understanding all types of herbal products
- Choosing the best standardized extracts
- Locating sources for your products
- Discovering tips for judging quality and value

What do you do if you want to experience the benefits of herbal medicine, but don't have any time to grow and harvest your own? That's where herbal products come in. You're fortunate today to have an amazing array of herbal remedies of all forms and descriptions. Liquids, tablets, powders, whole herbs, creams, salves, shampoos — all are available right from your local natural food store, herb shop, pharmacy, or herbal practitioner. That huge assortment of herbal products, though, may leave you wondering which kind is right for you.

This chapter answers all of those questions, giving you an overview of the best herbal products to answer your every need. (And if you want to save some money, turn to Chapter 6 for step-by-step instructions on how to make many of these herbal products at home.)

Discovering Herbal Products for Internal Use

An effective and convenient way to harness the healing power of herbs is to swallow some! On their journey through the digestive tract, many of the beneficial, biologically-active chemicals absorb into your bloodstream and are distributed to the tissues and organs that can benefit from their activity. Eating the fresh, whole herb is potent medicine but is often inconvenient, and some of the herbs are taste-challenged. As an alternative, try one of the many herbal products on the shelves of your local herb shop or pharmacy.

Herbal products that are taken internally tend to fall into one of the following categories:

Capsules

Capsules are probably the most popular and convenient way to use herbs. They have the advantage of being easy to swallow and they don't use binders or fillers the way that tablets do, so you're more likely to get nothing but the herb. Capsules (which I often refer to as *caps)* are made from gelatin — mostly from ground-up cows' hooves. They're also available as *veggie caps,* which don't contain any animal products. The most common sizes are the *00 (double-ought)* caps which holds about 400-500 mg (one-half gram) of powder. *Single-ought* caps are slightly smaller and easier to swallow — they contain about 300 mg. (Figure 2-1 shows an actual size comparison of the two sizes of capsules.)

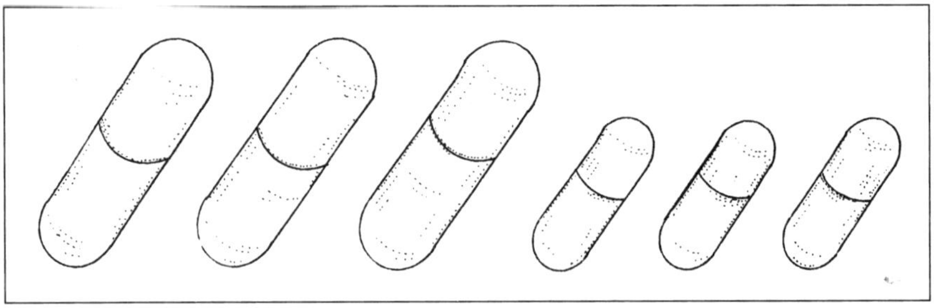

Figure 2-1: Capsules are a convenient way to take herbal medicines.

Capsules can hold powders of leaves, roots, and other parts of herbs, or they can contain extracts of herbs. Herb extracts are made from herbs by separating the active compounds from the inactive ones with the use of a *solvent* like alcohol. The manufacturer discards *inactive compounds* (like sugar, starch, and cellulose) and concentrates the active ones in a liquid form (called a *liquid extract*), or dried into powders (called a *powdered extract*).

Extracts are much more potent (up to five or ten times more concentrated than herb powders), and the body readily absorbs the active herbal compounds from extracts. I recommend taking most herbs in extract form (in capsules or liquids), especially when you have a specific health problem. When you're using herbs for prevention or for their health-promoting effects, using powders or teas is fine, because they don't have to be as concentrated. In the *Herb Guide* (located in the green pages near the end of this book), I give the ideal form of each herb, whether herb powder, tincture, or extract in capsules or tablets.

Tablets

Pressing herbs and other ingredients together with binders (like starch) creates *tablets.*

- Because the herbs are pressed under high pressure, you can get a higher quantity of herbs in a tablet than the same size capsule. A tablet the size of a double-ought cap can contain up to 1,000 mg of herbs — twice that of the capsule. This means that you only have to swallow half the number of pills — a wonderful idea for people who don't like to take a lot of pills.
- Many tablets are coated with a thin protective film that holds in freshness and makes the tablets easier to swallow. Tablets can have up to twice the shelf life that capsules have.
- Now the downside: To hold a tablet together, the manufacturer must add binders and fillers. Common ones include milk sugar (lactose), cellulose, gum arabic (a powdered tree gum), and starch. Some people are sensitive to ingredients, like lactose, that may be added to the tablets. Many tablets only contain small amounts of binders, so that the total herb content is still about twice that of a capsule.

Liquid extracts

When the active ingredients are removed from the whole herb through the use of a liquid solvent such as grain alcohol or glycerin, a *liquid extract* is created. A *tincture* is a particular kind of liquid extract that uses a combination of ethyl alcohol (grain alcohol) and water as the solvent. When the liquid is removed from a liquid extract, a powder is left, and the extract is called a *powdered extract.*

Liquid extracts have several advantages and a few disadvantages:

- They're easy to swallow — especially for people who don't like to down a lot of pills. With liquid extracts, unlike pills, you actually get to taste the herbs — herbalists feel that this makes the medicinal effects more potent. The taste experience engages all of your senses, stimulating the nervous, hormonal, and digestive systems.
- Tinctures have a good shelf life — up to three years if you keep them out of direct sunlight and in a cool place. You don't have to refrigerate them, so you can carry tinctures in your pocket or purse and take them anytime. I often keep a bottle of tincture in my pocket (depending on how I'm feeling), along with an assortment of herb flowers, seeds, and stems — great for smelling and tasting, but murder on my clothes when they go through the wash!

- One of the upsides of tinctures can also be a downside — the taste. Many people take time to get used to the taste of a bitter or sharp-tasting herbal preparation and may prefer pills instead.
- Most tinctures contain alcohol, which is a problem if you're an absolute abstainer or have had a problem with drinking alcohol. I don't like giving alcoholic extracts to people with liver ailments, either.
- Because of the alcohol content, some people are reluctant to give tinctures to children, although I think that tinctures can be excellent for children. They're potent, so only a small quantity is required, usually 20 or 30 drops. They're often a favorite of mothers and fathers because they're easy to hide in a sweet juice. Have you ever tried to get a kid to swallow a pill? I've found them under the couch and in other interesting places.

HERB TALK

Some liquid extracts are made with *glycerin* — a sweet liquid that is related to alcohol but has no effects on the mind and nervous system. *Glycerites,* as glycerin-based extracts are called, are often 50 percent weaker than the same amount of tincture and are drying to the mouth and throat. Yet glycerites with orange oil and other flavors are popular for kids.

Teas

When you add an herb to hot water and let it steep or soak, you make a tea. Teas are generally the strongest and cheapest way to go to get a daily therapeutic dose of herbs. Two major kinds of teas are infusions and decoctions.

HERB TALK

- Make an *infusion* by steeping either fresh or dry herbs in boiling water for 15 to 30 minutes. Infusions are the best way to use flowery and leafy parts of herbs, because the water can easily penetrate those parts.
- To make a *light decoction,* simmer seeds and thicker leafy herbs in water for 5 minutes, then steep the tea in a covered pan for an additional 15 to 30 minutes.
- For heavier plant parts like barks and roots, simmer the herbs for fifteen minutes to an hour, depending on the thickness and hardness of the plant material — this creates a *decoction.*

- You can also strain the liquid from the herbs after making a decoction, add fresh water, and simmer the herbs again for 30 minutes to make sure that you get all the active ingredients out (see Figure 2-2). This is a *double-decoction* and is useful when you're using expensive herbs like ginseng or astragalus and don't want to waste any of the herbal essence.

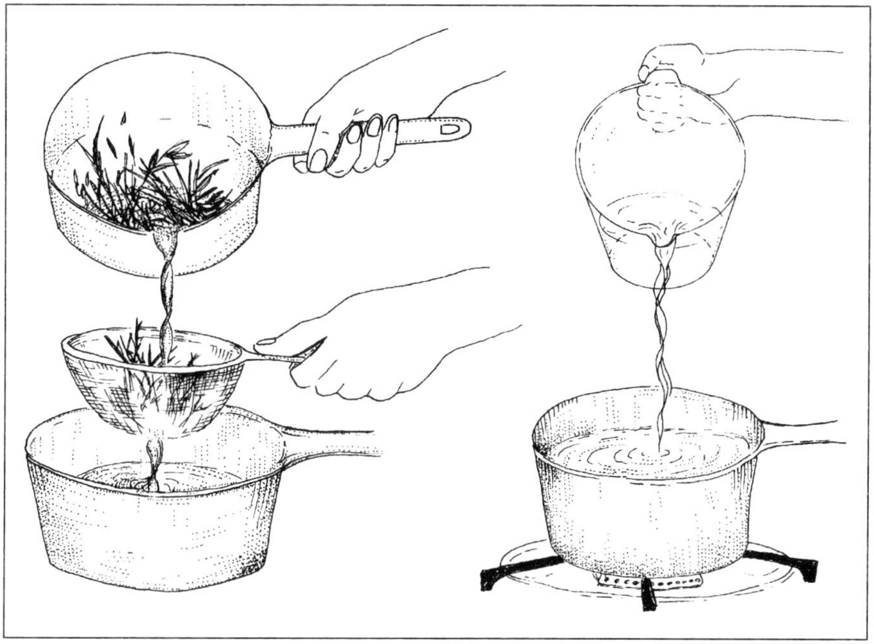

Figure 2-2: The double-decoction process is preferred for expensive roots, such as ginseng.

The downside of teas? Well, teas take time to prepare, and they can have a bad taste. I've seen dark, murky brews that would take the plating off a spoon. Making a tea that tastes good is an art in itself. To improve the flavor of your teas, try adding yummy herbs like ginger, cinnamon, orange peel, wintergreen, fennel, or any of the mints. Sweet herbs always help the medicine go down. My patients' favorites over the years have been licorice and stevia, which is often called "the sweet herb."

REMEMBER

You don't have to use dried herbs to make a tea. Fresh herbs right from the garden or picked in the wild work as well, or better, than dried. Fresh herbs, however, contain more water than dry herbs, so teas made with fresh herbs are usually somewhat weaker. To make a tea using fresh herbs, double the amount of dried herb that's called for in the recipe.

Syrups

Liquid herbal extracts added to a sweet, aromatic base, such as honey, make a *syrup.* Syrups are great for kids of all ages who like a pleasant, sweet, herbal preparation and are especially good for soothing coughs and sore throats. Syrups tend to coat the throat, delivering the herbal goodies right to the affected area.

Horehound syrup is among the best-known. Horehound is amazingly effective for stopping coughs cold, but the herb is so bitter that the only way to get it down is to add a lot of honey. Horehound is an easy herb to grow in your garden.

Make sure not to give honey to babies under six months of age.

Candies

Herbal candies are simple and easy to make from an herbal syrup. I often make herbal-tonic candies and throat-soothing, cough-stopping candies for children and adults. By sucking on the candy, the herbal essence lasts a long time — unless, of course, you crunch it down too fast.

Standardizing Extracts

Many extracts are *standardized,* which means that herb manufacturers guarantee that a product they make has the activity you expect. While this isn't a new idea, the ability to actually deliver on this promise based on our modern ability to look inside the plant with sophisticated sensing devices has only developed over the last twenty or thirty years. Standardization happens in two ways:

- Experienced herbalists know a good quality herb when they taste it. After years of touching, tasting, smelling, harvesting, processing, and giving herbs to sick people, herbalists develop a strong sense of exactly what specific population of herbs yields the best medicine. They also know which parts of the plant to pick, whether bark, leaves or flowers, and when to pick them, how to process them, and how to prepare the most effective medicines for their patients.

- In many parts of the world, however, a different kind of standardization is emerging. Medicinal plants are being cultivated on a grand scale — the plants are dug by harvesting machines and processed by massive, shiny extractors with the aid of industrial solvents such as hexane and chloroform. On this scale, the traditional relationship between trained herbalist, the healing plants, and patients is no longer possible. Modern herbalism is quickly emerging as big business — handling the herbs and marketing them is becoming a lucrative commodity.

  Many of these herbal extracts are products of modern scientific investigation and technology. Active ingredients are isolated from plants, purified, and tested in animal and laboratory studies. Finished extracts are designed to guarantee that a minimum amount of these compounds (the *active constituents*) is present. These active ingredients are identified, purified, and then added to unpurified herbal extracts to bring them up to specified levels. Many herbalists fear that these commercial extracts lead to the use of herbs as "magic bullet" medicines that have been so over-processed they don't contain the earth-essence that's vital to the success of herbal healing.

So, is there really any benefit to the modern approach of creating highly purified standardized extracts? I believe that both traditional and modern standardization methods can be used to help manufacturers make the strongest and most consistently active herbal medicines. Through the method of identifying specific patterns of chemical constituents that are unique to each herb, manufacturers can make a whole plant extract with herbs harvested and processed under the supervision of a trained herbalist. Through the understanding of science, manufacturers of the products that you buy can ensure that important identifiable active compounds are present. This is the best of each world, giving the benefits of both traditional standardization and modern standardization.

At present, these types of extracts (ones that meld traditional standardization with modern) are just beginning to appear. Table 2-1 gives a list of the most popular standardized extracts, with a brief indication of how each is used. I rate each extract for usefulness and purity, and tell you which ones that I prefer to use in tincture form, tea, or standardized extract form in capsules or tablets. A number of the extracts are equally effective in any of the preparations. Your choice should be based on what you prefer — and especially the kind of extract that you'll take consistently. The *potency* column refers to the biologically-active constituents that manufacturers identify in their extracts to help ensure their identity and consistency. These numbers are not the ultimate word on what extracts to buy, but are the common standards you find for the herbal extracts commonly available today. These standards will probably change as scientists identify and test other plant constituents for activity over the next decade and beyond.

Table 2-1 The Top 25 Standardized Extracts

Herbal Extract	*Main Uses*	*Potency*	*What's Most Effective?*
Bilberry	Visual problems, poor night vision	25% anthocyanidins	Standardized extract
Black cohosh	Menopause (eases hot flashes), PMS	2.5% triterpene glycosides	Tincture, standardized extract, or decoction
Boswellia	Arthritis	65% boswellic acids	Standardized extract
Cranberry	Urinary antiseptic	30% organic acids	Fresh juice, standardized extract, juice powder
Echinacea	Colds, flu, infections	5% echinacosides, 15% polysaccharides	Tincture made from fresh plants, standardized extract, decoction
Elderberry	Colds, flu	30% anthocyanins or 5% flavonoids calculated as rutin	Standardized extract (berries), infusion (flowers)
Feverfew	Inflammation, arthritis, migraines	0.7% parthenolide	Fresh leaves, tincture, infusion, standardized extract
Garlic	Antibiotic, prevention of heart disease	1,500 parts per million allicin	Capsules standardized to allicin, cold-extracted powder, garlic oil, other kinds of extracts
Ginkgo	Improves memory and circulation, antioxidant	24% flavone glycosides	Standardized extract in capsules, tablets, or liquid tincture
Ginseng	Energy stimulant, digestive aid	About 8% ginsenosides	Powdered extract, tincture, decoction
Green tea	Antioxidant	30-40% polyphenols	Infusion, standardized extract
Gugulipid	Lowers cholesterol	2.5% guggulsterones	Standardized extract

Herbal Extract	*Main Uses*	*Potency*	*What's More Effective?*
Hawthorn	Heart tonic	1% flavonoids	Flowers and leaves produce tincture, standardized extract
Horse chestnut	Injuries, varicose veins	8% aescin	Powdered extract, cream
Horsetail	Bone, nail, and hair strengthener	10% silicic acid	Standardized extract, decoction
Kava	Relaxant, sleep-aid	30% kavalactones	Standardized extract, tincture, infusion
Licorice	Ulcers, inflammation	2.5% glycyrrhizic acid	Standardized extract, DGL (deglycyrrhizinated licorice)*
Milk Thistle	Liver ailments, hepatitis	80% silymarin	Standardized extract or tincture; avoid tincture for long-term use
Olive Leaf	High cholesterol, herpes	6% oleuropein	Standardized extract, tincture
Saw palmetto	Prostate inflammation, bladder weakness	85-90% fatty acids and sterols	Solvent-free powdered extract, whole fruit in capsules
St. John's wort	Depression, insomnia, ulcers	0.3% hypericins	Standardized extract, tincture
Turmeric	Arthritis, inflammation	95% curcuminoids	Powdered extract, decoction, used in cooking
Valerian	Insomnia, nervousness	0.8% valerenic acid	Tincture of fresh roots, rhizomes; standardized extract
Willow bark	Fevers, headache	1% salicin	Standardized extract, decoction

*If you have edema, high blood pressure or other heart conditions, or you plan on taking licorice extract for more than several weeks, use deglycyrrhizinated licorice (DGL).

Using Herbal Products for External Use

A particularly appealing way to reap the benefits of herbs is to apply them to your skin. For example, you can use a rose face cream to prevent drying, rosemary shampoo to keep your hair healthy, calendula salve for a skin abrasion or for diaper rash, cayenne liniment to relieve arthritis pain, or St. John's wort oil for a stubbed toe or when you hit your thumb, instead of the nail, with a hammer. You can even make these products yourself — see Chapter 6 for instructions.

Creams

Creams are like herbal mayonnaise: Take an herbal tea concentrate, add an emulsifier (like borax) to make the oil and water mix together better, put it in the blender at high speed, and drip in an herbal oil until it turns stiff and creamy, and you have a cream. (See Chapter 6 for step-by-step instructions.) I like herbal creams because they aren't greasy — they go on easily, feel cool and moisturizing, and can carry many healing herbal constituents into your skin. Calendula cream is one of the all-time greats for helping to heal burns, bites, stings, rashes, and other skin problems.

Numerous cream products are available at your local natural food store or herb shop. To know if you're buying a high-quality herbal cream, smell it — if your herbal cream doesn't smell like herbs, it probably doesn't contain a high concentration of them. If the creams in your herbal shop are too expensive, take your own container and get your herbal creams in bulk. Many herb shops feature a wide variety for everything from chapped hands to sunburn.

Salves

The word *salve* comes from the Latin *salvere,* which means, "to heal." Salves are made by melting a wax, such as beeswax, in an oil (for example, almond oil). Herbs are often soaked in the oil beforehand. These healing preparations have the advantage of lasting a long time on the skin. They hold in moisture and protect the skin from harsh sun, wind, and water. While they feel greasier than creams, this feeling doesn't usually last long. Salves made from calendula, St. John's wort, plantain, and comfrey are all popular.

Shampoos

Herbal shampoos can help cleanse and protect your hair and scalp. I prefer herbal shampoos that contain horsetail and nettles extracts.

My favorite scent in a shampoo is rosemary, an herb that is revered for keeping the hair and scalp fresh and clean. Rosemary also has beneficial effects on dandruff and other scalp problems.

Liniments

Alcoholic herbal preparations, mixed with a little herbal oil and warming, fragrant essential oils like wintergreen, are called *liniments.* You can rub liniments onto sore and achy muscles, inflamed joints, and other painful parts of the body. Liniments are best for acute conditions with inflammation. Use a liniment for up to a week or two. Use herbal oils, discussed in the following section, for more chronic conditions due to weakness, such as on-going lower back pain.

Oils

Make herbal oils by soaking dried herbs in olive or almond oil. You can also use other oils, such as apricot kernel oil, but almond and olive oils are my two favorites, because they don't go rancid easily and they feel good on the skin. (Use almond oil when you want a lighter oil; olive oil for a heavier, but longer-lasting oil.) Calendula, St. John's wort, and arnica oils are always in my medicine chest.

- **St. John's wort.** The red, rich oil made from the flowers of this herb is effective for reducing the inflammation and pain of scrapes, burns, and rashes.
- **Calendula.** A gently healing oil made from the flowers for burns, bites, cuts, or wounds.
- **Arnica.** Although toxic when used internally, when used externally, the flowers of this herb make an extremely effective oil for reducing pain and inflammation of bruises, painful or inflamed joints, and other injuries.

  Don't apply arnica to an injury when the skin is broken — it can cause redness and irritation.

Judging the quality and value of herbal products

All those bottles and jars look a lot alike when you're walking down the aisle with your shopping cart, scanning for a particular herbal remedy for your head cold. How can you pick out the best quality product for your money? Here's insider information to help guide you.

- **Take the right herb for the right person.** Herb quality is important, but even more important is the art of matching the right herb or herb formula with the right person who has a certain set of symptoms.
- **Pay attention to how the herbs are grown.** Ideally, the herbs in your product are organically cultivated in living, vital soil without the use of toxic chemicals. The most potent parts of the plants are also harvested at the peak of perfection, carefully dried in the shade out of direct sunlight, and processed under conditions that don't compromise the balance and content of the plant's active constituents.
- **Look for the extracts.** Make sure your product contains extracts, not herb powders. If you're buying echinacea, the ingredient list should clearly state "echinacea extract" — if it says only echinacea, then it's just ground-up roots.
- **Compare total herb equivalents.** Multiply the milligram or gram total of the herbs in a product by the extract ratio. For example, if you buy a bottle of echinacea capsules that contains 400 mg of a 5:1 extract, you are actually getting the equivalent of 2,000 mg (2 grams) of echinacea root powder. Because the cells are broken down in the extraction process, and the active constituents are released and more easily absorbed, you're actually getting even more for your money than just the 2,000 mg. You probably get the equivalent of 7:1 or 8:1 times the 400 mg of echinacea root powder — 2,800 to 3,200 mg! Obviously, extracts are a much better value, especially if you don't like to swallow 10 or 15 capsules a day to get a good dose of herbs.
- **Look for the herbalist behind the product.** When a company has a trained herbalist on staff to oversee the production of the extracts, you're likely to benefit.
- **Keep in mind that what you see on TV isn't always best.** Some companies spend most of their resources on advertising and marketing and have little left over for buying high-quality herbs or a sufficient amount of high-quality extracts to help make their products effective.
- **Avoid buying the cheapest brand.** The cheapest brands contain extracts that aren't always what they seem — they may be made with inferior-quality herbs and may not be as thoroughly tested as the extracts in major brands.
- **When in doubt, ask.** Don't be afraid to ask a supplement department or herb shop worker if the brand that you're looking at has a good reputation. You can also call the company and ask where they get the extracts in their products.
- **Remember that what you take is what you get.** Even when you're taking the most potent extracts that money can buy, they won't work well unless you take them regularly, take enough of them, and take them long enough.

If you're like most people, you don't want to take herbs or supplements three times a day. Instead, I usually recommend taking 2 or 3 capsules or tablets in the morning and 1 or 2 in the evening (both around mealtimes). Take the largest dose of a liquid tincture in the morning before meals, and less in the evening. For stubborn symptoms, you may want to take herbs three times a day to make the herbs more effective.

Essential oils

These are nature's perfumes. Essential oils, such as peppermint oil, are actually made up of over one hundred separate chemical compounds. Each oil is a unique blend of these compounds, giving it its special flavor or taste. Essential oils are the highly concentrated essences of aromatic plants and give the fragrance and refreshing taste to toothpastes, mouthwashes, mint candies, and many other food and household products. The important plant compounds in essential oils are antiseptic and work on the digestion, the respiratory tract, and the urinary tract.

A few drops of peppermint oil in a cup of warm water is the best medicine for gas pains. It works fast and helps relieve cramping and pain when you need it most — for instance, in a restaurant at a big holiday dinner. See Chapter 3 for more on aromatherapy.

Finding Sources for Herbal Products

TIP

The following is a list of sources for herbal products. In this list, I include important tips to consider when deciding where to buy your herbal products and arrange the sources according to my favorites. (My criteria for picking favorites is whether or not the information about herb products is reliable and whether or not I can count on the quality of products.)

- **Herb shops.** Herb shops (if you're lucky enough to have one in your area) have a full range of traditional and modern herb products — a wide selection of high-quality products. You can find Chinese herb stores in larger cities — these ethnic shops are exciting places to visit for herb lovers. Because of wide selections at herb shops, you can easily compare prices. Salespeople are usually experienced and knowledgeable.

  When you go into a Chinese herb shop and ask for an herb by name, you may get a blank stare. This is because a Westerner's pronunciation of a Chinese herb name is often far from the correct Chinese pronunciation. You may want to take a Chinese book with you when you go to a Chinese herb shop. When you ask for your herbs, point to the Chinese characters to avoid a mistake. Before I figured out this trick, I had some big surprises. Once or twice when I went shopping for a Chinese herb, I thought I would be smart and practice my pronunciation. When I got to the store, I proudly asked for the herb with what I was certain must be perfect pronunciation. The shopkeeper smiled and nodded her head and immediately went off and brought a bag of the herbs. When I got home I opened the package, only to find a completely different herb inside!

- **Natural food stores.** Natural foods markets come in all sizes and styles — they can be small and focus only on pills and supplements, or they can be giant stores that carry everything from cleansers and carrots to pickles and pound cakes. Many knowledgeable consultants work in natural foods stores today. Prices are often quite good. The selection of products in larger natural food markets is usually the best anywhere.
- **Multilevel distributor.** Local distributors stop by your house or serve you by phone. Some salespeople are knowledgeable, but often they know only a few products, and their understanding of health is limited. Products are over-priced in my experience, and the quality is sometimes uneven.
- **Mail-order catalogs and online sites.** You can shop at home from a catalog or Web site, where many popular products are available. Today, many online Web sites have extensive and reliable information about the herbs and products from top herbalists and health researchers. Look for my research at `http://www.allherb.com`. One possible downside — if you have problems with products, they can be more trouble to return to these sources than a local store. See Appendix C for other Web sites and catalogs.
- **Drug stores.** Herbs have crept back into the place where they started — pharmacies — but most drug stores carry only the most popular standardized products. Salespeople and pharmacists may not be able to answer your questions, but many pharmacists are keenly interested in medicinal herbs and herb products and are quickly getting more training.
- **Supermarkets and discount stores.** Supermarkets and mega-sized discount stores are likely to have a very basic line of herb products these days, but it's rare to find anyone to talk with at all, much less someone who knows anything about herbs.

Chapter 3

Aromatherapy — Getting Well from the Smell

In This Chapter

- Discovering scents — what they are and how they work
- Discovering and using the top 30 scented oils
- Healing with scents — your aroma prescriber for common ailments

Scents stimulate memories and have the ability to act powerfully on emotions, taking you back to your early childhood or flashing you back to another time and place. The scent of cinnamon may bring on a wave of nostalgia for mom's apple pie, transporting you to the middle of her kitchen, your mouth watering for a bite. The experience is special because of the association with the nurturing, caring, and connection you feel with your mother. I remember all kinds of scents from my own childhood — I've always had a powerful connection with smells and take every opportunity to smell plants, fruits, and the breeze blowing off the ocean. Immersing myself in smells makes my life much richer and helps me access and appreciate my emotional life in many new ways.

Thirty years ago, when I began to formally study the healing power of plants, I realized that by picking certain plants and smelling them deeply, I could change my mood, enhance my energy, and stimulate my imagination and mental faculties. Today I still carry with me a variety of scented plant parts to scratch and sniff, as needed. For example:

- Scratching a eucalyptus fruit and inhaling deeply for a moment sharpens memory and alertness, and gives a feeling of safety.
- A sprig of rosemary helps settle emotions down when I'm excited or scattered.
- Lavender enhances creativity and lifts the spirits.

Mainstream use of aromatherapy

Essential oils are finding their way into the mainstream. How about these interesting uses?

- Real estate brokers add a dab of cinnamon oil to a light bulb to give the impression of hominess to prospective buyers.
- Nurses add essential oils to diffusers in hospitals to stimulate the healing processes of the body and pick up patients' moods.
- Managers add essential oils to air conditioning vents to stimulate creativity, increase energy, and improve productivity in the workplace.
- Nurses incorporate healing scents for the elderly in rest homes to invigorate and promote alertness and lift the spirits.
- Doctors and dentists diffuse relaxing oils like chamomile, rose, or orange into the waiting room to help reduce patient anxiety.
- Airline attendants use essential oils onboard in airplanes to help counteract jet lag and freshen the air — any improvement is a big help.
- Psychologists and psychiatrists use aromatherapy to help unlock emotional blocks.

Of course, you may not like having odd bits of plant material in your pocket. These herbal fragments often make a mess as they dry out and crumble — and people may think you odd and even label you as ec-*scent*-ric. My suggestion is to experiment and discover many other ways to receive the tremendous benefits of this science of scent, called *aromatherapy.* Hundreds of excellent products of all kinds — face misters, perfumes, soaps, cream, lotions, and inhalers — are as close as your local herb shop, natural food store, or pharmacy.

Making Sense of Scents

Most people don't appreciate their sense of smell. Sight, taste, touch, hearing — all these senses are considered irreplaceable, but the sense of smell gets a low rating. While the other senses are important, smell may have a greater impact on your well being than you realize. The sense of smell is an important aspect of health because it alerts you to toxins in the air, such as pesticides and herbicides drifting from a local strawberry field or food (like eggs or meat) that has gone over the hill. Remember that your smell also works with taste to bring you the full enjoyment of your food (which you know if you've ever tried to taste a fine meal while you had a stuffed-up nose).

Of the approximately 500,000 species of plants on planet earth, most are aromatic. With a little practice, you can detect and remember the unique smell of many plants. The scents of plants are highly complex and unique to each species. Technicians have identified over two hundred single chemical compounds from lavender alone. From a palette of thousands of possible compounds, each plant makes up its own unique blend, with the aid of an ancient genetic guide. Certain herbalists believe that humans have genes that respond to specific mixtures of these compounds. After all, incoming smells have a direct passage right into the brain. Many herbal plants create aromatic variants, called *chemovars.* Rosemary is a common scented garden plant and, while it is only a single species *(Rosmarinus officinalis),* it has many different scented chemovars, each with its own unique odor and unique makeup. While these different chemovars may smell the same to the uneducated nose, with a little practice, you can easily pick out and identify each one.

Only a few botanical families (or natural groups) create the most popular and effective fragrances, however. Knowing these groups and their families helps get you started with plant scents.

- **The mint family:** rosemary, lavender, thyme, lemon balm, the mints (peppermint, spearmint, apple mint, pennyroyal), oregano, basil, and hyssop.
- **The citrus family:** orange, lemon, and grapefruit (from the fruit rinds and leaves).
- **The laurel family:** cinnamon, camphor, and bay.
- **The eucalyptus family:** eucalyptus, clove, and tea tree.
- **The parsley family:** fennel, cumin, and angelica.
- **The daisy family:** tansy, yarrow, feverfew, wormwood, and southernwood.

Unlike tasting plants, smelling a new or unknown plant is unlikely to ever poison you. You may not like the smell, and it may temporarily put you in a bad mood if it doesn't agree with you, but it doesn't harm you. Remember — you *can* inhale.

Growing and harvesting a scented garden

You can grow many fragrant plants in your garden or in pots or planter boxes, even if you don't have a green thumb (see Chapter 5 for more on growing your own herb garden). I have peppermint, cinnamon, rose, and coconut geraniums growing right outside my office door, so that I can take a refreshing aromatherapy break during my workday. I either crush and smell the herbs, place a few leaves into a glass of water to give it an aromatic freshness and healing taste, or make a cup of hot tea by adding a few leaves to a cup of boiling water. I find that fresh herbal scents lift my spirits, melt away tiredness, and help me to be more focused and productive.

The following should help you get started:

- **Plant choices:** The best fragrant plants to grow include the scented geraniums, mints, lavenders, rosemary, lemon balm, citrus, and bay. Specialty nurseries sell a variety of scented geraniums by mail. The best scents include apple, nutmeg, rose, peppermint, and cinnamon. See Appendix C for names and addresses.
- **Climate:** The best climate for growing scented plants is a warm one. However, many plants can be cultivated in indoor pots throughout the year.
- **Parts of plants:** All parts of plants contain essential oils and are valuable in creating scents. Many single flowers (such as iris, orange, lemon, and rose) are scented as are some entire flowering spikes (for example, rosemary and lavender). Barks, like cinnamon and sassafras, contain large amounts of essential oils. Some underground stems and roots, such as valerian and calamus, contain large amounts of oils. The leaves and tender shoots of lemon balm, eucalyptus, and scented geraniums contain the highest percentage of oil.
- **Harvesting:** Many scented plants contain the highest amount of aromatic constituents during the summer. Pick flowers and leaves during a spell of warm weather at about mid-day. As the day progresses, and the sun beats down on the herbs, delicate constituents are volatilized by the heat and are lost. Some flowers, however, like the night-blooming jasmine, are at their peak of fragrance in the evening. Check out Chapter 5 for more on harvesting herbs. On the other hand, strip barks in autumn and dig roots during the early winter, before the ground is too wet.

Understanding Essential Oils

HERB TALK

Many of the *aromatic compounds* (chemical molecules) of plants are from classes of compounds that are *volatile* — they quickly dissipate into the air, even at room temperature. Many boil at about 180° to 240° and are carried off in the steam that's created when the herbs are simmered in water. This means that much of the healing essence of certain plants — peppermint, for example — is lost when you simmer them in an uncovered pot.

HERB TALK

Essential oils or *volatile oils* are the
molecules of plants that make smel
names comes from the word "esser
essence of many plants, and "volat
contain one or two hundred differe
pounds called *terpenes* or *hydroca*
unique blend of up to one hundre
palette, gives the plant the ability
their biological activity and mood
tial oils aren't true oils like almon
called *fixed oils.* Fixed oils don't
are much heavier.

Essential oils are super-concentrated. For example, it takes ab
pounds of fresh peppermint leaves to produce an ounce of essential oil. These oils constitute important active ingredients and flavor additives in many kinds of familiar, everyday products — candies, syrups, toothpastes, mouthwashes, cleaning products, skin creams, lip balms, shampoos, bath salts, and soaps. Essential oils even give flavor and aroma to the spices that you use to add zest to your cooking, such as cinnamon, allspice, and nutmeg used for apple cider, pies, and baked goods. Nutmeg, allspice, thyme, oregano, basil, and savory all contain essential oils.

They smell good, and they add zest to foods, but essential oils have many therapeutic effects you can put to work in many situations. For instance if you have a stomachache from indulging in a rich dessert, simply add 2 drops of peppermint oil to a cup of hot water and experience fast relief. Here's more about how the healing powers of essential oils work.

- The essential oils of plants are biologically active when the airborne molecules are inhaled, stimulating olfactory (sense of smell) nerves which in turn stimulate centers of the brain. The molecules may stimulate an immune response after entering the bronchial area and lungs, helping your body fight an infection. When you inhale essential oils, from the steam from a simmering pot of eucalyptus leaves for example, you can help your body dry up mucus secretions, lower inflammation, shrink swollen sinus membranes, and enhance airflow. All of these effects can help you breathe more freely during a cold or hay fever attack.

  Try diluting a little essential oil, such as lavender (1/4 teaspoon), with a fixed oil like sweet almond oil (6 tablespoons) and rub it on the skin. You may notice an immediate boost in your mood. The individual components of the essential oil penetrate the skin and the blood vessels, relieving pain and swelling, stimulating blood flow, and bringing healing to the area, or may enter the blood, ultimately affecting the brain, nervous system, and organs.

- Many essential oils are antiseptic and are among nature's most powerful protectors against bacteria and other infectious organisms. Thyme oil contains a chemical called *thymol* that is murder on bacteria and fungus. The compound is included in commercial soaps and antiseptics.
- Certain essential oils are toxic and a few are highly toxic when they're taken internally in amounts over a few drops. This amount varies, but as little as one-half ounce of pennyroyal oil has caused death. When used in products for external use and applied to the area undiluted, toxic essential oils are unlikely to cause a major problem, although they may cause redness and irritation of your skin. Be especially careful when using the extremely toxic oils listed in the section "Using essential oils safely."
- An alcohol-based preparation (such as a liquid extract or tincture) of a plant high in essential oils like eucalyptus or pennyroyal is much more potent than a tea made with water. This means that the teas made with these plants are extremely safe, but you need to be careful with the tinctures that contain the essential oil plants.

TIP

Look at Appendix C for mail order sources of high-quality oils. Also, many herb shops and natural food stores carry a line of natural oils — and natural perfumes. Ask at the body-products counter for guidance and read the label of any product you buy.

Start making scents — creating your personal scented products

So many exciting products are easy to make at home from plant fragrances and essential oils. You probably already use several right now — the refreshing scent of spearmint toothpaste, the antiseptic smell of pine cleaner and lemon furniture polish, cleansing herbal shampoos, and relaxing lavender bath salts. Many commercial perfumes contain not only essential oils, but also synthetic chemicals as fixatives and stabilizers. Instead of a commercial perfume, try using a natural blend of inviting essential oils, available from many herb shops and natural food stores.

Flip to Chapter 6 for your chance to branch out, experiment, and invigorate your senses with fragrant products of your own design. Working with essential oils is sheer delight — the products are full of exotic fragrances, are fun to use, attractive to others, and elicit responses of surprise and interest. The penetrating quality of essential oils adds a potent healing quality to many herbal products.

Uncovering how essential oils are produced

When you go to the store to buy essential oils, the oils you get vary in quality. Manufacturers may produce the oils with the aid of harsh solvents, while others are carefully extracted with pure steam or with a non-toxic fixed oil, like almond oil. You pay a little more for high-quality oils, but you get what you pay for. Essential oils that are extracted with solvents (like hexane) or synthetically-derived oils (usually from petroleum products) have a crude effect on the body. Don't expect wonderfully refreshing or positive changes in mood and emotions from these synthetic oils. Even the physical healing properties like the bacteria-killing effects are often not as strong as with pure essential oils.

All essential oils may not be what they seem. Manufacturers use five major methods to separate or extract the pure essential oil from plants. Some are made of pure essences of plants, created by extraction or steam distillation, while others are extracted with industrial solvents (like hexane) from flowers, leaves, and other plant parts. Solvent residues may occur in essential oils and may be present in trace amounts in the finished oils. Sometimes, essential oils are completely synthetic, made out of petroleum by-products.

Using essential oils safely

Many essential oils like orange or peppermint are mild and have a low toxic potential even with internal use. When used externally straight on the skin, some essential oils like thyme and sage may cause redness and irritation. Keep in mind, however, that essential oils are highly concentrated, and many are irritating to the throat and digestive tract. A few are toxic to the nervous system and have the potential to make you sick or cause death when taken internally in a high enough dose.

TIP

Using products that contain small amounts of essential oils isn't a problem for most people, but allergic reactions or skin sensitivity are possible. It pays to check for individual sensitivity by using only a small amount of essential oil or product containing significant amounts of essential oil on a small patch of skin overnight. If redness or irritation doesn't occur by then, you're unlikely to have a problem when you use the product. Here are a few guidelines to keep in mind when you use essential oils or products containing them.

- Always read and follow all label warnings and cautions.
- Keep oils tightly closed and out of the reach of children.
- Don't consume undiluted oils.
- Dilute the essential oil with a fixed oil like almond oil before applying it to your skin. A safe ratio is twenty or thirty drops per ounce.
- Sometimes very mild oils like lavender and tea tree don't cause skin irritation when applied undiluted, but I recommend diluting all essential oils. Dilute a small amount of the essential oil and apply it to the skin on your inner arm. Don't use the product if redness or irritation occurs.
- In general, avoid using essential oils during pregnancy. See the sidebar "Safe essential oils for pregnancy" for exceptions, though.
- Keep essential oils away from your eyes because they can cause irritation.
- Be moderate with alcoholic drinks when using essential oils therapeutically. By moderate, I mean not more than one glass of wine a day.

Be aware of these seven toxic oils — use them more cautiously or under the guidance of a qualified herbalist or aromatherapist (and never take them internally).

- **Pennyroyal:** An infusion of the leaves makes a safe digestive tea, but the essential oil has killed women who took it internally in an attempt to abort a fetus.
- **Calamus:** European calamus oil contains a cancer-causing terpene called *thujone* that is toxic to the nervous system. American calamus is free of it and is safe, but identity of any calamus oil isn't certain. Avoid using any calamus oil internally.
- **Wormwood:** Wormwood oil is the active ingredient of the infamous mind-altering drink (called *absinthe)* that was favored by artists at the end of the 19th century. It contains thujone. Don't use wormwood or mugwort (a related plant) tincture or essential oil internally without the advice of a qualified herbalist.
- **Tansy:** Tansy contains thujone. Another traditional *abortifacient* (used to induce abortions), tansy herb is toxic in all forms, including the tea. Tansy, shown in Figure 3-1, is a common pungent garden herb that looks a little like chrysanthemum and feverfew — both close relatives.
- **Wormseed:** Used traditionally to kill intestinal worms, the oil is highly toxic and has caused deaths in children who were given too much.

- **Wintergreen:** The fragrant oil contains a toxic terpene called *methyl salicylate,* which is from the same class of chemicals as aspirin. People often use wintergreen oil externally to help relieve the aches and pains of neuralgia and arthritis.
- **Camphor:** This essential oil occurs in a semi-solid buttery state at room temperature (not as a liquid like most essential oils). Camphor is a single compound, a *monoterpene,* which is toxic to the nervous system, causing mental confusion, nausea, and vomiting when taken internally at a high enough dose. Camphor is commonly used externally in products to clear the nasal passages, open up the chest, stimulate circulation, and relieve pain — it's the key ingredient in Vicks Vapo Rub and provides its pungent smell.

Before using any essential oils internally, seek the advice of a qualified herbalist.

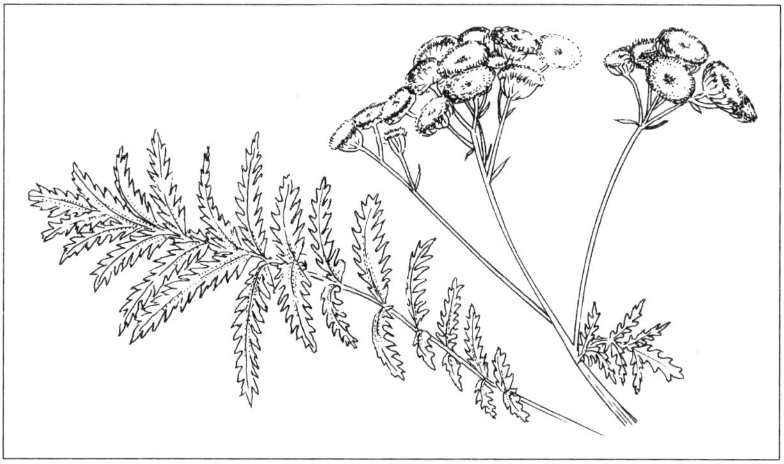

Figure 3-1: Tansy is a strong-smelling, toxic member of the daisy family.

Safe essential oils for pregnancy

The following oils are safe to apply on the skin during pregnancy:

- Chamomile
- Grapefruit
- Jasmine
- Lavender
- Neroli
- Rose
- Ylang-ylang

Inhaling fragrant oils through your nose and into the respiratory tract and allowing the essence to enter your blood stream activates centers in the brain, affecting your mood, emotions, and immune function. Here are simple and effective ways to wake up and smell the oils.

- The easiest and most direct way to use essential oils anytime, anyplace is to take the cap off the bottle of your favorite oil and inhale.
- When you feel stressed, apply 3 to 4 drops of lavender or chamomile oil to a handkerchief, then place it under your nose and breathe deeply. This practice was common in the last century and the early part of this century.
- Commercial aromatherapy inhalers are available in popular scents from many natural food stores or herb shops. Carry these in your pocket and inhale when needed. The inhalers are modeled after Vicks nasal inhalers, available from any pharmacy, which contain camphor essential oil, an effective ingredient for opening nasal passages.
- Here's a simple trick for men with mustaches. Whether you have a stuffed nose, are suffering from hay fever, or are working in a place with unpleasant background aromas, spread a small amount of Tiger Balm (available in most natural food stores and markets), or your favorite essential oil, onto your mustache and reap the benefits of the vapors. I often get the benefits from my own aromatherapy mustache for up to an hour.
- Another method of inhaling essential oils, shown in Figure 3-2, is to add about 6 drops to a bowl of steaming water, cover your head with a towel, and inhale the steam.
    - When you have a cold or hay fever, use eucalyptus and/or peppermint oil.
    - To perk yourself up at the end of a long work day, choose among clary sage, lemon, grapefruit, and peppermint or make a blend of your choice.
    - Enhance your sauna experience by mixing about 10 drops of eucalyptus, pine, or juniper oil in 1 pint of water. Throw the mixture onto the heat source of your sauna to get optimum cleansing and detoxifying for your body.
- Diffusers provide a safe and effective way of dispensing essential oils for environmental ambience. An aromatherapy diffuser, shown in Figure 3-3, is a device that continuously disperses minute particles of essential oils into the air with the aid of a small vibrating or heating element. You inhale the tiny oil molecules as they're floating into the atmosphere. Add about $^1/_4$ teaspoon of oil to the diffuser.

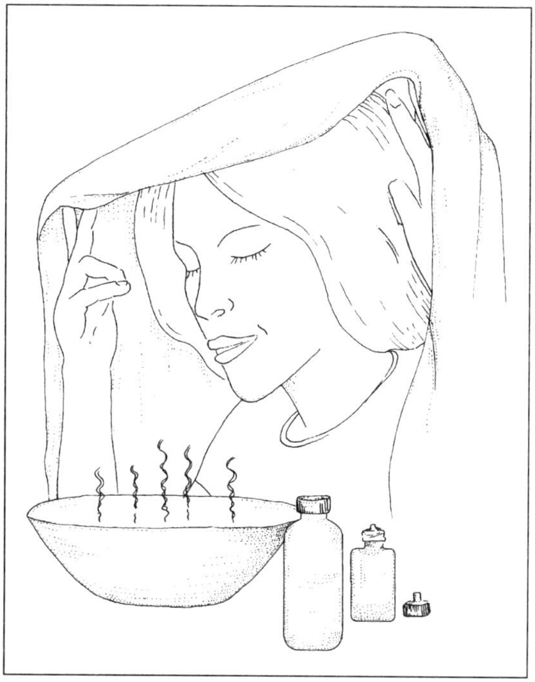

Figure 3-2: Inhaling the steam from essential oil-scented water relieves cold and hay fever symptoms and serves as a great facial.

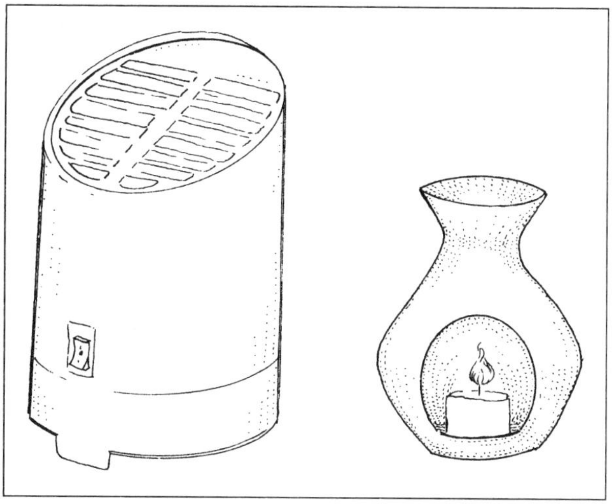

Figure 3-3: The aromatic diffuser is a popular tool for infusing a room with your favorite scents.

- A ceramic aromatherapy lamp is equipped with a small basin to hold a mixture of water and essential oil. The lamp is another device that makes good scents. A light bulb or candle is used to warm the basin. You can order aromatherapy lamps on the Web at www.naturesgift.com or by calling Moonrise Herbs at 800-603-8364.
- Incense is a gummy plant resin or other pleasantly-scented plant secretion that contains volatile oils and is burned to create an aromatic smoke. To make simple aromatic incense at home, buy pieces of gum resins like copal, myrrh, and frankincense from your local herb shop and burn them in a small porcelain dish or abalone shell. Incense produces fragrant smoke when it burns that purifies the air.

Thirty Titillating Scents

Perhaps you have your own favorite scents; if so, start using four or five of the essential oils that make you feel good. If you don't have a clue how to begin, here's a list of my favorite scents — tried and true ones that bring verve to your olfactory nerve.

- **Basil:** Essential oil of basil, or *sweet basil,* is used to clear the mind and strengthen the nerves. The oil is effective for relieving mental fatigue and the inability to concentrate. It has a refreshing, uplifting scent and a stimulating effect on the skin. One of my favorite ways to use essential oils is to put a drop or two of basil oil on my palm and then massage it into my hair after shampooing. It has a good effect on my spirit and makes my hair shiny. Basil oil is also used for headache, nausea, and head colds. Avoid use of this oil during pregnancy.
- **Bay:** Bay, which has a long history of use, has a pungent smell and is used most commonly as a liniment for sore muscles and sprains. The smell of bay helps relieve a headache and is useful for stimulating the immune response to help clear a cold or flu. As an oil that creates warmth in the body, bay increases circulation and helps unclog plugged sinuses.
- **Benzoin:** Oil of benzoin is made from the gum of the benzoin tree, cultivated in the Far East, and has a scent similar to vanilla.
    - It's often used as a fixative to increase the longevity of the oil and combines well with sandalwood and rose.
    - Oil of benzoin is used as an inhalation for asthma, colds, coughs, and bronchitis.
    - It's also beneficial for skin conditions, such as rashes, itching, dermatitis, and cracked or dry skin.
    - The oil helps lift depression and anxiety and picks your energy up when you feel tired or run-down.

- **Bergamot:** This highly popular oil is made from the rind of an Italian, orange-like fruit. (Many people are familiar with bergamot oil as the substance used to flavor Earl Grey tea.)
    - As an inhalant, bergamot oil is used for depression, nervous tension, and emotional imbalance.
    - In hip baths the oil is used for vaginal itching and urinary tract infections. To take a *hip bath,* fill the tub up just far enough so that the water just covers your abdominal area.
    - Diluted in a fixed oil, bergamot oil is effective for acne, shingles, eczema, and psoriasis.

  Bergamot oil increases photosensitivity of the skin. Avoid exposure to sunlight 4 to 5 hours after using directly on the skin.
- **Camphor:** Camphor oil has a eucalyptus-like scent and is cooling to the body, reducing inflammation.
    - Camphor is an ingredient in many pain-relieving salves for arthritis and sore muscles.
    - It relieves congestion and difficult breathing from coughs, colds, or flu and is a main ingredient of Vicks Vapo Rub.
    - Camphor is tonifying to the heart and nervous system in small amounts.

  Natural camphor is a main ingredient in rosemary essential oil. I recommend using rosemary oil, which is safer than pure camphor.
- **Cardamom:** Cardamom oil is a wonderfully musty-fragrant scent that acts as an aphrodisiac and is stimulating to the senses. The oil makes a good ingredient in pheromone blends and is often recommended for impotence.
- **Cedarwood:** Containing astringent and antiseptic properties, cedar oil is beneficial for many skin problems, including acne, dandruff, dermatitis, eczema, psoriasis, and insect bites. The oil is often recommended for mucus infections and congestion. Cedar oil has a clean, woodsy scent for use in personal scent and in pheromone blends — it's also a good insect repellent.
- **Chamomile:** Used for over 300 years, German chamomile oil contains a constituent called *azulene,* which is a potent anti-inflammatory agent.
    - Massage chamomile oil into sore muscles, swollen joints, and aching muscles of the back.
    - Chamomile is also famous for its sedative properties and is used for anxiety, insomnia, PMS, colic and intestinal spasms, and teething babies.
    - A good remedy for the skin, chamomile oil is applied to boils, rashes, burns, and dermatitis.

- **Cinnamon:** Cinnamon oil is strongly warming and is often added to liniments to loosen and relieve the pain of tight muscles. It's also used for indigestion and diarrhea.

  Use cinnamon oil as an inhalant to reduce stress and calm the nerves. The oil is helpful for respiratory mucus congestion when no acute infection is present.

- **Clary sage:** One of my favorite essential oils — a truly heavenly scent. Clary sage has many beneficial uses, invoking a feeling of euphoria and acting as an aphrodisiac. Used in an aromatherapy bath, clary sage oil is warming and relaxing and is reputed to help preserve smooth and youthful skin. It's tonifying to the uterus and is used for menstrual cramps, PMS, and hot flashes.

- **Clove:** Clove oil is hot and spicy and is often added to liniments for arthritis and sore muscles. The oil has a numbing effect and is used for easing toothaches. Apply a drop or two with a cotton swab to the gums around the sore tooth.

  TIP: Always dilute clove oil, because it often causes skin irritation.

- **Eucalyptus:** Eucalyptus oil isn't widely used in perfumes but is excellent as a steam inhalant for coughs and sinus infections, for cleansing mucus from the respiratory tract, and as a chest rub. The oil has cooling properties and is good for fever. Eucalyptus oil is a strong antiseptic and is used on boils and wounds and for urinary tract infections.

- **Gardenia:** Gardenia oil contains mood uplifting and antidepressant properties. Few scents top this one for sheer sensuality — try it in a bath or in a mist spray. Gardenia is one of the most potent of the pheromone herbs, as the popularity of the well-known perfume, Jungle Gardenia, attests.

- **Ginger:** Ginger oil is warming and activating to the digestion and helps to relieve nausea and an upset stomach. Try adding a few drops of ginger oil to your favorite ginger ale. Commercial brands often don't have enough gingery punch to do the job.

- **Grapefruit:** Grapefruit oil is used for obesity and depression. Aromatherapists often recommend it as a cleanser for the lymphatic system. This oil is useful for preventing and treating skin problems. It increases energy and is a good to use in a diffuser in the afternoon.

- **Jasmine:** Jasmine oil has a strong effect on the emotions, acting as an antidepressant and provoking a feeling of optimism. The oil works on the sexual centers and is a popular aphrodisiac. Jasmine is used in massage oil to help alleviate menstrual pain, but it's pretty expensive.

- **Lavender:** Lavender oil is one of the most versatile of all essential oils, adding a light floral note to almost any preparation.
  - The oil is effective for the nervous system and the respiratory and digestive tracts. One or two drops of lavender oil added to 1 cup of ginger tea is an effective remedy for quelling nausea or upset stomachs.
  - A lavender inhaler, bruised flower spike, or a good whiff from a small bottle of essential oil quickly lifts the spirits. Inhaling lavender every few hours works well taken in conjunction with St. John's wort for mild to moderate depression.

    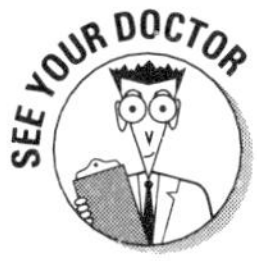

    If you have chronic or severe depression, see your doctor.
  - Lavender products are good to use if you have chronic infections with weakened immunity.
  - Try a lavender oil bath when you feel run-down, tense, have sore muscles, or during a period when you're experiencing chronic sinus or respiratory tract infections. See Chapter 6 for a lavender bath preparation.
  - Lavender reduces the itching of insect bites and helps relieve migraine and other headaches.
- **Lemon:** Lemon is a cooling and purifying oil that works well in air fresheners. Lemon oil is used in facial products for oily skin types. It has cleansing properties, especially to the liver and gall bladder, and immune-activating powers, providing protection against bacterial and viral infections.
- **Orange:** Orange oil is one of the least expensive, yet most useful of the essential oils. It has a cooling, purifying effect and is used for colds, flu, and hypertension. Aromatherapists consider the oil an effective nervous system relaxer, for reducing nervous tension. Orange oil (diluted) works great to rid your kitchen of ants and your dog of fleas.
- **Patchouli:** Patchouli oil has a strong earthy scent that's healing to the skin — it's used for acne, eczema, and cracked skin.

  Patchouli oil acts as an aphrodisiac. In the late sixties, patchouli oil with its earthy, sensual aroma was a favorite with hippies everywhere — and it is still. The oil works well as a minor note in perfumes and personal scents, especially for attraction.
- **Peppermint:** This popular essential oil is used for the following:
  - Indigestion, nausea, and motion sickness, as well as for colds, flu, and fever.

  - Peppermint is available in *enteric-coated capsules* as an effective remedy for irritable bowel syndrome. These capsules are specially-coated to allow the oil to move through the stomach, releasing its contents in the intestines.
  - I like to keep a vial of peppermint oil in my pocket for an instant breath freshener, which also serves to perk me up.
  - Add a drop or two in a cup of hot water anytime you have gas pains for fast relief.
  - One of the most useful oils, peppermint contains menthol, a strongly cooling terpene that is the active ingredient of many toothpastes, mouthwashes, and facial fresheners.
  - Add potency to calamine lotion by adding about one-half teaspoon of the oil to a four-ounce bottle. Rub the new, improved lotion on poison oak, poison ivy, or other itchy, burning skin rashes. The results may amaze you.

- **Rose:** Rose oil is perhaps the most revered of all the essential oils. It acts as a digestive, vascular, and nervous system tonic and is renowned as an aphrodisiac. Rose is recommended by aromatherapists for keeping all skin types young and wrinkle-free, and as an addition to douches for its freshening, soothing properties. It's pricey, though.
- **Rosemary:** A favorite garden herb the world over, rosemary is one of the most reliable gentle energy stimulants. The oil contains natural camphor, a nervous system activator. I find that a good smell of it picks me up when I'm feeling down, gets my mind going in the morning, and helps anytime that I feel sluggish. Despite its uplifting effects on the spirit, rosemary seems to ground me when I'm unfocused.

  Rosemary oil is commonly found in shampoos and is one of the best herbs for healthy hair. See the section "Producing a hair rinse" for a recipe to make a healing hair rinse with rosemary oil that is good for your hair and scalp. The oil is excellent for improving circulation, memory, and bringing on slow or late menses.

  Use rosemary sparingly if you have high blood pressure.
- **Sage:** Sage oil is a strong antiseptic and is used for bacterial infections, bronchitis, sore throats, and mouth infections. Women use small amounts of sage oil to relieve menstrual pain, regulate the cycle, and suppress lactation. Aroma-therapists recommend sage for lifting depression and mental fatigue and for slowing secretions like excessive sweat and mother's milk.
- **Spearmint:** Spearmint oil is used in many of the same ways as peppermint — for nausea, indigestion, colic, fever, intestinal cramps, and gas. I recommend the oil for relieving headaches, refreshing the nervous system, and relieving mental strain. Spearmint freshens the breath and uplifts the mood.

- **Tangerine:** The smell of tangerine oil is likely to get your digestive juices flowing. I used to pick fresh ripe tangerines in the Palm Springs area where I grew up, often eating ten or twenty in a day. I would peel them just for the aromatic smell, which always reminded me of the beautiful open desert with its purple mountains and fresh air and wide-open spaces.

  I recommend the oil for painful, weak digestion and for easing intestinal spasms and flatulence. Aromatherapists often use it for relieving nervous shock, tension, hysteria, and grief. Tangerine oil is great for flavoring alcohol- and glycerine-based liquid herbal preparations for kids and adults.

- **Thyme:** Thyme oil is the most potent antiseptic of all the essential oils, containing the active compound *thymol,* an ingredient in soaps and disinfectants. Thyme oil is used for bacterial, viral, urinary tract, and bronchial infections. The oil creates a warming effect in the body and is used in liniments for sore muscles and achy joints.

  Always dilute the oil, because it irritates sensitive skin. Thyme is the favorite herb of one of my close herbal friends. A few years ago, he purchased a bottle of the essential oil and decided to add it to his hot bath to relax his muscles and heal a small skin infection. He poured half of a bottle into the bath and then eased in. He slid down with a contented sigh, but a moment later he roared and leaped up out of the bath feeling a powerful burning sensation all over his body. He ran to a shower and tried to wash it and towel it off. Fortunately he was not hurt, but learned a valuable lesson — essential oils are highly concentrated, especially to sensitive tender skin and those extra special areas.

- **Vanilla:** The familiar scent of vanilla enlivens the senses and makes a great addition to attractive pheromone-like personal essence blends.

- **Vetiver:** This oil has a comforting scent and is used for nervousness, insomnia, arthritis, and tight muscles. Vetiver is an earthy and spicy scent that helps relieve spaciness and poor concentration. It's healing to the skin and is sometimes used as a fixative to prolong a scent.

- **Wintergreen:** Wintergreen oil is a familiar scent in chewing gum and breath mints. It contains the compound *methyl salicylate,* which is related to aspirin and helps relieve the pain of sore muscles, joints, and body aches.

  Wintergreen is an ingredient of many commercial preparations for easing aches and pains, but be careful with the pure essential oil — it's toxic. Never use it internally, and keep the bottle out of reach of children.

To love, honor, and smell for the rest of your life

Scientists recently confirmed the existence of human pheromones — sexual attractants. Without smell, how could you identify that special someone? Finding the right person among millions of possible partners is hard enough (as divorce rates show) and doubly so without your sense of smell! This process is mostly unconscious. Someone you're attracted to often smells attractive to you even when he or she isn't wearing any perfume. Lovers understand the importance of scents — like flowers, humans also want to be attractive and sexy to potential mates, partners, and friends.

An Aroma Prescriber

Use Table 3-1 to choose one or more of the following essential oils for your every need, then blend them into your own creations.

REMEMBER

All the oils are for external use only, except grapefruit, lemon, orange, tangerine, peppermint, and ginger.

Table 3-1 Aromatherapy For Common Symptoms

Condition	*Essential Oil*
Arthritis	Camphor, grapefruit, juniper, helichrysum, vetiver
Asthma	Benzoin
Athlete's foot	Tea tree
Burns	Lavender, peppermint
Circulation problems	Rosemary
Colds	Basil, benzoin, camphor, eucalyptus, peppermint, thyme (inhalation), orange, peppermint, sage
Concentration problems	Rosemary
Congestion	Camphor, eucalyptus (as inhalation or vaporizer)
Constipation	Basil (dilute with oil and massage into abdomen)
Coughs	Benzoin, eucalyptus, thyme
Cuts	Tea tree, myrrh, lavender
Dandruff	Cedar, rosemary

Condition	***Essential Oil***
Depression	Benzoin, bergamot, gardenia, grapefruit, jasmine, lavender
Digestive weakness	Ginger, lavender, rose, tangerine
Fatigue	Rosemary
Fever	Lavender, peppermint, spearmint
Fungal infections	Tea tree
Gas, flatulence	Ginger, peppermint, spearmint, tangerine
Hair and scalp problems	Rosemary
Hay fever	Eucalyptus (inhalation), bay
Headache	Basil, bay, lavender, peppermint
Immune system weakness	Bay, lavender, bergamot, thyme, sandalwood, lemon
Infections	Bergamot, cedar, eucalyptus, lavender, lemon, sage, thyme
Insect bites	Cedar
Insect repellent	Eucalyptus, citronella, tea tree, pennyroyal, orange
Insomnia	Chamomile, lavender, vetiver
Intestinal pain or cramps	Chamomile, peppermint, spearmint, tangerine
Itching	Benzoin
Liver and gall bladder cleansing	Lemon
Menses that's late or sluggish	Rosemary
Mental fatigue and fuzzy thinking	Basil, rosemary
Motion Sickness	Ginger
Mouth and breath freshener	Peppermint
Muscle pain or soreness	Bay, camphor, chamomile, cinnamon, lavender, thyme, wintergreen
Muscle strain	Ginger
Muscle tension	Clary sage, vetiver, wintergreen
Nausea	Basil, ginger, lavender, peppermint, spearmint

(continued)

Table 3-1 *(continued)*

Condition	*Essential Oil*
Nervous tension	Bergamot, chamomile, cinnamon, clary sage, lavender, orange, tangerine, vetiver
Nerve weakness	Rosemary
PMS (premenstrual syndrome)	Chamomile, rosemary
Rashes	Benzoin
Sex drive that's low (attractants)	Cardamom, cedar, clary sage, gardenia, jasmine, patchouli, vanilla
Sinus congestion	Bay, cinnamon, eucalyptus, lavender
Skin problems (acne, eczema, psoriasis, rashes)	Bergamot, cedar, chamomile, grapefruit, patchouli, peppermint, vetiver
Skin protection and wrinkle aid	Rose
Sore throat	Tea tree, niaoli, sage
Sprains	Bay
Stomachache	Peppermint, ginger
Sunburn	Lavender, peppermint, spearmint
Sweating too much	Sage
Teething (for babies)	Chamomile
Toothache	Clove

Chapter 4
Herbs for Everyone

In This Chapter

- Discovering herbs for women
- Getting to know herbal remedies for men
- Checking out herbs for kids
- Staying young with herbs
- Using herbs for athletic achievement
- Keeping your pets healthy with herbs

Recipes in This Chapter

- Chocolate Soy Delight
- Castor Oil Pack
- Apple-Peel Cure
- Ginger Compress

Herbs are universally used, but thinking of specific herbs for particular types of people with special needs also makes sense. By focusing on a small group of herbs that herbalists know work well for your individual needs, you can remove some of the confusion associated with herb selection and get going on your own herbal program. After you feel the benefits of certain herbs for specific needs, you can branch out and try others that may be commonly used for other groups of people.

In this chapter, I discuss herbs for women, men, children, senior citizens, athletes, and finally, pets.

Herbs for Women

Women have special needs and health concerns that respond well to herbs. Over the centuries, many herb products have been created with the hormonal balance and menstrual difficulties of women in mind. Many of the most famous North American herbs, such as blue cohosh (CO-hosh), black cohosh, false unicorn root, partridge berry, beth root, and cramp bark are primarily known as women's herbs.

This section contains herbal programs for women, many of which have been time-tested for generations.

Anemia

Anemia — called blood-deficiency in Traditional Chinese Medicine — is associated with loss of blood or a deficiency of iron, folic acid, or vitamin B12 — or a combination of these factors. (Sometimes, as in the case of a bleeding ulcer, the blood loss is so subtle that you don't notice it.)

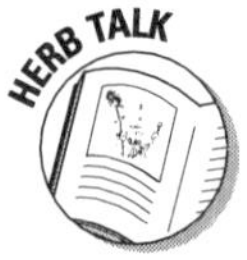

- Women of reproductive age are more prone to iron-deficiency and other types of anemia because they lose blood during the menstrual flow each month.
- Elderly women are also more likely to develop the condition because of poor nutrition and lowered ability to assimilate and utilize nutrients from their food.
- Vegetarian women who eat lots of whole grains, but no red meat, are at increased risk, because some molecules from grains, called *phytates,* can interfere with iron absorption.

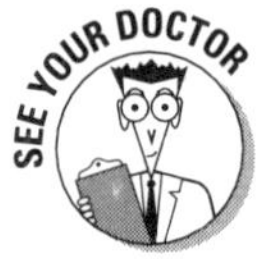

Mild anemia can be subtle and can affect your memory, learning ability, mood, immune status, and energy levels. However, if you experience chronic fatigue and your tongue and cheeks are pale, or if your menstrual flow is slight or stops altogether, see your doctor for a diagnosis.

To improve the symptoms of anemia, try the following:

- **Eat iron-rich foods.** If you find that you have a blood-deficient condition or if you feel a little run-down and have pale cheeks and a pale tongue, add more iron-rich foods to your diet. If you eat meat, I recommend adding 3 or 4 ounces of red meat each week. Liver is a particularly rich source of iron. Eat more green leafy vegetables, almonds, and almond milk.
- **Take nutritional supplements.** Take an all-inclusive dietary supplement that gives you from 15 to 20 milligrams of iron a day. A comprehensive nutritional formula for building strong blood contains iron, folic acid, vitamin B12, pantothenic acid, pyridoxine, riboflavin, thiamine, vitamin A, vitamin E, and copper.
- **Keep your digestive system strong.** According to traditional systems of healing, like Traditional Chinese Medicine, strong blood is built with the aid of a strong digestive system. If you have any digestive symptoms (such as gas after eating) or if you're overweight, you're more likely to have digestive weakness. I recommend adding a bitter tonic formula to your daily regime to enhance the uptake of nutrients necessary for building strong blood — you can find bitter tonic formulas at your local herb shop or natural foods store (and some information on bitter tonics in Chapter 1).

Estrogen-replacement therapy

One of the biggest, and in many cases, most difficult and controversial questions facing women is whether to take estrogen pills or use patches. This is especially true of women over 50 who start to produce less estrogen on their own. Today, doctors and drug companies are promoting estrogen pills for women going through menopause more than ever. Some doctors tell you that if you're a woman over 50, you should be taking estrogen for the rest of your life. Other doctors, like Dr. Susan Love, a breast surgeon, are concerned about women taking extra estrogen. She says that by taking estrogen after menopause, you're not replacing something that's missing, but adding something that's not naturally present.

Traditional estrogen-replacement therapy does the following:

- Reduces the risk of osteoporosis.
- May reduce the risk of heart disease.
- Decreases hot flashes.
- Keeps some women looking young.

TIP

If you do decide to take estrogen, use a product containing estrogens that are natural to your body. Good formulas are available containing estradiol, estriol, and estrone — the major estrogens. Premarin is the most widely prescribed estrogen. (Be aware that Premarin is produced from pregnant mares that are kept caged and catheterized in small stalls, and given little water to concentrate their urine. The foals are sold to the meat industry for pet food. This may weigh on your concience.) Natural estrogens are produced in a chemical laboratory from vegetable sources, mostly wild yams and soybeans.

Side effects of estrogen-replacement exist, however:

- The most well-studied and documented side effect of estrogen supplementation is an increased risk of uterine cancer. Adding progesterone or a progestin to estrogen reduces, but probably doesn't completely eliminate, the risk.
- The most controversial potential side effect of estrogen supplementation is an increased risk of breast cancer. Many studies show an increased risk, but no one knows the exact extent of it. This depends on your health habits, immune strength, genetics, and other factors.

Although many doctors tell you that the potential risks of estrogen replacement outweigh the benefits, this is your decision. Many women tell me that they would rather have heart disease or risk having a broken bone at 70 or 80 than even slightly increase their risk of breast cancer. Women often feel that at least heart disease and osteoporosis are within their control, whereas breast cancer is not.

The bottom line is that estrogen supplementation can be useful for a year or two when a woman is having severe hot flashes, depression, or other symptoms during menopause. It may be necessary for women who have had their ovaries removed at an earlier age. Always take natural estrogen, and always take it *with* natural progesterone.

An increasingly viable and empowering option is natural estrogen therapy and the decision to avoid estrogen pills or creams. New natural products that help relieve symptoms from lowered estrogen levels are available in natural-foods stores, by mail, from the Web, and from pharmacies (see Appendix C).

An exciting development in natural medicine is the recognition that protective, estrogen-like substances, called *phytoestrogens,* occur in food and are abundant in some herbs. (*Phyto* means plant-based.) Phytoestrogens (FI-toe-ES-tro-gens) are thought to stimulate estrogen tissue like that found in the breast, gently supporting a woman's own estrogen, while protecting the tissue from over-stimulation from more powerful estrogens. Estrogens from your own fat tissue and potent estrogen-like toxins from the environment, such as certain pesticides, are known to increase the risk of developing breast cancer and other cancers. Scientists have identified several kinds of phytoestrogens, but only two have any research to show their effectiveness. These are the — *lignans* (LIG-nans), which occur naturally in flaxseed meal and *isoflavones* (eye-so-FLA-vones), such as genistein (gen-ISS-teen) and daidzein (DYED-zeen) that are abundant in many legumes. The isoflavones, especially genistein, are among the most powerful.

If you're currently taking estrogen or if you're considering taking it, here are some practical ways to try the natural (and potentially safer) way:

- **Consume phytoestrogens.** Drink 2 cups daily of an herbal tea containing phytoestrogens, like red clover or alfalfa. Or take a powder, tablets, or capsules daily that contain an herbal extract containing phytoestrogens. Some products are labeled right on the package, indicating how much phytoestrogen they contain. Several exciting new phytoestrogen products are now sold in natural-foods stores and pharmacies, including a red clover extract tablet. I use a soy protein powder that offers a specified amount of genistein with each spoonful. Yes, men also eat foods with phytoestrogens in many traditional cultures, like China. Prostate cancer is almost non-existent in China, and some scientists point to the abundant quantities of phytoestrogen — rich soy products and other beans that Chinese men consume — as a likely factor.

My friend Jim Duke, an internationally-known herbalist and scientist says, "I would rather enjoy my medicine." With this spirit in mind, check out the recipe for Chocolate Soy Delight, a phytoestrogen treat — it's really as good for you as it is delicious.

- **Add more beans to your diet.** Beans are the best natural source of phytoestrogens. Soy products like soy milk and tofu are the most talked-about and heavily promoted dietary sources of phytoestrogens, but beans from other parts of the world, including ones that grow in your own area, are well-worth adding to your diet. I recommend that women who need extra estrogen (or protection from breast cancer) eat beans in some form daily. In my house, we have bean soups and stews at least three or four times a week, especially during the winter months — my wife and I also eat a lot of tofu, tempeh, and other soy products.
- **Take an herbal hormone-balancing tea or extract product.** The most popular and proven herbs are black cohosh, which is especially helpful to reduce hot flashes, and vitex (VY-teks), for menopause and PMS. The two herbs are often blended together in herbal products.
- **Add two tablespoons of flaxseed,** ground to a powder in a coffee grinder or blender to your morning cereal or other dishes.

Chocolate Soy Delight

This rich, creamy chocolate drink provides phytoestrogens, antioxidants, and mood-enhancing properties from the chocolate.

Preparation time: *10 minutes*

Yield: *1 cup*

2 tablespoons soy protein powder

1 to 2 tablespoons unsweetened cocoa powder

1 cup soymilk

1 ripe banana, peeled

1 teaspoon vanilla extract (optional)

1 Put the soy protein powder and unsweetened cocoa powder together in your blender.

2 Pour in 1 to 2 cups of soymilk, depending on how thick you like your shake. Place the banana in the blender. Add vanilla, if desired.

3 Blend until creamy. Enjoy!

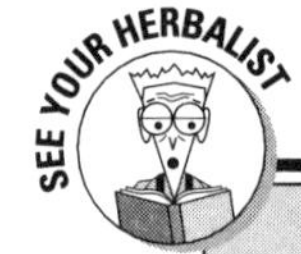

Antibiotics? Probiotics!

Recent studies show that when you take antibiotics for some common infections like bladder infections, you can have symptoms longer than when you didn't take them. You may also contribute to the growing numbers of drug-resistant strains.

For many kinds of mild to moderate infections, try seeing your herbalist or natural health care provider for a check-up and herbal formula. Bacteria and other disease-causing organisms have trouble adapting to herbs because they contain many types of effective compounds.

Here are some helpful hints if you decide to use antibiotics to help get rid of an infection.

- If you have a very mild infection, try taking probiotics instead of antibiotics! Probiotics are beneficial organisms (such as acidophilus) that, when taken orally for a week or so, can discourage bacteria and other disease-causing agents from proliferating, eliminating the infection. Take 3 capsules a day of an acidophilus or other strains of probiotic organisms with meals.
- Take the antibiotics as directed. If you stop before you finish the prescription, the bacteria can sometimes adapt to the drug and develop resistance.
- Many antibiotics are stressful to your liver. Take 2 or 3 capsules or tablets of a milk thistle product for extra protection.
- Take an immune stimulant like echinacea to help your body deal with the infection. Use 3 to 5 droppersful in a little water, 4 or 5 times daily.
- After finishing with the antibiotics, continue taking the echinacea for another five days and add an acidophilus supplement daily for two to four weeks. I recommend capsules containing up to 3 billion active beneficial organisms like various kinds of acidophilus.

Fibroids and cysts

Uterine fibroid cysts occur commonly in women of all ages, especially before menopause. After menopause, declining estrogen levels often lead to a reduction in size and numbers of fibroids. Fibroid cysts in the uterus are not usually life-threatening, but they can be painful and can interfere with pregnancy. Herbalists often recommend blood-moving herbs to help prevent the formation of cysts and immune stimulants to assist the body in removing the cysts. Phytoestrogens (see the section "Estrogen-replacement therapy") can help reduce overstimulation of the uterus by too much estrogen. I know women who have been able to eliminate uterine fibroids with the complete program that I recommend in this section.

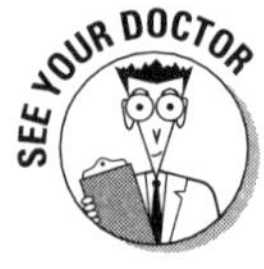

Have an ultrasound examination if you suspect you have fibroid cysts. Excessive menstrual bleeding is a possible sign.

Blood-moving herbs, such as motherwort, cayenne, and ginkgo, are traditionally recommended by herbalists to open up blood vessels to tissue in the body that has a stagnation of blood and vital energy. When these two life-giving substances are not moving properly, such as during times of stress or inactivity, the flow of nutrients and oxygen is restricted, and wastes build up. When this happens, you may feel pain in the pelvic area, and cysts and tumors are more likely to form.

- **Blood-moving herbs:** Make a tea or take an extract in tablet or capsule form of one or more of the following herbs: dong quai, cayenne, or turmeric. Take the herbs morning and evening every day for several months, or until pain disappears and cysts are improved.
- **Hormone-balancing herbs** like vitex and black cohosh taken regularly are a key part of a uterine health program.
- **Immune stimulants:** Castor oil is one of the most powerful herbal aids for resolving tumors and cysts. The noted healer Edgar Cayce recommended placing a castor oil pack over tumors and cysts and reported many successful treatments. The use of castor oil packs is a renowned and favored treatment of many herbalists.

Castor Oil Pack

Use a castor oil pack two or three days a week — more for stubborn cysts. I know women who've use the pack for months with great success. Combine the pack with healthy dietary habits and lots of exercise (such as daily walking) to help circulate the blood and remove wastes.

Preparation time: *30 minutes*

Yield: *1 pack*

1 cup castor oil

Linen cloth, folded to about 6" x 8"

Glass baking dish

1 Pour the castor oil into a glass baking dish. Soak the folded cloth in the oil and place in a 300° oven.

2 After 15 to 30 minutes (or when the pack is hot but not scalding), take the dish from the oven.

3 Place the cloth over the lower abdomen (or other area with a cyst or tumor). To prevent the oil from leaking, cover the cloth with a plastic bag.

4 Cover the pack with a hot water bottle or heating pad. Keep the pack hot, but comfortably so. Leave the pack in place for 30 to 40 minutes.

Menstrual discomfort

While some women have painless and predictable periods, others experience symptoms such as back pain, nausea, and cramping. For many women, herbs can help ease both physical and emotional symptoms.

- **PMS:** Most women know all too well what premenstrual syndrome is all about. According to modern medicine, PMS is a collection of symptoms that come and go in relationship to the menstrual cycle. About a week after ovulation and just before menstruation begins, a woman's hormone levels drop precipitously. Mood-regulating chemicals in the brain like serotonin also drop. These changes can dramatically affect a woman's mood and disposition, leading to sugar cravings, acne, a feeling of tension, and constipation, all of which are generally relieved when the menses start flowing. The hormonal changes that happen during a woman's cycle are delicately balanced. Many factors can disrupt this balance, especially stress and strong emotions, but also diet and lack of exercise. Fortunately, herbs such as vitex, dong quai, evening primrose oil, and skullcap can help.
- **Cramping:** Many herbs are useful for easing the cramps associated with the premenstrual phase, even when they continue into the menses. Antispasmodics help relax the uterus, and prostaglandin-inhibitors can ease cramping and pain.

  Herbal prostaglandin-inhibitors include evening primrose oil, feverfew, and meadowsweet. Evening primrose oil (in capsules) can be helpful for some women when taken during the cycle, along with freshly-ground flaxseed meal. Sprinkle a tablespoon or two of freshly ground flaxseeds on cereal or other foods. About a week before your period is expected, begin taking a teaspoon of the tincture of meadowsweet or feverfew, in a little water, 3 or 4 times daily, away from meals.
- **Late periods:** You may or may not be worried if your period is late, but either way, the feeling of expectation is sometimes difficult. Tension builds up, and symptoms of bloating or fullness and irritability can rule your life for a time. Herbalists recommend a class of herbs called emmenagogues (em-MEN-uh-gogs) to get things flowing. In my experience, the most reliable emmenagogues are yarrow, black cohosh, blue cohosh, and feverfew. Use them as a tea, drinking 3 cups a day. Or, when you're in no mood to brew up the herbs, take them in convenient tincture form, up to 1 teaspoon in a cup of hot water, 3 times daily. (See Chapter 2 for more on tinctures.) These herbs are available in capsules and tablets, but they don't work as well as a liquid preparation for late periods.
- **Irregular cycles:** Herbal hormone regulators are helpful when your cycles are not like clockwork. When this has you wondering and adds stress to your life, try a hormone-regulating herb throughout several cycles. Vitex, the small, spicy, brownish-red fruits from a common Mediterranean shrub, is often the answer. I've recommended it to women for helping regulate hormone balance for 15 years.

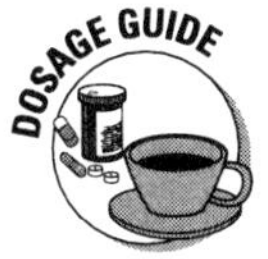

Science shows that vitex works on the pituitary gland, the master regulator of all your hormones, to increase progesterone production from the ovaries. The extract can also regulate other hormones to help make the menses a more enjoyable, or at least tolerable, experience. Take vitex liquid drops, first thing in the morning before breakfast — 2 or 3 droppersful, depending on your size.

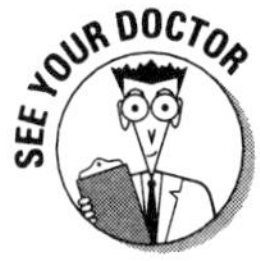

- **Amenorrhea:** When your periods stop (called *amennorhea*), the problem can vary. Women athletes who reduce total body fat to a low level produce less estrogen and can experience increases of testosterone. This can stop the period temporarily. When your period stops and it is a concern to you, or if you are trying to get pregnant, reduce the intensity of your workouts for a month or two to see it they start. If you're blood deficient (anemic) or protein deficient, the period often stops or is lighter than normal. If you don't exercise intensively and your period stops, make sure you're getting adequate protein and blood-building nutrients. If this condition persists, you may want to see your doctor. See the section called "Anemia," earlier in this chapter. If a hormone imbalance is to blame, try two or three months of vitex liquid drops.

Osteoporosis

Hip fractures and the thinning of bones can reduce the quality of life and even lead to death in many older women. Strong bones are created early in life with the help of a nutritious diet rich in minerals and low in refined sugar. Exercise is another important ingredient for strong healthy bones all through life. After menopause, *estradiol* (ess-truh-DIE-all), the most potent estrogen your body makes, declines. Because estrogen is a bone-growth stimulant, your bones can start a thinning process that can continue for decades. Adding extra estrogen can help slow this process for up to ten years after the onset of menopause, but not much after that. Estrogen can also increase your risk of developing some cancers later in life and can sustain your menstrual cycle for years. New studies, while not conclusive, show that natural phytoestrogens can provide some of the benefits of oral estradiol or Premarin with even more benefits and none of the risk.

- **Herbal bone-builders:** Sea vegetables such as wakame (WA-kuh-may), nori (NOR-ee), and kombu (KOM-boo) are nature's most potent bone-builders. Add a nettle and horsetail extract and you have a powerful addition to a healthy diet. Horsetail extracts help increase the body's uptake of calcium. Horsetail is a plant rich in the bone-building mineral silicon.
- **Phytoestrogens:** Herbal phytoestrogen sources include red clover and alfalfa. All beans contain these substances in abundance. Add foods like hummus dip and the traditional fermented soy product, tempeh to your diet on a regular basis — a great way to protect your bones *and* enjoy your medicine.

REMEMBER

If you're pressed for time, but still want your protective phytoestrogens and minerals, take about 3 tablets of a complete nutritional system with at least half of the daily requirement of vitamin D, calcium, magnesium, and other important bone-building nutrients. Add 2 or 3 tablets of a horsetail extract. For dessert, pop 2 tablets containing a red clover extract or drink a strong cup of alfalfa and red clover tea. Because it's dessert, add a little stevia herb or a few licorice slices to make it sweet.

Pregnancy and birthing

Whether you're planning a pregnancy or are already pregnant, herbal remedies are a time-honored and safe way to go. Several herbs are recommended widely by midwives and are considered safe to use during pregnancy. Others are controversial and still others are known to be unsafe to use during pregnancy (see the sidebar "Avoid these herbs while pregnant or nursing"). The following six herbs are your best bet during pregnancy. See the *Herb Guide* in the green pages near the back of this book for complete dosage information on these helpful herbs. I recommend starting with a standard dose and varying it slightly, depending on your height and weight.

- **Ginger:** Morning sickness is an unwelcome challenge for millions of pregnant women. Ginger tea is a natural alternative to settle the stomach and reduce nausea. Studies show that it's as effective as leading anti-nausea medicines and that ginger is completely harmless, with a 3,000-year track record of safety. Use only fresh ginger, organic if it's available, from any market or natural food store. Crystallized ginger is sweet and yummy, convenient, and can work as well as the tea.
- **Nettle leaf:** The leaf of the nettle plant is nature's vitamin pill. Revered by herbalists for centuries, nettle tea is a nutritious and pleasant-tasting brew for women, whether they're pregnant or not. Simmer 1 cup of the nettle leaf for 20 to 30 minutes, and drink several cups daily. Add red raspberry leaf for regulating your bowels and tonifying the uterus, or chamomile flowers for its relaxing qualities.
- **Red raspberry leaf:** This good-tasting herb is the safest and most widely recommended herb for toning and preparing the uterus for birth. Drink 1 or 2 cups daily throughout the pregnancy.
- **Yellow dock:** Many women are iron- and blood-deficient during pregnancy. This can make you tired and deliver less oxygen to you and your baby's cells and tissues. Widely recommended by midwives, using the root of this common weed is the best way to enhance iron uptake and utilization during pregnancy. Yellow dock tea, tincture, or capsules act as a mild bowel regulator, helping to keep you regular. Add nettle leaf tea or natural iron supplements in capsules or tablets to yellow dock.

Avoid these herbs while pregnant or nursing

Although certain herbs are beneficial during pregnancy and can prevent anemia or help with a smooth delivery, the following herbs should be avoided during this time:

- Aloe vera
- Angelica
- Anise
- Arnica
- Asafetida
- Ashwaganda
- Barberry
- Basil
- Bee balm
- Black cohosh
- Bladderwrack
- Blessed thistle
- Bloodroot
- Blue cohosh
- Blue flag
- Borage
- Buchu
- Bugleweed
- California poppy
- Camphor
- Cascara sagrada
- Cassia
- Castor oil
- Catnip
- Celandine
- Celery
- Coltsfoot
- Comfrey
- Corydalis
- Dong quai
- Elecampane
- Ephedra
- Fenugreek
- Feverfew
- Goldenseal
- Guggul
- Horehound
- Hyssop
- Ipecac
- Juniper
- Kava
- Lemongrass
- Licorice
- Lobelia
- Mace
- Motherwort
- Mugwort
- Myrrh
- Nutmeg
- Oregon grape root
- Osha
- Parsley
- Pennyroyal
- Pleurisy root
- Prickly ash
- Quassia
- Red clover
- Rosemary
- Rue
- Sage
- Senna
- Thuja
- Turmeric
- Uva Ursi
- Vervain
- Vitex
- Wild indigo
- Wormwood
- Yarrow

Avoid the following herbs during nursing unless under the care of a qualified health care practitioner:

- Aloe vera
- Basil
- Black cohosh
- Bladderwrack
- Borage
- Bugleweed
- Cascara sagrada
- Coltsfoot
- Comfrey
- Elecampane
- Ephedra
- Kava
- Licorice
- Male fern
- Senna
- Queen's delight (stillingia)
- Wormwood

Vaginal infections

The top three vaginal infections are associated with the disease-causing agents (pathogens) trichomonas, candida, and chlamydia and are responsible for about nine-tenths of all vaginal infections. Gonorrhea is no longer as common as it once was because of antibiotics, but resistant strains are making a comeback.

Candida

Candida is a yeast-like organism that lives in the vagina and intestinal track. If your immune system is strong, and your vaginal and intestinal environments are balanced with beneficial organisms and generally healthy, candida is often well behaved. When these environments get out of balance from taking antibiotics or from stress, poor nutrition, and a host of other factors, candida can run amok, creating a vaginal yeast infection. Symptoms include a white, cheesy discharge with a yeasty smell and a red and irritated vulva.

Tried and true herbal treatments for candida include echinacea drops, taken internally, and tea tree oil used as a douche. Here are the herbs that I find most effective for preventing and easing vaginal yeast infections from candida overgrowth. Consult Appendix B for the standard doses that I recommend. Vary the dose slightly, depending on your size and needs.

- **Garlic:** Take 2 to 3 capsules of a garlic product. Aged products with no odor are not effective for infections. If you don't mind the odor, fresh garlic is even more potent. Cut the cloves into slices and swallow 1 sliced clove several times a day with a little fennel tea or water. Chewing a little parsley can help eliminate the garlic odor on your breath.
- **Echinacea:** One clinical study from Germany supported this traditional American herbal remedy as an effective treatment and preventative for candida yeast infections. Take a standard dose as given in the *Herb Guide* in the green-colored pages near the back of this book.
- **Tea tree oil:** You can use a potent herbal douche to help discourage candida growth. Tea tree oil, a distilled essence from an Australian tree, is popular, safe, and effective for killing candida yeast. Make a tea with Oregon grape root or barberry by simmering 1 tablespoon of the herb powder or coarsely-cut herb in $1^1/_2$ cups of water for 15 minutes. Let the tea cool, strain until clear, and add about 6 drops of tea tree oil. Use once a week for prevention if you're experiencing on-going yeast infections or daily for up to five days for an acute infection. Drink 2 cups of a mild Oregon grape root or barberry tea, 2 to 3 times daily, for persistent infections.

Dilute tea tree oil to prevent irritation to your delicate vaginal tissues. I recommend adding 6 drops for every cup of tea, but you can reduce this dose if you experience any sensitivity or irritation.

- **Yogurt or apple cider vinegar douches:** You can alternate the tea tree oil/Oregon grape root douche with a yogurt or mild apple cider vinegar douche to support the health of the vaginal intestinal flora. This discourages candida growth.

Other vaginal infections

If you have a vaginal infection with a fishy or foul smell, you may have a vaginal infection associated with chlamydia or trichomonas. Consult your doctor or gynecologist for a diagnosis. Some vaginal infections can lead to more serious infections.

If you have a vaginal infection other than candida, for instance trichomonas, gardnerella, or chlamydia, your doctor will most likely prescribe antibiotics. Huang lian (hwang lee-EN) tablets, available from Traditional Chinese Medicine practitioners or from health food stores, are an effective alternative to antibiotics. Refrain from taking antibiotics when you can — many researchers are concerned that after years of overusing antibiotics for every sniffle or sore throat, new antibacterial-resistant and dangerous superbugs are proliferating. Visit your herbalist or natural health care practitioner for some alternatives.

Herbs for Men

Men don't buy herbs and use them as often as women, but in my experience, many men are keenly interested in natural medicine and are becoming more interested in exploring new health options. Like everyone, men can benefit from herbs for treating common ailments as diverse as on-the-job injuries, upset stomachs, poor digestion, headaches, and fatigue.

Like women, men also have particular needs. Here are some of the most important men's health issues today.

Prostate inflammation (BPH) and cancer

The prostate is a small doughnut-shaped gland wrapped around the urethra. It secretes nourishing and lubricating substances that form part of the semen. Enlargement of the gland is associated with symptoms like painful urination and frequent urination, especially at night, which can interrupt sleep. This ailment occurs in over 40 percent of men in their 50s and about 90 percent who are in their 80s! Treatments from modern medicine include drugs (such as Proscar, which is also called finasteride) and surgery, but both can have significant side effects such as hormone imbalance, lowered sex drive, and permanent impotence.

I see significant results with saw palmetto for men in my Santa Cruz clinic. My dad swears by the herb. He had unpleasant effects and no benefit from Proscar and decided to switch to natural medicine. He was able to sleep through the night without trips to the bathroom after three months of regularly using saw palmetto. We were both interviewed on a PBS show on health recently to attest to the benefits of this beneficial men's herb.

Other prostate herbs that are popular today include nettle root, pumpkin seed oil, kava, and pygeum (pie-GEE-um). These herbs are included in formulas to support prostate health. Pygeum is considered rare and endangered in Africa — I recommend avoiding products that contain it for now.

For men over 55, I recommend regular prostate checkups, preferably every year or two. Because prostate cancer is increasingly common among men over 50, pay attention to the health of this important organ.

Why wait until symptoms, such as difficult urination, happen? Getting at least 20 minutes of daily exercise helps prevent prostate problems. Get a complete checkup and herbal program from your herbalist or natural health care practitioner. Add lots of fresh vegetables and fruit, whole grains, and beans to your diet. If you eat red meat, I recommend cutting your intake to once a week. Eating fish can also improve prostate health.

Impotence

The failure of men to achieve an erection has many causes. A man may not be in the mood or have emotional blocks to prevent him from relaxing and experiencing true intimacy. However, because most men have hardening and blockage of the arteries to some degree, blood circulation to the penis is often increasingly impaired as they age.

Speaking of circulation, news of the new men's drug Viagra is circulating around the globe. Some men seem to get good results with the pill, which helps the penis hold blood and maintain erection. The latest reports show that taking Viagra with certain heart medications, like nitroglycerin, can be fatal. Herbalists and doctors don't know much about the long-term safety and effectiveness of the drug, while herbs have been around for thousands of years. While this "men's pill" is hyped to the heavens, as an herbalist, I emphasize the importance of good diet, counseling, exercise, clear vessels, and herbal medicine as a lasting and healthful approach to impotence — even if Viagra does work for you. Here are the herbal remedies that can really help when you take them regularly:

- **Calming herbs to help get in the mood:** Helpful herbal remedies include calmatives, or relaxing herbs, like California poppy extract, valerian (va-LEHR-ee-an), passion flower, and kava.
- **Circulation means motivation:** With good circulation through all the vessels of your body, you will live a longer, healthier, and happier life. Your brain and memory will work better, and for some men, "the second brain," will be performing much better. A healthful diet low in fats and high in whole vegetables, fruits, beans, and grains, in addition to regular exercise are the most important elements of a successful program. Good circulation herbs include ginkgo, hawthorn, garlic, and cayenne. Use them regularly every day for helping to "let it flow."
- **Hormone support:** Sexual function and desire are intimately linked with the body's hormone balance. Steroid hormones like testosterone and estrogen help regulate your sexual desire and ability. Ancient Chinese herbs like ginseng are renowned for helping to balance hormones and support sexual function. The most useful men's hormone support herbs include red ginseng, a mushroom called cordyceps, cistanches, psoralea seed, dodder seed, and for men who also have high blood pressure, the bark from the eucommia tree. Many of these popular herbs are available from an herb supplier and in larger natural food stores. Chinese *patent* (pre-made) formulas in pill and liquid form are available containing blends of several of these herbs — you don't have to take them separately. A traditional formula is balanced with other herbs to reduce possible side effects and enhance the effects of the formula.

  I recommend visiting a practitioner of Traditional Chinese Medicine (TCM) for a complete diagnosis and treatment plan, including a traditional herbal formula to support hormone health and balance.

The original Viagra — yohimbe

For years, doctors have been prescribing a drug derived from the bark of an African tree, yohimbe *(Pausinystalia yohimbe)* to increase circulation to the penis and help men achieve and maintain erections. Studies show that yohimbe (yo-HIM-bee) works for some men. The whole herb is available in numerous men's products found in natural-foods stores, drug stores, and herbs shops. The herb is also a central nervous system stimulant, so taking it regularly can interfere with your sleep and lead to nervousness in some cases. I recommend avoiding the herb altogether if you feel nervous, have trouble sleeping, or have high blood pressure.

Always consult with your herbalist and doctor if you are taking pharmaceutical drugs like MAO inhibitors for depression — dangerous interactions can occur.

Baldness

A thick head of beautiful hair is a sign of health and vitality, but just because you don't have one, don't feel that you aren't healthy or vital. Sometimes the genes play tricks on you, and many men watch in anguish as more hair falls out week by week. Unfortunately, no magic herbal bullet exists for preventing hair loss.

You *can* help slow down the process and increase the health of your scalp and hair by improving circulation and nutrition to the hair follicles. Brush your hair and scalp regularly and apply alternating hot and cold washcloths (a process called *hydrotherapy*) or hot and cold shower sprays right on the scalp. This increases circulation and removes waste products.

Try the following tips:

- **Try using silica — nature's hair strengthener.** The best nourishing silica-containing herbs for the hair are nettle and horsetail. Extracts of these strengthening herbs are available in capsule and tablet products. Take these herb extracts internally for several months (up to one year) and use a strong tea of nettle and horsetail to rinse your hair. For even better results, add $^1/_4$ cup of apple cider vinegar and 20 drops of rosemary oil to each cup of herb tea. Rinse your hair with the blend and work it into the scalp with vigorous massaging motions for a few minutes each time you shampoo.
- **Increase circulation to nourish hair follicles.** To increase circulation to the scalp, take 3 cayenne caps twice daily with meals. Or add a hot, spicy meal to your diet once or twice a week. A ginger compress is an excellent circulatory stimulant. Make 2 cups of strong ginger tea with 5 or 10 slices of fresh ginger from the market and add a few sprigs of rosemary or 10 drops of rosemary oil. To make the compress, dip a washcloth into the warm (but not scalding) tea, wring it out, and place it over your scalp and hair. Allow the tea to come in contact with the scalp for best effectiveness, and repeat several times with fresh tea.

  Regular exercise can also help increase circulation and remove wastes through the lymphatic system.

Herbs for Kids

Because herbs can help relieve common complaints in a gentle, effective way, they're a natural for treating children's ailments. The following list contains the most common children's health challenges and remedies to treat them.

- **Colds:** An excellent tried and true herbal formula for colds is made up of equal parts yarrow, elder, and peppermint, and it's safe for kids. Also try adding ginger tea or powdered ginger to baths at the onset of a cold. Echinacea tincture, which rallies the body's defense system, is safe for children and can be given in 5- to 30-drop doses, several times a day, depending on the age, size, and robustness of a child. (See Chapter 2 for more information on tinctures.)
- **Congestion:** To help ease nasal congestion, which is often worse at night, add a few drops of eucalyptus essential oil to a vaporizer and let it fill the room while the child is sleeping. Try an herbal *glycerite* (liquid preparations of herbs in vegetable glycerin that are especially designed for kids) and herbs like eyebright (a decongestant) to open the nasal passages.
- **Conjunctivitis (pink eye):** To cool and soothe infected eyes, use freshly grated potato to make a poultice (herbal pack) for the eyes. Place a handful of the grated potato in your hand, lean your head back, and place it over your eyes (keep eyes closed). Leave the poultice on for five to ten minutes. You can repeat the process as often as you like. You can also make an eyewash with goldenseal tea, but strain the tea thoroughly before applying it to your eyes. Wash your eyes with the cooled, strained tea or place the tea in an eyecup. To soothe itchy red eyes, place a cool and moist chamomile tea bag over the infected eye or eyes for up to five minutes.
- **Coughs:** Make a tea with 1 teaspoon marshmallow leaf and mullein (MULL-en) leaf, 1/4 teaspoon licorice, and a few anise seeds added for flavor for each 2 cups water. Give in 1 tablespoon doses frequently, as needed. A few sage leaves added to the tea make it more effective, but not as tasty. Good herbal cough syrups are available at natural-foods and herb stores, including the effective loquat (LOW-kwat) syrup from China or a native American Indian favorite, wild cherry bark.
- **Cuts:** Use a healing salve containing plantain, calendula, echinacea, and/or St. John's wort. Apply a small amount to the affected area several times daily.

- **Diarrhea:** Black walnut tincture or blackberry root tincture in a little water work wonders for diarrhea. Take 10 to 30 drops, 3 times daily. Additionally, you may want to put your child on a diet that's easy on the digestion — bananas, rice, applesauce (sprinkled with cinnamon), toast, and yogurt — for a day or two. Check out the recipe for Apple-Peel Cure, which follows this list.

- **Diaper rash:** Creams or salves from calendula flowers or chamomile flowers can help clear up diaper rash quickly. They are readily available in natural-foods stores, or you can make your own (see Chapter 6).

- **Earache:** Use mullein and garlic ear oil, which are available at natural-foods stores or from mail-order sources listed in Appendix C. You can also give echinacea tincture internally, 2 to 3 droppersful, 3 to 4 times daily.

  Cutting out dairy products often relieves the symptoms of earache and can even stop the infections from recurring in chronic cases. Over the years, I've seen great results from this simple dietary change from cow's milk to flavored soy, rice, or almond milk.

- **Fever:** Make a hot tea with peppermint, catnip, and elder and have your child drink 3 or 4 cups during the day. Apply cool compresses of elder flower tea to hands and feet to help lower fevers. For higher fevers, bathe the child for 10 or 15 minutes at a time in a cool bath with a few cups of added elderflower tea with 5 drops of lavender oil. If it's more convenient, give your child echinacea and goldenseal tincture blended 50/50 with meadowsweet tincture every half-hour. Aspirin can bring fevers down quickly, but meadowsweet tincture has similar compounds and may work without the risk of aspirin. Remember that fever is nature's way of eliminating disease-causing organisms and waste products.

  When the fever persists for more than 48 hours or it gets higher than 104°, call your doctor.

- **Gas:** Make a tea of equal parts fennel, caraway, peppermint, and chamomile and have your child drink 2 or 3 cups of it. For small babies, you can give teaspoonful doses of anise or caraway tea. Simple peppermint tea, a cup every few hours during the day, works fine.

  Don't give honey to infants under 6 months of age. Instead, use stevia or licorice tincture or tea.

- **Hyperactivity and restlessness:** My favorite herb for kids who can't slow down is California poppy. Tinctures, glycerites, and tablets that contain the herb are available. California poppy is effective and safe for kids. In my experience, even kids taking drugs like Ritalin often do well on the herb and can sometimes reduce their dose of the drug.

Make sure to consult your professional health care provider if you want to try California poppy while a child is taking pharmaceutical drugs.

- **Insect bites:** The best remedy for bites, stings, cuts, and minor burns is fresh plantain, chewed and placed right on the spot. Turn to the Herb Guide in the green pages of this book to find out more about this amazing, healing plant — a common weed in many yards everywhere. If you don't have plantain nearby, collect seed from a vacant lot or field or order from one of the seed companies listed in Appendix C. Spread the seeds in an open area in your yard, cover with soil, and keep moist.

  In addition, for insect bites, apply echinacea tincture directly to the area. A salve of plantain, calendula, or comfrey also works well (see Chapter 6 for information on making your own salves). A little St. John's wort oil applied right to the bite is effective.

- **Irritability:** When your child is particularly fussy, which sometimes occurs at the end of the day, give him or her a cup of catnip, chamomile, or linden tea. While you're at it, you may want to have one yourself!
- **Sleeping problems:** Giving a child a bath of linden flowers, chamomile flowers, lemon balm herb, or lavender flowers is excellent for calming before bed. Make a strong tea and pour it into the bath. Baths are a painless way of getting herbs into kids. They also love massage, so add a few drops of relaxing chamomile or lavender essential oils to massage oils and use them just before bedtime. Make an effective sleep pillow by filling an 8" square cloth with hops, lavender, and lemon balm.
- **Stomachache:** Warm peppermint and/or chamomile tea works well given in small, frequent doses. Also, massage the stomach with lavender massage oil. When the child has a stomachache along with nausea or vomiting, give ginger and chamomile or peppermint tea, $^1/_2$ to 1 cup, up to 5 times during the day.

  If the child is throwing up for more than an hour, call your doctor. Either way, give the vomiting child plenty of fluids, and replace electrolytes with 1 teaspoon of Dr. Bronners Balanced Amino Bouillon, which is available in most natural-foods stores, in 1 cup of water every 2 hours (or other rich source of electrolytes as directed by your doctor) if vomiting continues.

- **Sunburn:** Use fresh aloe leaf gel or bottled aloe vera gel (or both). St. John's wort oil and lavender essential oil also work wonderfully to take away the pain of burns and to encourage healing.
- **Teething:** Two homeopathic preparations, chamomilia and belladonna, have a high success rate in treating teething babies (see Chapter 1 for more on homeopathy). You can also gently rub St. John's wort oil onto the gums to provide relief.

Apple-Peel Cure

This classic recipe is for healing diarrhea. The natural pectin in the apples firms up the bowels and kids love the sauce.

Preparation time: *25 minutes*

Yield: *1 cup*

4 apples

1 teaspoon honey, or to taste

Cinnamon to taste

1 Peel the apples and add the peels to 1 cup of water. (Set aside the apples for some other use.)

2 Simmer the peels with the honey for 20 minutes or until a sauce forms.

3 Sprinkle with cinnamon and serve.

Getting kids to take herbs

Kids don't want to hear about how herbs are good for them. They only want to know one thing: do they taste good? Unfortunately for parents, not all herbs are palatable to kids. Here are time-tested ways to get your kids to dose up with health-promoting herbs.

- Capsules are suspect right away. The last thing a kid wants to see is a parent holding out a pill. The answer? Try dipping a capsule or tablet in a little honey-water, or in stubborn cases, a little sugar. You can add a few drops of your child's favorite flavor into the sweet solution by adding a drop of essential oil. Kids usually like orange oil, but some also go for cinnamon or mint.
- Alcoholic tinctures (see Chapter 2) are easy to hide in juice or sweet tea. In small doses, I rarely see problems with the alcohol in tinctures for kids. Infants under 6 months old only need a few drops. Here are the average doses I recommend:

Age	Dosage
Under 6-months old	2 to 10 drops
6-months to a year	10 to 20 drops
One year to five years	20 to 30 drops
Five years to ten years	30 to 40 drops
Ten years to 15 years	1 to 2 droppersful
Over 15 years old	Adult dose

Herbs for Staying Young

Feeling and looking young has a great deal to do with attitude. When you look for opportunities to keep learning and growing personally, you create youthfulness. Paul Bragg, the founder of health food stores and my teacher, was a major inspiration to practice a healthy lifestyle; he called himself a life-extension specialist. He lived past 95 and was still swimming and active until he died. He considered the most important elements of a healthy life eating high-quality whole foods and eating moderately. Bragg believed in fasting and cleansing on a regular basis. He also exercised daily.

HERB TALK

Modern science is identifying many protective compounds, called *phytonutrients,* in your foods. These include the following powerful *antioxidants* (that deactivate and protect you from harmful chemicals targeted as one of the common causes of aging, called *free radicals*):

- **OPCs (oligomeric proanthocyanidins):** Found in grapeseeds, chocolate, and green tea
- **Flavonoids:** Found in many vegetables and greens
- **Phytoestrogens:** Found in all beans

Ongoing research continues to prove that many of the foods that your ancestors considered an important part of a healthy diet can protect you from cancer and heart disease and prolong your life.

Herbs are storehouses of life-extending chemicals that can help keep you healthy well into old age. Of the many exciting discoveries in nutritional and herbal science over the last ten years, the potent anti-aging constituents called antioxidants are worth a closer look. According to the free-radical theory of aging (a widely-accepted theory about why people age), active free-radicals react with vital components of many of your cells, wreaking havoc with the life processes of your body. Free radicals are thought to play a major role in skin wrinkling, heart disease, and cancer. The body produces protective chemicals, but often too little, too late to protect your tissues and organs.

Fortunately, mother nature provides numerous antioxidants in foods, among them, vitamin E (the most widely researched of all the antioxidants) and vitamin C, which you're probably familiar with. Herbs also contain high concentrations of free-radical fighting antioxidants, and antioxidant herbs offer specific protection for important organs or for the entire body. Well-researched herbal antioxidants, such as milk thistle, turmeric, and ginger are worth taking regularly for even more protection. The following list is a youth-promoting top ten lineup of the major herbs that can play a powerful role in keeping you feeling young and healthy.

- **Milk thistle** is a rampant weed that grows in California and other parts of the United States and Europe. An herbal extract of milk thistle protects the liver and helps it regenerate and also improves digestion, which is often a challenge for the elderly. Milk thistle has a powerful antioxidant effect specifically for the liver. Its active ingredients are flavonoid-like compounds, commonly found in many fresh vegetables and fruits, particularly in the peels of lemons and oranges. Milk thistle concentrates in the liver cells and provides surrounding tissues with powerful, protecting antioxidants. The liver is one of the major organs in the body that is impacted by toxic waste products and is exposed to high doses of free radicals every day. If you drink alcohol or take pharmaceutical drugs (antibiotics are stressful on the liver), then milk thistle is appropriate for daily use. The dosage is three 60-mg capsules of a standardized extract daily as a preventative.

  Note that recently the U.S. Food and Drug Association (FDA) has begun requiring manufacturers of pain medications like acetaminophen (Tylenol) and non-steroidal anti-inflammatory drugs like aspirin to disclose on their labels that these compounds are significantly toxic to the liver. People have sustained liver damage with therapeutic doses of aspirin and acetaminophen, especially if they are used with alcohol. If you take these products, take milk thistle along with them.

- **Turmeric** contains a potent anti-inflammatory and antioxidant compound called cucurmin (coo-CURR-min). Turmeric has beneficial liver-protective and digestion-enhancing properties and is used in traditional Chinese and east Indian medicine and cooking. Turmeric adds zest and color to curries and sauces and is helpful for arthritis, irritable bowel syndrome, or any type of inflammatory disease as a supplement. It's available in capsule and tablet form as a standardized extract (see Chapter 2 for information on extracts) and also a dried powder. You can add it to your food or place the powder in empty capsules (available at natural-foods stores) and take 3 capsules, 3 times per day. Cooking with turmeric also has a positive, protective effect on the liver.

- **Ginger** stimulates the digestive vitality. Maintaining the digestion in good working order is extremely important as aging occurs. As you get older, all the body fluids start cooling off and slowing down, causing you to produce fewer hormones and digestive enzymes. Ginger stimulates the blood flow to the digestive organs and enhances assimilation, which is important as you age. In Chinese medicine, the digestion is considered to be the central point from which your vitality and daily energy come. The immune system is also intimately linked with the digestive tract, so keeping your digestion in optimum working order makes you more resistant to colds and infections. In all its forms — ginger tea, ginger powder, or ginger extract — this herb is fantastic for any digestive symptoms, especially during the winter months.

- **Hawthorn** leaves and flowers contain important antioxidants, including OPCs, which are flavonoid-like compounds. Hawthorn is especially good for the heart and vascular system — it dilates the coronary arteries, which feed blood to the heart. Taking hawthorn on a regular basis causes more blood to perfuse through the heart muscle, giving it more oxygen and strength. The leading cause of death in most developed countries in the world, including the United States, is cardiovascular disease, so this potent antioxidant herb is an important herb to take as you age. My dad has been taking the herb extract for nearly 20 years, and he is a true believer in the herb's benefits. It can be taken in standardized extract or in tincture form (see Chapter 2 for more on tinctures and extracts). A good tincture of hawthorn is bright red, showing all of the coloring compounds.
- **Ginkgo** is an ancient tree, grown today on streets all over the world. German researchers identified powerful antioxidant and memory and circulation-enhancing compounds in this herb in the 1940s and 1950s. Ginkgo remains one of the top-selling drugs in Europe and is now one of the best-known anti-aging herbs in the United States.

  Studies have shown that the ginkgo compounds concentrate in the brain, the inner ears, and the retina, making it especially good for protecting the eyes and ears, for macular degeneration, and for other types of eye and ear problems. Ginkgo extracts are widely prescribed for poor circulation in the legs, declining memory and alertness in the aged, and is showing promise for prevention and as part of a treatment program for Alzheimer's disease. Ginkgo increases blood circulation to the brain and has potent antioxidant effects. As you age, the tiny vessels in the brain start clogging up and hardening and lose their elasticity, so you don't get as much oxygen in the brain as you need. Ginkgo improves alertness, concentration, and memory, because it enhances the blood flow and protects the vessels in the brain and enhances neurotransmitter activity. It's one of the best herbs for protecting the mind, alertness, and awareness during the aging process.

  Daily intake of ginkgo is also appropriate for protecting the hearing. As you age, the little hairs in the inner ear become susceptible to free radical damage, reducing hearing acuity. The herb is also used for ringing in the ears, known as *tinnitis.* If tinnitis is of less than one year's duration, chances are that ginkgo can help reduce the ringing sounds. You have to take it for three or four months before it really starts working, so don't give up if it doesn't work right away.
- **Grapeseed** extract is another important antioxidant. Research shows that the skin of purple grapes contains a compound known as resveretrol (rez-VERR-uh-trahl), one of the most potent cancer fighters

ever identified. In the seed of purple grapes is a fantastic supply of the OPCs that are strong antioxidants. If you don't have a ready supply of concord grapes, you can buy grapeseed extract. It's not only important as an anti-aging supplement, but it's also beneficial for chronic inflammatory conditions, such as arthritis and irritable bowel syndrome.

- **Green tea** has strong healing properties and is the second most popular beverage in the world. (What's the first most popular beverage? If you said Coke or coffee, like most of my students, guess again — it's water.) Green tea contains a rich storehouse of OPCs. Men and women in Asian countries consume a lot of tofu and green tea and have a lesser incidence of heart disease and cancer, especially prostate cancer. Green tea protects the blood vessels and the heart.

  I recommend keeping caffeine in any form to a minimum, because it can weaken your nervous system and digestion and increase nervous tension in your body. If you *do* drink coffee, tea, or soft drinks for your caffeine energy fix, why not switch to green tea? It tastes great, and unlike the other drinks, you actually get major health benefits along with moderate amounts of caffeine. My motto is "Get the benefit with the buzz." When you switch from coffee to green tea, you can still get your stimulation as well as the beneficial compounds that strengthen the immune system, prevent inflammation, and lock up free radicals. If you don't like the taste of green tea, it is also available in capsule form. Green tea has a pleasant refreshing flavor that many people enjoy.

- **Gotu kola** is a famous plant from India. In Thailand you can buy gotu kola juice from street vendors — it is said to slow aging and make your memory and mind sharper. Although it doesn't have as much scientific research proving its activity as ginkgo, gotu kola has been used for thousand of years, and you often find it with ginkgo in formulas for memory. I like to add a sprig of rosemary for flavor and to increase the antioxidant power.

- **Rosemary** is a beneficial brain and nervous system herb. It contains natural camphor and is one of the most potent antioxidants in the vegetable kingdom. Rosemary extracts are used in the food industry to keep oils and fats from going rancid.

- **Red Korean and red Chinese ginsengs** are ancient treasures for helping to stay young and active. Red ginsengs are appropriate herbs to "warm you up" as you ease into middle age and beyond. After 50, production of hormones like estrogen and testosterone slows down, cooling your ardor for certain activities — ginseng is thought to enhance estrogen and possibly testosterone levels in the body. It's also the number one energy herb — besides coffee and tea. But unlike these stimulant drinks, which don't actually *give* you energy but instead *use up* deep energy resources by overstimulating your adrenals and nervous system, ginseng can actually enhance energy production. My Chinese herb teacher always said not to take ginseng when you're young, because then what are you going to use when you're old?

A bitter pill to swallow

As you age, take herbs that can increase the fire of the digestion so that you can completely burn your food, facilitating the release of vital energy and elimination of waste by-products. My experience tells me that weak digestion is the basis for chronic inflammatory diseases like arthritis, as well as chronic fatigue, allergies, and general weakness. So promote powerful digestion by taking digestive bitters daily. In Europe, millions of people take bitters every day.

A good digestive bitter product contains a bitter herb like wormwood, mugwort, or artichoke leaf to increase the secretion of hydrochloric acid in your stomach and all your digestive enzymes. Wormwood tea is excellent for people recovering from illness. Bitter herbs can strengthen immune function, release vital energy, and help your body build strong blood that's so vital to youthfulness and health.

Besides bitter herbs, a good bitters product also contains aromatic herbs, like cardamom, ginger, or cinnamon, to increase digestive fire and blood flow to the digestion organs. It may also contain carminatives (gas-relieving herbs), such as fennel or caraway. Bitters have to be taken every day to have the best effects, preferably 15 minutes or so before your biggest meals of the day. After a few weeks, you'll probably notice that your digestion is much stronger and that you're likely to have more energy and recover faster from illness.

Herbs for Athletes

Steroids and nervous system stimulants like ephedra are notorious performance-enhancers for athletes and are banned from competition. Many of these drugs are at the very least not conducive to health, and at the worst can be downright dangerous to your health.

Herbal extracts are the perfect choice for athletes who want to enhance their performance, increase endurance, reduce muscle soreness, and minimize feelings of fatigue.

Enhancing performance

The most effective herbs for enhancing performance in my experience are eleuthero, red ginseng, and caffeine-containing herbs like kola nut, guarana, black tea, and ephedra. These stimulants can increase your metabolism and make more reserve energy available to the body. If you're in good health, a mild dose of stimulants, such as kola nut extract, isn't really harmful, as long as you burn off the extra energy with a workout. Keep in mind that they are stimulants for the nervous system and metabolism, so long-term use can promote digestive, hormonal, and nervous system weakness. Caffeine- and ephedrine-containing herbs are banned in officially-sanctioned sports events.

The following is a review of other herbs that are commonly found in sports products:

- **Eleuthero** (el-LOO-thur-oh), also called Siberian ginseng, is the best-known herb for increasing endurance and speeding up recovery time after exercising. Professional athletes, Olympic athletes, and weekend warriors commonly use it to enhance their workouts.
- **Red ginseng:** A mild stimulant to the body's nervous system and metabolism. The herb may help build up muscle mass when used in conjunction with a good diet and regular weight-training program.
- **Wild yam:** Forget it, save your money — as far as it is known, wild yam doesn't contain any steroids that the body can use and it has no history of use as a sports herb. Wild yam contains the plant steroid diosgenin, which shows a weak estrogenic effect only in animals.
- **Sarsaparilla:** The rhizome and roots of a vine that grows in the Caribbean, Mexico, and Central America are traditionally used as a cleanser and flavor ingredient in beverages. A few reports coming from Mexico say that the herb can increase testosterone in men, but this is unlikely based on my experience, its history of traditional use, and its known chemical constituents.

Treating injuries

Herbs can be effective when sports injuries, such as sprains and strains, occur. Stock your first aid kit with the following herbal remedies:

- **Arnica oil or cream:** Arnica is the premier herb for sports injuries. Apply it directly to sore muscles 2 to 3 times daily. Arnica is also excellent to accelerate the healing of sprains and strains. You can take a homeopathic preparation of arnica internally at the same time.

  TIP: Don't use arnica preparations on any areas where the skin is broken.
- **Ginger compress:** An effective, time-honored, herbal remedy that works wonders for strains, sprains, bruises, and other injuries when applied 2 or 3 times a day for several days. I prefer fresh ginger, but powdered ginger works if you're out of the fresh. Add a tablespoon of cinnamon powder for extra warming and dispersing action. See a recipe for Ginger Compress, following this list.
- **Horse chestnut cream:** This product, which is widely used in Europe, is excellent for sports injuries, such as strains and sprains. Horse chestnut cream is now available in North America. Apply the cream as needed.

- **St. John's wort oil:** This oil works quickly to relieve pain and reduce inflammation — it is excellent for muscle pain, strains, and sprains. Apply the oil externally and take the tincture internally for best results.
- **Tea tree oil:** Tea tree oil is an effective anti-fungal agent and works wonderfully when applied directly for athlete's foot.
- **Wintergreen oil:** This pleasant-smelling oil can be rubbed on sore muscles or a tennis elbow. It relieves pain and inflammation. Never use wintergreen oil internally.

Ginger Compress

Try this ginger compress for back strains, sprains, bruises, and other injuries. You gain the most benefit with this herbal treatment by using it several times a day for a few days.

Preparation time: *20 minutes*

Yield: *2 cups*

$^{1}/_{2}$ cup fresh ginger rhizome

2 cups water

1 Grate the ginger rhizome into a small saucepan.

2 Add the water and simmer for 5 minutes.

3 Let steep for 15 minutes.

4 Soak a washcloth in the strong tea and apply to painful or stiff muscles until the compress cools. Do this 3 to 4 times and then repeat the process 2 or 3 times per day.

Vary It! For inflamed muscles and strong pain, try alternating the ginger compress with a cold or even icy compress (1 minute of the cold to 4 minutes of the hot).

TIP

Right after an injury, apply a cold pack to the area for 10 to 20 minutes, several times during the day. After the first day, alternate hot and cold, or use only hot if the pain is not too severe. Cold controls tissue damage and pain right after the injury (for the first 24 to 48 hours, depending on the severity of the injury), but afterward restricts blood flow and the healing process.

Herbs for Pets

You can save your pets needless trauma and save yourself expensive veterinary bills by using your herbal medicine chest or herb garden as a pet pharmacy. To start using healing pet herbs, try these common and safe remedies. Your furry friends will benefit.

- **Cuts and scratches:** Make a tea of calendula flowers and spray it on the affected area. Or apply calendula salve, though be aware that animals are apt to lick it off — you may want to wrap the area with a cloth.
- **Ear infections and ear mites:** Use garlic-mullein ear oil, 3 to 4 drops, 2 times daily.

  Dogs and cats have especially long ear channels, so it's good to massage the ears to get the oil to go down. Animals often like to have their ears massaged anyway, especially when they're having trouble with them. If your pet is sensitive to touch, and if the sensitivity persists, call your vet.
- **Eye infections or watery eyes:** Use a well-strained goldenseal tea as an eyewash. Be sure to buy cultivated goldenseal, as the wild populations have been seriously overharvested. Eyebright herb tea is an effective second choice.
- **Disease prevention:** Give your pets proper nutrition, adequate opportunities for exercise, and plenty of tender loving care. Most pets like stroking and petting, which definitely have an immune-enhancing effect.
- **Fleas:** To prevent fleas from hopping on pets, you can make an herbal flea collar by dipping a string into a combination of essential oils containing eucalyptus, citronella, and sage and tying it around your pet's neck. Yarrow tincture sprayed onto affected areas can discourage fleas.

  Use orange oil to kill fleas when your pet does get an infection. Add a 1/2 teaspoon orange oil to a quarter cup of people shampoo. Then shampoo the animal, covering them with suds. Start at the neck and work down, so that too many fleas don't end up right on your pet's face. Then, rinse it off. If it's a really bad case, do it again in two days and vacuum the house thoroughly at the same time.

  Note that I don't recommend applying undiluted essential oils directly to the skin where they can be licked off and make your cat or dog sick. For troublesome areas, though, you can mix 20 drops of eucalyptus oil in 2 ounces of almond oil to apply directly. Work the blend well into the hair.

- **Foxtails:** If your pet gets objects caught under the skin or between the toes, you can make a fresh plantain poultice or comfrey poultice by putting fresh leaves in a blender with a little water and blending it up. Apply the poultice to the area. This remedy even works for foxtails, the stickery type of grass seeds that often plague animals.
- **Hyperactivity:** Makers of modern designer personality drugs bring "Prozac for pets." The drug is actually reported to moderate animal behavior such as compulsive barking or licking. Before you go for such drastic measures, try adding calming teas or a few droppersful of a relaxing tincture like valerian, chamomile, or California poppy to your pet's water dish. Capsules and tablets are available if you can get pets to swallow them.

  My recommendation is to use St. John's wort for pets. For a small dog, use about $^{1}/_{4}$ to $^{1}/_{2}$ teaspoonful of the liquid tincture added to water or food, 1 or 2 times daily.
- **Infections:** When your pet gets an infection, you can often help them heal quickly by giving them low doses of echinacea tincture (5 to 10 drops, 3 to 4 times daily, for one week). In general, when using tinctures, adjust the dose for the animal's size — the label dosage is generally meant for a 150-pound human.
- **Lung problems:** Make a mullein tea and put it in the water bowl or pour it over your pet's food.
- **Skin problems and hair loss:** Calendula salve is a good healer for skin problems, but give an internal blood-cleansing herb, such as red clover flowers or yellow dock root, at the same time. You can also make a tea of burdock root and sarsaparilla root for skin problems. Horsetail herb and nettle leaf tea are both used to prevent hair loss. You can also massage the skin with a few drops of rosemary oil diluted in almond oil.
- **Urinary tract infections:** You can use soothing urinary tract herbs that help reduce infection and strengthen tissue. Besides echinacea, which is a must for any infection, try some beneficial herbs that have a special affinity for the urinary tract like pipsissewa (pip-SISS-uh-wah) or uva-ursi (OO-vah URR-see). If you have an herb garden, brew a little fresh yarrow or plantain leaves and add it to your pet's water.
- **Worms:** Garlic is a good preventive for parasites. Chop it into your pet's food or use a powder. If you start this practice when your pets are young, they develop a taste for it. If prevention fails, and they actually get worms, you may have to use garlic capsules to get rid of the parasites.

See Appendix C for a listing of books and journals on the subject of herbal pet care.

Giving herbs to pets

You can sprinkle fresh or dried herbs onto the animal's food, add a tea to dry food, or put herb tea by the water bowl. For internal use, a lot of herbal remedies can be used the same as for people, and they have to be cut down proportionately according to the animal's weight.

When giving tinctures to your pets, don't give them straight — put the drops in their water bowl instead. (For dogs, however you can put the tincture mixed with a little water straight on the dog food or on favored tasty treats.) When administering pills, stick the capsules or tablets down the animal's throat, close the mouth, and then rub downward on the throat, which causes a swallowing action.

Keep in mind that herbs don't always work the same in animals as they do in humans, but in many cases, the effects are similar.

Part II
Growing and Brewing Your Own Herbs

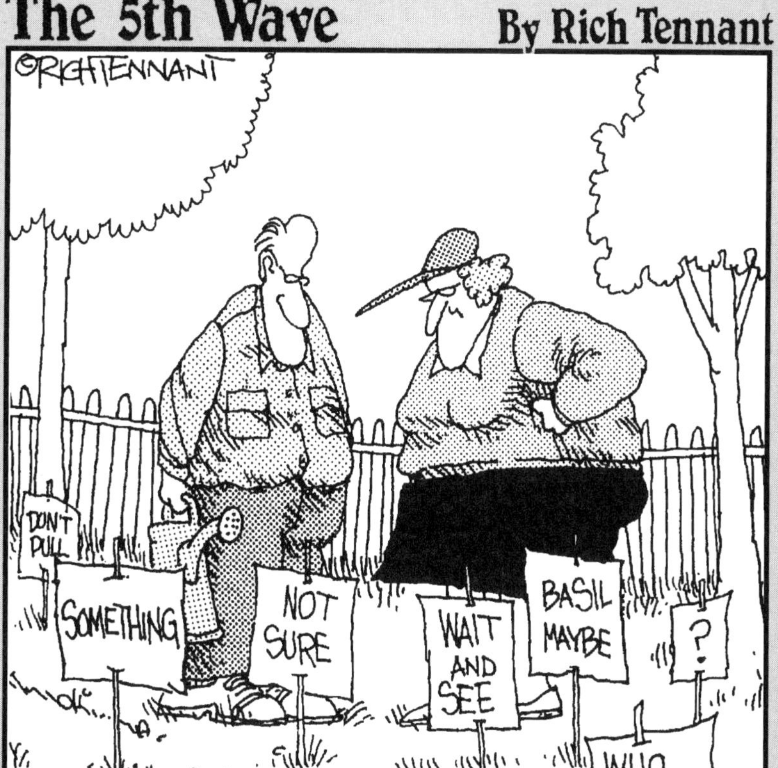

"That should do it."

In this part . . .

What image comes to mind when you think about herbal medicine? A bottle of tablets or tincture? Or a garden full of fragrant flowers of all colors and shapes? Maybe a remote and wild place where you can pick medicines from the earth? As an herbalist, I hope your image involves a connection with the herbs themselves rather than with just the finished product.

In times past, a community herbalist, who had years of experience, harvested and prepared herbal medicines by hand. Today, however, multinational corporations harvest vast acres of plants with tractors, cut them up with powerful grinders, and remove the essence with industrial solvents in huge gleaming extractors. The extracts are pressed into tablets and stuffed into capsules. The product you reach for on the store shelf is far removed from the wild plants that your ancestors depended on for their health and their lives.

Much of the healing power from plants is subtle. It can't yet be measured and is difficult to study. But the true healing essence of plant medicines is imparted when you sit in an herb garden or wild spot. Growing, harvesting, smelling, and working with plants in the kitchen is even better. This part shows you how to grow your own herbs, cook with them, and make your own herbal products.

Chapter 5

Growing, Drying, and Storing Herbs

In This Chapter

- Planning your herb garden
- Creating healthy soil
- Discovering the benefits of composting
- Using containers to grow herbs — indoors and out
- Finding sources for seeds and plants
- Getting tips for harvesting herbs
- Understanding how to process and dry herbs
- Finding tips for storing herbs

Herbs are a diverse group. A lemon tree, an oregano plant, garlic, ground covers such as thyme or chamomile, and even weeds — all are defined as herbs. Herbs are generally quite hearty by nature and tolerate a wide range of conditions. Compared with many fruits and vegetables, herbs are easy to grow — in pots (as houseplants), in borders around your house, or in garden beds. And you don't have to be highly skilled at cooking or making things with your hands to practice the art of harvesting herbs. Try the practical suggestions in this chapter for harvesting and processing your herbs, and each year you will probably find that you get more of a feel for the herbal way of life — and are amply rewarded with healthful medicines, fewer doctor's bills, more energy, and a positive outlook that working directly with nature can bring.

REMEMBER

Many natural food stores have high quality fresh dried herbs available in bulk, but in many cases they sit on the shelves for months. Commercially-grown herbs, especially spices like dill, may be irradiated or grown in foreign places with chemicals that aren't allowed in the United States (such as DDT) — a far cry from going right outside your door and picking oregano leaves fresh to add to spaghetti sauce or gathering fresh mint leaves for an after-dinner cup of tea.

Still not sure about whether or not to try growing your own herbs? Here are enticing reasons to give it a try:

- **Grow your own living home medicine chest.** This may be the best reason of all to plant herbs. People have been planting healing herbs in and around their homes for thousands of years, and you can carry on the tradition with your own medicine-chest garden. Home-grown herbs are the highest-quality that you can possibly find — and you did it yourself. Many healing traditions emphasize that having a connection to your medicine makes it that much more powerful.
- **Spend less of the green stuff on your green stuff.** Prepackaged herbal products are convenient, but are usually your most expensive option. Even bulk herbs can be expensive to use for long periods — echinacea root can cost $40 or $50 a pound or more. Grow it at home, and the cost is only a fraction of what you pay at the store. Chapter 6 is filled with information on making your own herbal products.
- **Create a feast for the senses.** By growing your own herbs you increase the aesthetics of your environment. Many herbs have beautiful, brightly-colored flowers with provocative aromas. Imagine having your own aromatherapy garden that's available any time you need a pick-me-up or a relaxing stroll (see Chapter 3 for the scoop on aromatherapy).
- **Attract birds and butterflies.** Herbs with brightly-colored flowers bring a varied and colorful array of life into your garden. Anise hyssop, buddleia, the mints, and many of the sages provide nectar sources that birds and butterflies can't resist.
- **Keep your cats happy and entertained.** Catnip herb and valerian rhizomes are the herbs of choice for your feline friends — they love them. If your cats are lying around the house, bored out of their minds, these herbs are for them.
- **Spice up your life.** Herbs can be used in soups, stews, salads, and even desserts to add flavor, preserve food, and increase their healing and protective qualities. See Chapter 7 for more on kitchen medicine.
- **Brewing with herbs.** If you like to brew your own beers, festoon your fences with different varieties of hops. Hops add relaxing qualities to the beer, as well as flavor and character. Another aromatic herb, mugwort, is the original brewing herb. Its name is derived from "mug," a large cup, and "wort," which is an old word for plant or herb.
- **Keep pests away from your garden vegetables and fruits.** Discourage earwigs, aphids, leafhoppers, and other hungry insects and animals by planting aromatic herbs at the ends of your garden beds or by interspersing them with your valuable vegetables. I plant marigold, anise hyssop, epasote, garlic, and chives abundantly — and enjoy the herbs in cooking.

Edible bouquets

The enjoyment of making up your own herbal bouquets is one of the beneficial aspects of having fresh herbs for the picking at your fingertips. They smell great, look beautiful, and you can eat the whole thing! You can create your bouquets with basil, borage, oregano, mint, parsley, rosemary, feverfew, dill, fennel, anise hyssop, or whatever combinations are particularly appealing to you. Pick the flowers off and add to salads or sprinkle over pasta dishes and other dishes to add color, interest, and flavor to your epicurean delights. Give an herbal bouquet to a friend — it can make a delightful gift.

- **Cut flowers for the home.** Plant sages, anise hyssop, echinacea, valerian, and other herbs to add uniqueness to your floral arrangements.
- **Relieve stress.** Gardening is a wonderfully relaxing activity and a nice escape from the technological and fast-paced lives that many people lead.

Gardener, Spare That Dandelion!

HERB TALK

Before starting your garden, you may want to determine which herbs already exist in your garden, or in your ungarden. An *ungarden* is the waste area around your house and yard where plants of dubious reputation — weeds — grow. What people call weeds, however, are highly medicinal and useful plants. Most herbalists will tell you that the weeds are the most healing plants of all. I harbor a wide variety of herbal weeds in my yard, and I collect new weed seeds to plant in my garden everywhere I go.

Healing weeds don't require much water, care, or cultivation but have highly nutritious and healing qualities.

- **Burdock:** The young tender roots of this plant are called *gobo* in Japanese culture, where they slice them and add them to soups and stews. Gobo is thought to impart strength and vitality when eaten regularly. I recommend a decoction of the root tea to help cleanse the body, relax and regulate the liver, and improve digestion. A tincture or decoction of the seeds is a favorite remedy to help relieve skin eruptions like acne.
- **Dandelion:** The leaves are highly nutritious as a wild green and added to a soup or stir-fry. The leaves are also nature's gentle diuretic. Use them dried, sprinkled on foods, in soups or other dishes, or to make a tea. The root is a great liver cleanser and cooler for helping to prevent acne and other skin ailments. Dandelion is traditionally used for spring cleansing.

- **Mallow:** The round, kidney-shaped leaves are excellent in salads and with stir-fried vegetables. Decoct the entire above-ground parts of the plant to make a soothing tea for any kind of irritation or mild infection of the urinary tract or bowels.
- **Mustard:** Another mustard family member, this plant always has yellow flowers and is a common weed in fruit orchards. The seeds are ground up and combined with vinegar, garlic, and other spices to make a brown, spicy home mustard.
- **Purslane:** After this gets going in your garden, watch out — it can really spread and take over vegetable beds. I allow it all the room it needs, because it produces a great-tasting, green vegetable that has a sour twist. The tangy leaves and stems are an important item in traditional Greek and middle-eastern cooking. The plant contains important fatty acids that may help reduce the inflammation of arthritis.
- **Sheep sorrel:** A small, sour-tasting plant with arrow-shaped leaves from the buckwheat family. It is useful in teas and salads to help the body eliminate toxic waste products. Sheep sorrel is a key ingredient in the popular folk remedy Essiac, which is recommended for the prevention of cancer.

  Sheep sorrel is a rich source of the acid-tasting chemicals called oxalates, so avoid using it as a tea or in salads if you have kidney stones or have a concern about them.
- **Spurge, peplys:** Any member of the spurge group of plants is excellent for removing warts. Over the years, I've seen this remedy work many times. Dab a little bit of the white milky sap directly on the wart twice daily for several days. The wart easily peels off and leaves no scar. Any garden spurge, like gopher spurge, works.

  Don't take any spurge internally. It is highly irritating — some species are poisonous. It can cause irritation and redness when applied to sensitive skin. Don't get it near the eyes. Use only the white milky sap directly on a wart.
- **Wild carrot:** The wild form of the domesticated carrot grows commonly in many parts of the world. It is also known as *Queen Anne's lace.* The seeds, which make a traditional tea for preventing kidney stones and gravel, are reported to have diuretic qualities and are helpful to get the menstrual period going when it doesn't come smoothly. The seeds are known as a powerful carminative for relieving gas.
- **Wild lettuce:** A bitter relative of the common garden lettuce, its young, tender leaves add interest to a salad. The juice of the plant has significant relaxing and sleep-promoting qualities. The dried milky sap, known as *lactucarium,* was an official drug in the U.S. and other countries in the late nineteenth century and early part of the twentieth century.

- **Wild radish:** A common weed from the mustard family, with spicy green fruits that can add relish to soups and salads. Pick them when they're young and tender. The small brown seeds are commonly used in Chinese medicine as a tea or condiment to help promote complete digestion.
- **Yellow dock:** A common plant of fields and yards, the fresh spring greens of yellow dock are delicious and mildly cleansing. The yellow root can be simmered in water to cleanse the bowels and help build up the blood. The root tincture is recommended by midwives to help strengthen the blood during pregnancy. Yellow dock tea is a good preventative for women who are prone to vaginal yeast infections and bladder infections.

Designing a Medicine Chest Garden

You first need to decide which herbs you want and/or need in your medicine chest garden. If you often have trouble sleeping, you probably want to include California poppy, passion flower, hops, and valerian in your garden. Or if you or any of your family members have lung problems, you may want to plant mullein, horehound, and thyme. You can do theme sections in your herb garden, like herbs for digestion, for the nervous system, and so on. To help plan your medicine chest garden, look at the *Symptom Guide* and pick out the most useful healing herbs. Herb seeds and plants are available from any of the suppliers listed in Appendix C.

After you decide which herbs you want in your garden, draw up your plan on paper. Make sure to plan enough room for trees, shrubs, and all the perennial herbs. Find this information in *Gardening For Dummies,* by Mike MacCaskey and the Editors of the National Gardening Association (IDG Books Worldwide, Inc.) or from your nursery worker. Keep the following factors in mind when making your plan:

- **Grow healing trees:** Place medicinal trees in areas where you want to add shade to make a home for plants that don't like full sun. Remember that small trees eventually become big trees, so allow plenty of room. Under trees, I like to grow sun-tender plants like violets, angelica, and sweet woodruff and any of the classic medicinal plants from the eastern United States like goldenseal, wintergreen, and the cohoshes in shady areas. Medicinal trees you may want to consider include witch hazel, slippery elm, ginkgo, and fringe tree.
- **Plant perennials:** Decide where to put perennial herbs (which grow back year after year) such as vitex, elderberry, the sages, the mints, thyme, rosemary, and lavender first, but leave room for annuals (that die at the end of every year) such as basil, cilantro, and parsley.
- **Consider the height of the plants:** Place tall herbs like angelica, foxglove, mullein, vitex, and echinacea in the back of your herb beds.

- **Watch the width of the plants:** Certain herbs, including wormwood, mugwort, coltsfoot and lavender, can spread out and grow quite large.
- **Know the creepy plants:** A few plants turn out to be downright nuisances when you plant them in a nice rich bed along with your favorite medicinals. Peppermint, bergamot, yarrow, St. John's wort, mugwort, coltsfoot, and the dog rose have underground runners that spread rapidly in certain climates and must be dug out and removed. I've given up entire beds to bergamot and spearmint — it was easier than trying to control them.
- **Create wide paths for easy access:** Consider making the pathway wide enough for ease of movement of garden equipment, like wheelbarrows or garden carts. Design your herb bed so that you can comfortably reach all the plants without having to step on the bed. You can accomplish this with the use of stepping stones, like flagstones or wooden rounds. If you plan to eventually give garden tours or classes, you may want extra wide pathways.
- **Use pleasing and practical shapes:** A garden with specific designs, like a wheel with spokes, can be beautiful but is difficult to work in. Think of appearance when designing garden shapes, but if your garden ends up not being comfortable to work in, you probably won't spend much time there.
- **Keep friends in the family:** Think of grouping plants with similar necessities, such as water and sunlight, together. Even if your yard is already landscaped, you can often sneak in an herb plant here and there between existing plants or set aside one part of your landscape to be your herb area. If you have an existing vegetable garden, incorporate herbs as bed ends or as borders.
- **Think a few years down the road:** Consider how long you plan to reside in the place where you're creating a garden. If you're only staying a limited time, consider growing annuals or shrubby plants that can be easily transplanted or containerized. If you'll be there long-term, plant long-lived trees and shrubs, such as ginkgo and hawthorn.
- **Keep water resources close by:** After your herb plants are established, you won't need to water them much. However, if you live in an area that doesn't get much rain in the summer, you have to do a little watering. If your water resources are limited and you don't get much summer rain (like in California), find out about native plants in your area. In all parts of the country, native herbs have acclimated both to the soil type and the weather conditions of particular regions. Nurseries all over the country are beginning to specialize in native regional plants, and their staff members can help you choose plants for your garden. Local and regional gardening books can also be quite useful — even if they're mostly about vegetable growing, these books can inform you about first and last frost dates in your area, potential crops, and soil types.

Figure 5-1 shows a small, perennial, herb garden.

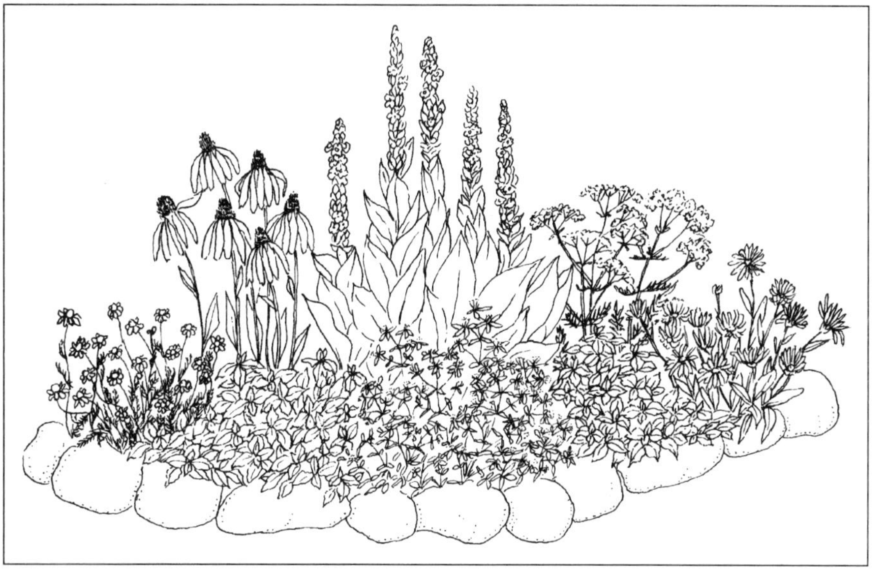

Figure 5-1: A medicine cabinet bed with lavender, mullein, valerian, and echinacea in the back, and chamomile, lemon balm, St. John's wort, and calendula, in the front, along with a little thyme.

TIP

If you have gopher problems or you like the appearance of herb beds enclosed in wooden boxes, build frames with rot-resistant woods. The two most resistant and long-lasting woods are redwood and cedar. Both are scarce resources and expensive; however, plastic is now an option. Another option is recycled plastic lumber for making raised beds. Pressure-treated wood is toxic and is unsafe for growing plants that you are ingesting. My feeling is that raised beds in boxes are often a waste of resources unless you particularly desire the aesthetic aspect of it, or if you have health problems that make it difficult for you to bend. Raised beds can make gardening more comfortable for elderly or disabled gardeners.

Building Healthy Soil and Growing Healthy Plants

In addition to sun and a moderate amount of moisture, many herbs prefer a well-drained soil that has lots of organic material in it, like compost. To grow healthy plants with optimum healing potency, the soil in which they're growing needs to be healthy, strong, and balanced. Like people, a plant's immune system is at maximum strength when the environment (in this case, soil) in which they're growing is healthy. A plant with a strong immune system can resist pests and viral infections, which sidesteps the need to use toxic chemicals on your herbs. After all, when using herbs for healing, do you really want to take even small amounts of pesticides and herbicides into your system?

Soil, like humans, needs air, water, food, and even shelter (mulch). Two common types of soil are *sandy* and *clay*. Sandy soil is a weaker soil and can't hold nutrients or moisture well; clay is stronger, inherently, but more bound up, so that water and nutrients have trouble reaching the roots of the plants.

Not sure which type of soil you have, or what nutrients it is lacking, and which ones to add? If you're going to be developing a large garden, invest in a soil test. Find out about county extension services in your area and send them a sample of your soil. A few gardening supply companies can also send off your sample for you (see Appendix C for more information). Soil tests that you conduct yourself aren't generally worth your time or money, so if you're really interested in getting information about your soil, send a sample away to a professional soil-testing company. If you decide not to do a test, you can glean information about the soil in your area from local nurseries, your agriculture extension agent, local farmers and gardeners, and by looking at soil surveys done by the U.S. Geological Service available at Soil Conservation Service offices.

Be sure to assess the potential toxicity of your soil. For example, houses painted before the 1960s may have lead or mercury in the paint, which can fall off the house and into growing areas, if they are within five feet or so from the house. If your house fits this description, import soil and grow your plants in raised beds or containers. If you're unsure if this is the case with your soil, have it tested for lead and mercury. See Appendix C for labs where you can send your soil to have it tested. The presence of spiders is a good indicator that little or no toxic materials have been sprayed over the soil, because spiders tend to accumulate poisons such as lead or pesticides in their systems and die out.

Scratch and sniff — an aromatherapy garden

Consider creating your own aromatherapy garden. You can grow many scented plants in indoor pots or outdoors around walkways, in formal beds in the garden, or at the ends of vegetable beds to help keep away pests. My favorites are lemon balm, lemon verbena, the many scented geraniums, mints, rosemary, lavender, anise hyssop, and thyme. See Chapter 3 for more on aromatherapy.

Using organic amendments and fertilizers

If your soil is inherently deficient in a nutrient, you can add that nutrient into your soil through amendments or fertilizers. *Fertilizers* work by feeding the plant roots directly, skipping over biological processes through which nutrients are slowly released from the soil. Adding an *amendment,* on the other hand, is a practice of feeding the soil so that the soil in turn is able to feed the plant. Amendments include compost, rock phosphate, green sand, kelp meal, and ground rock dust — all available at your local nursery. Compost, otherwise known as "gardener's gold," is invariably my first choice due to financial and ecological reasons (see the "Compost happens" section, for more information on composting). Compost that's made up of plant materials is full of everything you need to grow plants — and also has disease-suppressing organisms, biological activity, microbes, and soil-enhancing properties.

Healthy soil produces healthy plants that are resistant to pests and disease. Herb plants in general tend to be quite hearty and relatively pest-resistant. However, consider trying to attract beneficial insects, such as trichogramma wasps, lacewings, and ladybug beetles, by planting flowers in your garden — especially those in the carrot, parsley, and sunflower families. These flowers provide nectar and pollen for the beneficial insects that prey on plant-eating insects, such as aphids. If, instead, you start spraying pesticides whenever you see a few holes in the leaves of your plants, you risk disrupting ecological balance and killing the beneficial insects as well as the detrimental ones. The surviving herbivorous insects tend to be quicker at reproducing and often get a jump on the beneficial ones, throwing your garden even further out of balance.

Compost happens

Compost — a mixture of decaying organic material, such as grass, leaves, and manure — is a crucial component in creating biologically active soil. Compost is a complete fertilizer — it's made up of plant material and it gives plants everything they need to grow.

Here are a few benefits of home composting:

- Reduces the impact of waste disposal on the greater environment. Composting is an ideal way for residents of both urban and rural areas to begin taking responsibility for their waste. You can even compost and detoxify materials like newspapers, cardboard, and office paper. A good compost pile will literally sterilize itself by heating up to an amazing 150°!

- Lessens the need for the fossil fuels that home garbage pickup requires.
- Minimizes the amount of organic matter entering the landfill.
- Creates a highly beneficial product that you can use in gardens or houseplants.

Keep the following in mind when composting:

- When building your compost pile, balance equal parts of wet ingredients (food scraps) with dry ones (straw).
- If you have a problem with varmints, avoid putting meat scraps and milk products in your compost pile. In general, it is okay to add small amounts of meat and milk if you bury them deeply.
- Layering your compost pile is a way to blend the materials and to know how much of each material you're adding. For example, add a bucket of food scraps, then add straw or grass clippings on top of that, watering it as you go.
- Your compost pile needs moisture to thrive. A general rule is to keep the contents of a pile as moist as a wrung-out sponge.
- Continue watering every week after that if you live in a dry climate; if compost dries out too much, the activity that breaks it down will stop. Err on the side of adding more of the drier ingredients, because too many food scraps by themselves create a smelly pile.
- To prevent a potent-smelling compost pile, cover the heap during heavy rains and balance out the addition of wet materials with drier ones.
- You can get a finished compost pile more quickly and greatly accelerate the process by turning it — or flipping it over — at least once a week with a pitchfork; in essence, the more time you put in, the quicker you can get finished compost.

  Turning is also a great way to take a peek inside the pile and assess what's going on and determine whether the pile is getting enough or too much air, water, and so on.
- Compost is finished when a majority of the ingredients in the pile can no longer be identified. Finished compost looks, feels, and smells a lot like rich garden soil but is lighter and spongier. After the compost is completely done, cover it during heavy or prolonged rains — the nutrients can leach out.
- A bin protects piles from domestic and wild animals as well as from foul weather. A bin also insulates the pile so that heat can build up quickly, helping the raw organic materials to break down; contains the pile to make it easier to build and to turn; and improves the appearance of the pile. Whether piles are free standing or in bins, try to have a pile that is at least three feet cubed. If possible, locate it in a partially shaded area that's protected from prevailing winds.

Mulching's a must

Mulching is the layering of coarse organic material around plants to help keep moisture in and weeds out. I like weeds, but some will take as much space and nutrients as you allow. Too many weeds around your herbs can compete for nutrients and other resources. You can manage weed growth with mulch. Mulching is the best way to conserve water, especially in areas with low summer rainfall. Mulch helps reduce soil compaction from irrigation or rainfall — it's a long-term strategy for managing the health of the soil, and it creates a beneficial habitat for soil organisms. Here are some good, inexpensive mulches.

- Shredded newspaper
- Cardboard
- Wood chips
- Bales of rice straw (other straws may bring in unwanted weeds to your garden)

Small-particle mulch, like sawdust, tends to provide fewer hiding places for slugs, snails, and other injurious insects than straw.

Growing Herbs in Containers

From lettuce to apple trees, almost any crop that you can grow in the ground, you can also grow in a container. Keep in mind, though, that a container holds a limited amount of soil for plants, so the soil in containers dries out faster and heats up more quickly. This makes mulching and regular watering particularly important.

Growing herbs in containers makes a lot of sense for the following reasons:

- Containers can be easily moved from location to location.
- You don't need much yard space.
- You don't have to worry about gophers and other garden pests.
- In colder climates, you can bring the plants in during the winter.
- You have an easier time planting and tending to the herbs.
- You need only a minimal investment of time and money.

Understanding container types

The most common containers for potting are plastic, clay, and wood (see Figure 5-2).

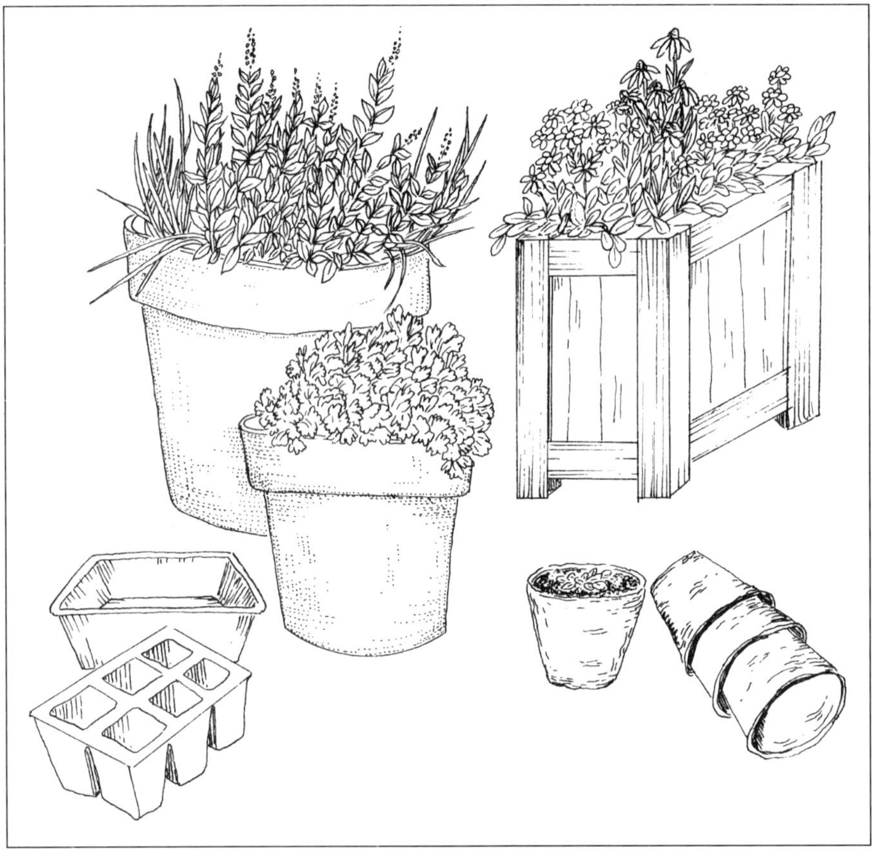

Figure 5-2: Herb containers come in all shapes, sizes, and materials.

- **Clay:** Pots breathe, causing the plant to lose moisture.
- **Plastic:** Black plastic and other plastic pots retain moisture the best, are the cheapest, and are the most durable.
- **Wood planter boxes:** Boxes are attractive, although they're a little expensive.

Buying a soil mix or making your own

When buying a soil mix, look for a diversity of ingredients. Avoid mixes made by chemical companies and those made primarily from barks — organically produced mixes are superior. The soil needs to provide ample drainage, yet must also be able to hold moisture well, and it must be fertile.

Soil mixes differ from potting mixes in that they contain materials such as clay, silt, and sand that don't break down after one season of use. When you make your own soil mix, you can continue feeding and replenishing it during the growing season. If you use the proper ingredients, the mix can be maintained for a lifetime of use, just like the soil in non-container gardens.

A purchased potting mix, on the other hand, tends to be more like a throw-away mix — it's good for a little while, but in a season or two it will be depleted of nutrients. A bagged potting mix is a good bet, though, if you are only growing a few containers in one season.

Here are the six essential ingredients for making a good soil mix. See Figure 5-3 for a look at how these ingredients work together.

- **Sand:** Use builder's sand or play sand available at landscape supply stores — it's extremely cheap when purchased in bulk.
- **Compost:** An invaluable addition to soil mix, compost increases biological activity, enhances the holding capacity of nutrients and water, and serves as both a short- and long-term source of fertility. If you don't have a source of good compost, you can also use well-aged manure in addition to, or in place of, compost.
- **Lighteners:** A term applied to any materials such as perlite, vermiculite, or peat moss that add bulk to a mix without adding any significant weight. All lighteners eventually need replacing because they decompose in the soil mix or lose their fluffiness.
- **Fertilizers:** Ammonium sulfate, blood meal, bat guano, and well-aged chicken or cow manure are products that feed the plants directly, often circumventing soil processes.

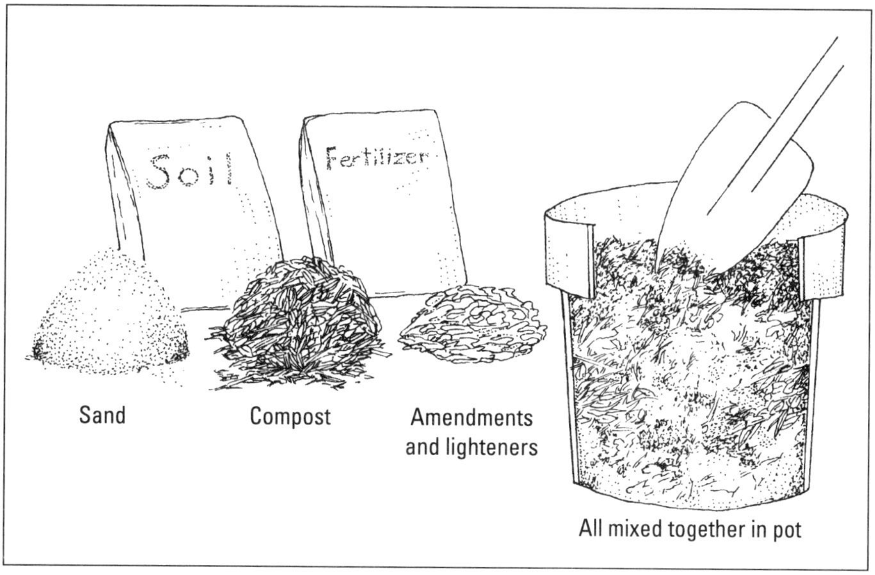

Figure 5-3: How the ingredients in a good soil mix work together to nurture your plants.

- **Amendments:** Made up of compost, earthworm castings, kelp, and bone meal, amendments actually feed the soil itself, ensuring that it feeds the plants with which it lives in symbiosis. Amendments are a long-term strategy for sustainable soil fertility.
- **Soil:** The best type of soil to use is healthy garden soil. If you don't have access to any soil, you can buy it at landscape supply stores.

Include equal parts of sand, soil, compost, and lightener and about a half part of fertilizer or amendment in your mix. When preparing your soil mix, remember the desirable characteristics you want for your plants — good drainage, high biological activity, diverse particle size, good water retention, and high fertility.

HERB TALK

For perennials you can *mulch* (top-dress) the soil with a thick layer of compost, coffee grounds, or earthworm castings. With annuals, dump out the containers after the plant has finished producing for the season, and the soil mix can be replaced or replenished with compost, earthworm castings, or other organic amendments. At this time you can even do a bit of root pruning which stimulates growth.

For more information on growing herbs in containers, check out *Container Gardening For Dummies,* by Bill Marken & the Editors of the National Gardening Association (IDG Books Worldwide, Inc.).

Acquiring Seeds and Plants

Before you can grow herbs in your garden, you need to find a source for seeds, cuttings, root pieces, and other parts of plants that grow and create new plants. Small herb plants are available from your local nursery, on the Web, and by mail order. (See Appendix C for sources.) You can often collect wild seeds, plant cuttings, and even cuttings and seeds from a friend, neighbor, or local botanical garden. That's an exciting aspect of herbal medicine — plants are growing everywhere you go, and they will gladly come into your garden with little invitation.

Visiting nurseries

Local nurseries can be good places to buy your herb plants and seeds. Native plant and other specialty nurseries are sprouting up in many communities. You may want to inspect the plant's roots by popping it out gently — and discreetly — from the container. If the roots are brown and encircling intensively throughout the pot, you can speculate they have been in there too long. White, vibrant-looking roots are still in good health.

Hungry and homeless plants

One of my joys is giving a home to hungry or sick plants that I find by the roadside or local development site. Plants run-over by tires in parking lots, in the path of bulldozers, by the sides of freeways, or ones that are getting just enough water to survive are all fair game. I carry little brown coin envelopes (found in many stationery stores) with me wherever I go, looking for wild and weedy seeds. Believe it or not, I take plants that many people are trying to get rid of such as dandelion, chicory, clover, and alfalfa seeds. I want all of them right here on the land, where I can discover more about how they grow, and so they're at hand to harvest and brew as healing teas. Many wild plants and weeds are amenable to small cuttings and seed collections. Many plants transplant well and flourish if moved in the early spring when the new roots and shoots are just starting to form.

In addition to finding your own wild plants, you may want to call your local botanical garden for seeds and cuttings. The gardeners there are often happy to provide this material, because their most important mission is to protect and disseminate the plants — especially when they're rare and endangered.

I have to leave my credit card at home when I go to nurseries; I'm on restriction and am not allowed unsupervised nursery visits. This started with an impromptu trip to southern California after Beth (my wife) and I finally bought our 15-acre dream farm, which we call the Living Farmacy. I acted out all the pent-up energy and frustration of moving my herbs from place to place over the last 20 years and not having a place where I really felt I could put down my roots for good. Because I couldn't find a good selection in northern California of the semi-tropical plants that I wanted to grow, I decided to go to southern California to buy them. I flew down to San Diego, home of many amazing nurseries. I rented a moving van and started hitting nurseries. I was in heaven. Two days later, the van was full, and I was still trying to fit in a few last plants. I'm happy to say that these wonderful plants are in and doing well — except the ones that the gophers feasted on. A word to the wise: If you have gophers, cage your plants to give them a good start. That was the end of my nursery-visiting days — for now.

Propagation

HERB TALK

Because I'm not allowed to purchase plants these days (after the nursery incident), I find plants from other sources, with a process called *propagation*. Now that I take seeds, cuttings, and divisions from plants that I already own or that I find in the wild (or in other herb gardens), I know my herb garden will grow — without the use of my credit card.

I list a number of excellent mail-order companies where I buy my plants and seeds in Appendix C, arranged by specialty area. Many companies ship live plants in good condition right to your door.

- **Propagation by seed.** You can start seeds (purchased from a store or catalog) in containers on a sunny windowsill, in a greenhouse, or in a cold frame. A *cold frame* is a small wooden frame box covered with clear plastic and oriented toward the sun to keep the soil and plants warm during cool months. This can make the process of seed germination simpler and more controlled. Starting plants indoors also allows you to get a jump on the outdoor growing season, and it helps you avoid insects or organisms that may eat the seeds or the young sprouts. At the stage when the plant is small, it is the most sensitive to variations in water application and susceptible to insect attack, so transplanting a healthy, container-grown seedling helps it survive in your garden.

  Here are specific guidelines for successful seed propagation.

  - Plant the seeds to a depth 2 to 3 times the diameter of the seed.
  - Keep soil consistently moist until sprouting (also called *germination*) occurs.
  - Keep the soil consistently warm before, during, and a week or two after germination (when the seed sprouts).
  - As the plant begins to grow, you can slowly back off on watering.

  Herbs that grow well from seed include basil, catnip, chives, dill, coriander (cilantro), fennel, marjoram, and oregano.

  One of the best sources of information about seed propagation and specific seedling requirements is from the seed catalogs or seed suppliers. You can also check out *Perennials For Dummies,* by Marcia Tatroe & the Editors of the National Gardening Association and *Gardening For Dummies,* by Mike MacCaskey & the Editors of the National Gardening Association (both by IDG Books Worldwide, Inc.).

- **Propagation by cuttings.** *Cuttings* generally consist of small pieces of branches from existing plants that range anywhere from 3 to 12 inches long. Cuttings are especially successful with perennial plants that are difficult to grow from seed or when you want to be sure of the variety (for example, a particular type of lavender or rosemary). Some cuttings, called *stem-tip cutting,* are taken from new growth before flowering has occurred but after the new growth has matured and stiffened somewhat (half-ripe wood). You can take hardwood (fully mature wood that is hard) cuttings on deciduous plants (for example, elder, willow, and lemon verbena).

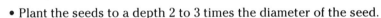

Here's how you take a cutting:

- Cut a piece of the stem of the plant you want to propagate with six nodes. Nodes are the places where the leaves attach and the new buds sprout from. If you take six nodes, you want to place three below the surface and three above. Pinch off any leaves, buds, or other growth on the part of the cutting that will go underground, so that they don't rot. Check out Figure 5-4. Because cuttings have no root system, they can't draw water into their stems and leaves. So, remove a majority of the leaves from the top of the cuttings, leaving only a few small ones.
- Keep the rooting soil mix for the cuttings sterile, consistently humid or moist, and protected from direct sunlight. Because cuttings are sensitive, don't put any organic materials like organic chicken manure in the rooting medium, because they can rot. A commonly used rooting medium is a mixture of half vermiculite and half perlite.
- Rooting hormones, such as Dip and Grow, can help increase the likelihood that your cuttings survive but aren't necessary for most plants.
- If you want to go organic, try soaking pieces of fast-growing willow shoots and stems in a gallon of water — they contain natural rooting hormones. Soak your cuttings in the willow water overnight before planting out.
- Keep the soil warm when planting a cutting — don't let soil cool off below 70° or so at night. Electrical heating wires or pads to place under the plants are available from suppliers in Appendix C.

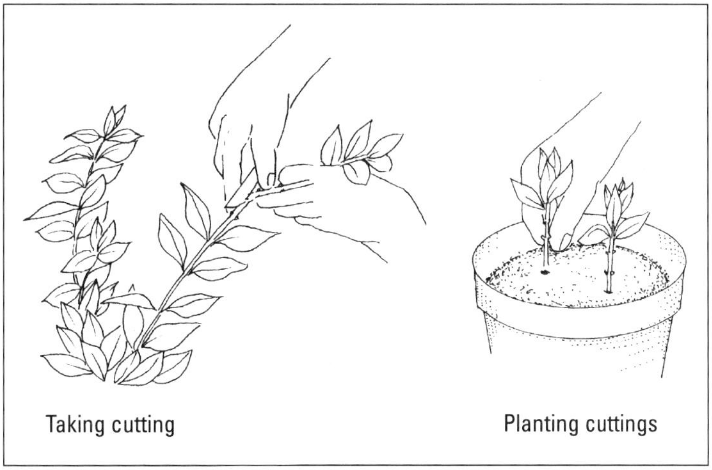

Figure 5-4: Make a cutting with six nodes, snip the leaves off the lower three nodes, and remove the larger leaves from the upper three nodes.

  • Don't expect 100 percent success in cuttings — it's a trial and error process. Different plants have different subtleties.

  You can get advice from your local nurseries and from garden books (see suggested reading in Appendix C), but experimentation is often the best teacher.

  Herbs that grow well from cuttings include just about any member of the mint family (like garden sage) and any other sages; mints like peppermint, spearmint, or bergamot; scented geraniums; lavender; lemon balm; lemon verbena; rosemary; and thyme.

- **Propagation by divisions.** Many perennial herbs spread outward as they grow; plants such as echinacea, feverfew, and valerian exhibit this growth pattern. During the fall as the plant's energy begins to draw back down into the roots, you can dig up these perennials and divide the tops of the root masses (crowns) into more clumps (see Figure 5-5). You can either dig up the whole root mass, take off a piece, and have that be your new center, or take a part of the newer growth from the root mass and plant that. You can also plant root divisions in containers to put in a protected area or use as a houseplant.

  Herbs that grow well from divisions include *Echinacea purpurea,* comfrey, feverfew, valerian, coltsfoot, lamb's ear, mints, thyme, oregano, wormwood, and yarrow.

  Certain plants, such as comfrey and mint, are too tough to divide by hand and may require you to cut the root with a spade or pruning shears.

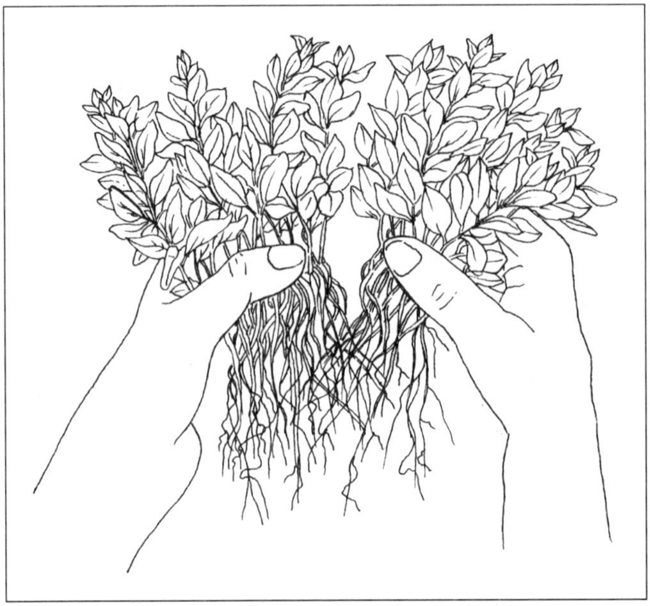

Figure 5-5: Break off pieces of the root mass of plants like St. John's wort, valerian, or feverfew, to grow new plants from a mother plant.

Harvesting Herbs

Identifying plants, knowing exactly when to harvest them, and processing plants into potent medicines is a time-honored art. People have passed this skill from generation to generation for hundreds of years. In fact, what you're finding out now as you read this book brings you into the time-honored practice of herbalism. Your ancestors probably harvested medicinal plants, perhaps drying yarrow and St. John's wort in the kitchen, and created the medicines that kept people healthy.

Parts to harvest — roots, stems, or seeds?

Certain parts of every healing plant hold the most potent medicine; in fact, several herbal remedies can be harvested from a single plant. Consider, for example, the common mullein. The bright yellow flowers are plucked individually from the stout main stalk during the early summer and soaked in olive oil to make potent ear drops for preventing and helping to heal ear infections. The leaves are harvested and used to make infusions for soothing and strengthening the upper respiratory tract and as an expectorant for bronchial mucus congestion of colds. The two remedies are completely different.

To determine which part of a plant to harvest for your particular needs consult the *Herb Guide,* located in the green pages near the back of this book.

Protecting environmentally-sensitive herbs

Certain medicinal plants need your help to survive. With the explosion of interest in herbal medicine and destruction of habitat due to encroaching development, a few popular healing herbs have become scarce due to commercial overharvesting. Consider joining United Plant Savers, the herbalists' UpS, which is working to ensure the rich diversity of medicinal plants. A chart in the Cheat Sheet that comes with this book acquaints you with the most common, at-risk, North American plants compiled by United Plant Savers. I recommend using these plants for short periods only for your specific needs or substituting other herbs with similar properties until they're available as organically-cultivated.

To join United Plant Savers, call 802-479-9825, e-mail `info@plantsavers.org`, or write to P.O. Box 98, East Barre, VT 05649.

Although each plant differs considerably in its qualities, distinct properties relate to each plant part (see Figure 5-6):

- **Flowers:** Herbal flowers and flowering parts (flowering tops) often contain essential oils, which are the aromatic essence of herbs, explored in Chapter 3. These plant constituents are antiseptic, antifungal, and can either relax or stimulate the emotions and nervous system. Flowers are often used in preparations to help heal and protect the skin.
- **Leaves and leafy shoots:** The leafy parts of plants hold many kinds of plant compounds and activities. Most contain chlorophyll, which can detoxify and cleanse, as well as several vitamins and minerals.
- **Barks:** The stem and trunk barks of plants often contain sugars and mucilage, which sooth the digestive tract and nourish body processes.
- **Roots and rhizomes:** The underground parts of plants tend to hold bitter and starchy constituents. These parts are cleansing to the blood and body tissues, and many have strong nourishing and sustaining qualities, especially to the immune system.
- **Seeds:** The seeds of plants are nutritive and calming to the nervous system. They contain fats, oils, and starches.

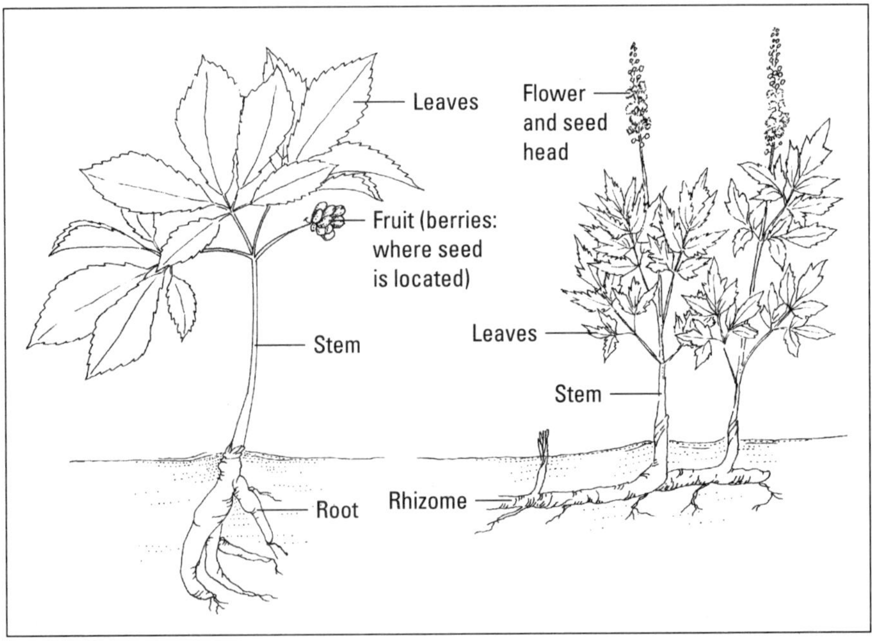

Figure 5-6: You can use several parts of the same herb for different healing effects.

The herbal experience — not all a bed of lavender

Although I usually recommend hand-harvesting, one exception is nettle herb. Years ago, a friend and I harvested a batch of stinging nettle with our bare hands. After picking a bag or so, our hands were red and felt like they were on fire. Why did we do it? You may say we were fools, and I wouldn't argue the point. But this process is part of becoming an herbalist. We have to hurt ourselves sometimes to really get the true essence and experience of the herbs. It teaches us that herbs are powerful and sometimes unpredictable in certain situations — much like nature itself. And we have stories to tell, often slightly embellished, of course. By the way, the easiest way to harvest nettles is with a pair of protective gloves on your hands.

Using the right tool for the job

No matter what herbs you're harvesting, the right tool makes the job more enjoyable and reduces injury to the plant. The most convenient tool for harvesting is your bare hands. I keep a slightly longer thumbnail on my right hand for pinching off shoots, stems, and flowers. I pinch with the nail, and for stiffer branches, snap at the same time, to avoid tearing or disfiguring the plant. Some herbal purists like the idea of keeping their herbs away from metal or other tools. I have an affinity for this idea — harvesting herbs with your own hands is simple and direct.

Hand-harvesting seeds and flowers makes sense because with your bare hands, you can easily remove these parts from the plant. I've also harvested roots by hand (by pulling up a plant), but many plants break off at the ground level before their roots come up. Roots are easier to pull after the first good autumn rains, when the soil is moist and loose.

Harvesting harder stems, barks, and most roots, however, requires other tools to do a good job. When not harvesting by hand, use pruning clippers, a sharp knife, or scissors to harvest leaves or flowers — this ensures a clean cut on the stem. Heavier branches require a pruning saw. When digging up roots, use a shovel or a garden fork.

Timing is important

Herbalists watch plants closely and always consider the health and vitality of the plant in each season. I've found through many years of observation and practice that the best medicine from any particular part of the plant comes when the plant is in its most scented, flavorful, colorful, and vital stage.

- **Flowers** are gathered at the peak of their blooming period, just before or immediately after they have fully opened. Examples include St. John's wort, mullein, calendula, violets, and honeysuckle.
- **Seeds** are gathered at the period of their full maturity as they begin to dry on the plant.
- **Barks** are stripped or sliced from the tree during the fall. Examples of useful tree barks include witch hazel, white willow, cascara sagrada, slippery elm, and sassafras. I like using the second- and third-year growth, because these twigs are covered by the most potent barks. Strip all the bark when still fresh; the bark is difficult to remove after the stems and branches are dry.

  For harvesting trunk barks like wild cherry or slippery elm, the best tool to use is a *drawknife,* a special, long knife with a handle at each end. Pull the knife down, cutting a three to five inch strip from the outer bark. Then carefully strip the inner bark. If you don't have a drawknife, harvest smaller stems and branches from a tree or shrub. If you're using pruning shears, cut out two or three medium-sized stalks from a shrub or branches from the main trunk of a tree.

  Be mindful of the possibility of killing a tree or shrub by removing too much bark from around a trunk or main stalk (called *girdling*). I try to always be aware of how much bark I can safely remove from a tree or shrub without causing severe injury to the tree. For most trees, don't remove more than a vertical strip one to two feet long and six to eight inches wide, depending on the size of the tree.
- **Roots** that you harvest can come from perennial plants such as trees, shrubs, and herbs that grow back year after year from the same roots like barberry or Oregon grape root. Dig roots of these perennials in the fall or early spring. Harvest the roots of annual plants, such as California poppy, during the time of flowering. You can collect the roots of biennials, such as burdock and chicory, in the fall of the first year (after the above-ground vegetation has died back) or in the spring of the second year (when the above-ground vegetation is just beginning).

  Perennial roots such as echinacea and yellow dock are generally not picked until the plant is two to five years old. Otherwise, they can be harvested at the same time of the year as biennials.
- **Rhizomes** are underground stems that often spread out from the original plant right under the ground. Roots often come off of the rhizomes. Common examples of *rhizomatious plants* (plants that have rhizomes) include valerian, coltsfoot, and mugwort. These plants aren't always well-behaved and can need lots of room — my Chinese mugwort plant is slowly eating the entire bed, overtaking its neighbors. Harvest rhizomes at the same times as the roots of plants, because the two are connected — when you dig up a mass of valerian, for example, you find the highly-branching rhizomes and roots.

- **Leaves** are gathered just before their full development, often before the flowers are in full bloom. Young, tender shoots of plants are often potent, because they contain all the protective chemicals the plant produces to discourage hungry animals and insects. These young, tender shoots are full of sugars for the growing plant and are a sweet treat for deer and other browsing animals, sometimes despite bitter and acrid plant components. If you pick from plants that are more fully developed (later in the summer), try to pick the youngest, healthiest shoots and leaves.

REMEMBER

You want your herbs to be in a healthy, vital state when you harvest them. Sometimes, the harvest of particular plants continues throughout a season. For example, I harvest calendula flowers as they mature, place them on a screen, and continue adding to my screen of calendula flowers throughout the season — this way, I have enough flowers to make tea, salve, and oil. Certain plants, such as calendula and roses, are actually stimulated to produce more flowers after being harvested.

Independent of the season, the best time of day to harvest herbs is in the morning after the dew has had a chance to dry and before the sun is very bright. Volatile oils are at their peak at this time, so the herbs are cooler and less likely to deteriorate after cutting. After you cut the herbs, get them ready for drying as soon as possible to preserve good quality (see the section "Drying Herbs" for more on the drying process).

HERB TALK

Join the garbling party

The process of carefully picking the flowers and leaves from the stems of plants is called garbling. Trimming roots and cleaning out the dirt from large root crowns and removing dead leaves from a plant is also garbling. So, *garbling* is preparing your herbs for drying and/or storage by hand.

For example, if you harvest and carefully dry a bunch of oregano from your garden, you begin garbling by spreading out the herbs on cloth or newspaper placed on a table top. Then, strip off the small flowers and leaves from the larger stems. (The easiest way to do this is to grasp the bottom of the stalks and strip all the small stems, flowers, and leaves. Try to strip against the angle of the branches. If most of the branches are angling upwards, grasp the top of the stem and strip downwards.) Then, pick through the pile of leaves, flowers, and stems to pull out the larger branchlets, leaving mostly leaves and flowers. Don't worry about having a few small stems in your finished batch of herbs.

You may find that garbling is an enjoyable way to get to know your herbs — their smell, feel, and presence. How about a garbling party with friends and family members? Kids usually love to garble.

Drying Herbs

After you harvest your herbs, keep them out of the direct sun, because sunlight darkens their color and evaporates important essential oils. Remove any discolored or unhealthy-looking leaves. A dark, warm place out of direct sunlight and with good air circulation is optimum for drying herbs. Dry your herbs rapidly to preserve color and freshness, but without going above 100°. Here are tips for successful drying.

- **Fit to be tied.** Tie herbs, such as lavender, yarrow, and mugwort, in bunches and hang them from rafters in an attic or garage. See Figure 5-7.
- **Screen your herbs.** Herbs too small to be tied into bundles can be laid on screens. Window screens work well — I buy old window screens from a recycled building supply house for little money. You can make your own by stretching stainless steel screening (available from a hardware store) over a wooden frame. Stack your screens at least six inches apart using wooden blocks or bricks (see Figure 5-8).

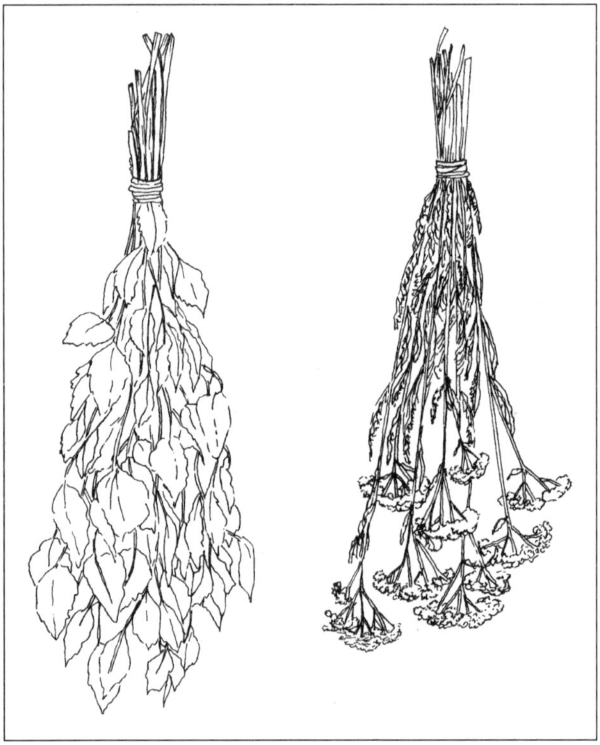

Figure 5-7: Dry herbs by bundling them and hanging them upside down in a room with good air circulation.

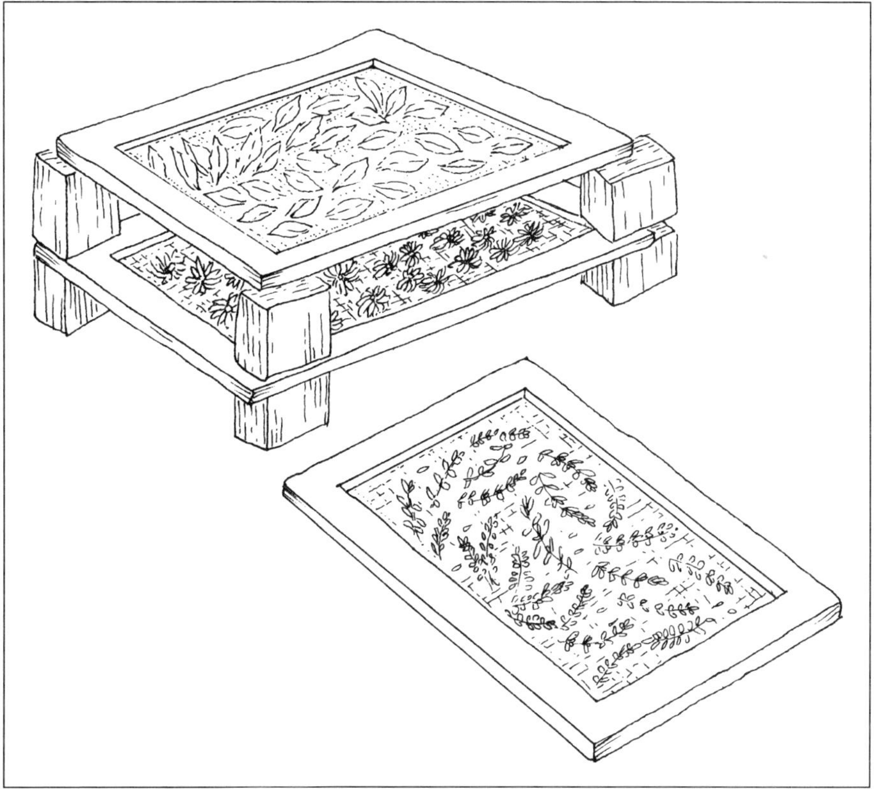

Figure 5-8: Drying herbs on screens works well.

- **Dry and collect seeds.** When drying seeds, hang the plants upside down inside a paper bag, as shown in Figure 5-9, so that as the seeds ripen, they fall right into the bag.
- **Separate leaves.** Take leaves off of the stems and loosely spread the leaves on a drying surface, like a screen. Stir them occasionally until they're dried.
- **Don't over-dry leaves and flowers.** Look for lighter herbs that are brittle, but not so crisp that they turn to powder when they're crushed.
- **Handle with care and keep them whole.** Keep in mind that the less herbs are handled and processed, the better they maintain their flavor and color. Package leaves whole and don't crush them until you're ready to use them. Store any herbs in their whole state whenever possible until you're ready to use them or make an extract.

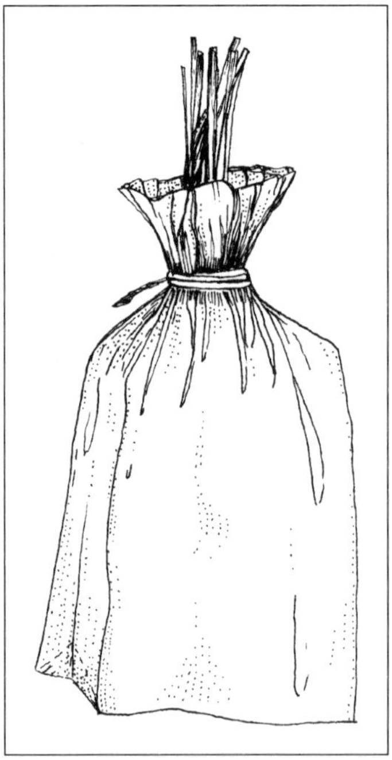

Figure 5-9: Use paper bags to catch herb seeds.

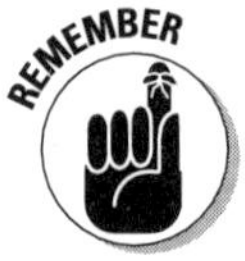

- **Dry roots and barks.** Roots and barks can be dry on the outside, but moist on the inside. I've lost several batches of root slices to mold by placing them in jars before they were completely dry inside. Because they *looked* dry, I was fooled. Snap root slices and barks to make sure they're dry all the way through before you store them.
- **Keep air circulating.** Drying herbs need ample air circulation, so don't place them too close together on a screen or tie them in bunches that are too tight. An ideal herb drying spot is a warm shed or room out of the direct sunlight with plenty of warm air flowing through. When drying on screens or racks, arrange herbs horizontally above each other so that the air current is able to pass over and through every part. You may want to stir the herbs a bit every day or two to encourage the herbs to dry evenly and to prevent molding.
- **Fast, but not too hot.** Flowers need careful and rapid drying to preserve their color, but at temperatures under 90°. Spread them loosely on the drying surface and stir occasionally until they're dry.
- **Set the temperature.** Most herbs collected in the warm months and during dry weather may be air-dried in a dark, well-ventilated room. In cool, damp weather, artificially heat the room or area at a temperature between 70° and 100°.

Understanding the art of wildcrafting

Wildcrafting, or harvesting plants from the wild, is a term for conscious harvesting that's in tune with the natural resources of the earth. Wildcrafting is a time-honored way to supply your needs and those of your family and friends for high-quality plant medicine.

Here are important rules for wildcrafting:

- **Harvest with thankfulness.** Herbalists know that the most important aspect of wildcrafting is harvesting with reverence and thankfulness. At the very least, maintaining a constant mindfulness of the gifts you're receiving from the earth is important. This is in contrast to carelessly or greedily ripping the plants (or bulldozing them) from the ground.
- **Harvest selectively and sparingly.** When you see three plants in a population, don't pick any of them, unless you're only taking some flowers and leaves — not the entire plant. If you see ten plants, harvest only one or two; if you see twenty, harvest three or four. Prune above-ground parts of plants and allow them to grow back. Some flowers are actually stimulated to produce more flowers after being picked — they can be harvested more thoroughly. Remember that harvesting roots kills a plant. In addition, never harvest the old plants or the very young ones. Pass these plants by and collect plants of medium size and age.
- **Harvest away from roads and factories.** Plants can take in heavy metals and toxins from their surroundings. Never harvest plants close to a road — harvest plants that are at least 100 to 200 feet from busy roads, fifty feet from moderately frequented roads, and use your judgement on roads with only a few cars a day. Be conscious about lead and other toxic compounds that come from automobile exhaust. Avoid plants next to factories or in fields where spraying has occurred. Check to see if plants are shriveling up and appear to be dying, have widespread yellowing, or are distorted — they may have been sprayed with pesticides.
- **Find out about local populations.** When you go into a population of plants to harvest, know if the plants are abundant or rare in your area. A good plant identification book can supply this information. Additionally, government offices may provide a list of the plants that are rare in your state.
- **Don't harvest rare and endangered wild plants.** A few medicinal plants are highly sought-after in many countries of the world and have become severely reduced in numbers. Avoid picking these plants from the wild, except when you have plenty in your local area and you're using them for your family's use (not for commercial sale). Check out the table on environmentally-sensitive herbs in the Cheat Sheet that comes with this book.

Storing Herbs

For the most luck storing your herbs, keep the following tips in mind:

- The better they're stored, the longer herbs last.
- As long as they look fresh and maintain their aromas, the herbs are still useful.
- Flowers and leaves maintain their potency for one year; roots and bark for up to two years.
- Airtight containers (such as glass jars) are ideal for storing herbs. Keep them in a kitchen cabinet or cupboard, away from light.

  You may be tempted to place herbs and spices on an open shelf above the stove — unfortunately, this is where they deteriorate most rapidly, because they're exposed to excess heat and humidity. Of course a closed, dark cupboard above the stove is fine.
- You can store your dried herbs in brown paper bags stored inside a large, sealed plastic bag.
- Keep the herbs labeled with their names, the harvest dates, and the location where you harvested the herbs.
- If you have dried herbs left over, you can always add them to your compost pile.

Chapter 6

Making Herbal Products at Home

In This Chapter

- Stocking up on tools, equipment, and ingredients
- Understanding how to make teas, tinctures, infused oils, salves, creams, cough syrups, and elixirs
- Blending your own aromatherapy scents and healing products

Recipes in This Chapter

- An Infusion of Calmness
- Elderflower Tea
- Immune Vitali-Tea
- Pass-on-Gas Tea
- Echinacea Leaf and Flower Tincture
- Horehound Hack-Free Cough Syrup
- High-Energy Elixir
- Fabulous Moisturizing Cream
- Quick and Easy Aromatherapy Cream
- St. John's Wort Oil
- Muscle Pain Oil
- Heaven-Scent Massage Oil
- Bath Salts
- Rosemary Hair Rinse
- Nature Scent Freshener
- Facial Mist
- Rose Petal Potpourri
- Ginger Compress
- Protective and Healing Salve
- Ease-Up Liniment

Harvesting wild or cultivated herbs and creating wonderfully-scented aromatic balms and potions fulfills a basic human desire — to find allies for preserving health and vitality and promoting long life. A special bond exists between herbalists of all ages and those who feel the call to experience these colorful, aromatic herbal potions, elixirs, and salves. This chapter shows you how.

An effective way to even find out more about creating effective herbal products is to visit herb shops, natural-foods markets — even pharmacies — to smell and taste their products, feel the texture, and observe the coloring. You can be guided by seeing how the experts do it. A salve maker who has made thousands of jars of calendula salve or a tincture maker who has created thousands of bottles of echinacea both know how to make a product that tastes good, looks good, and works well. And soon, you will too!

A Little Jargon to Get You Started

Most capsules, tablets, liquid extracts like tinctures, salves, creams, and even herbal shampoos contain extracts (see Chapter 2 for the lowdown on extracts). When you make a tea on your stove, for example, you're making an extract — by placing the herbs in a pan with water and simmering them, the active ingredients are released from the plant into the tea. As you strain the tea from the herbs and drink the tea, you take the vital healing essence of the plant into your body. What you discard with the spent herbs are compounds that make up the bulk of the plant but are not as active. The following list helps clear up some of the mystery behind this process:

- **The solvent:** When you make a tea, you add water to the herbs. The water is the *solvent,* also called the *menstruum.* A solvent is a liquid that can selectively remove certain active ingredients (often called *active compounds*), like alkaloids, from herbs. Think of a cup of coffee as a liquid extract and freeze-dried coffee as a powdered extract. Think of Mr. Coffee as an extractor that removes the active ingredients from the herb (ground coffee). Besides water, other solvents include alcohol, glycerin, and liquid carbon dioxide. The art of extraction is choosing the right solvent system for each herb to maximize its effectiveness.
- **The marc:** After a batch of herbs is extracted with water or other solvent, the liquid is thoroughly pressed from the spent herb. All the liquid is then collected and bottled or further processed. The dry, spent herb material is known as the *marc.* The marc is usually composted to make fertilizer for growing more herbs (see Chapter 5 for more on composting).
- **Maceration and percolation:** The process of soaking herbs in a solvent for a period of time, often about two weeks, is called *maceration.* Pouring or forcing a solvent through the herbs packed into a large funnel to pull out active ingredients is called *percolation.* Herbalists use either of these two methods to make herbal extracts.

Tools of the Trade

To make herbal products at home, you need a few pieces of basic equipment, such as a blender, a coffee grinder or seed grinder, and a double boiler. You can often find these items in natural-foods stores, department stores, or kitchen shops. Consult Appendix C for equipment sources.

Blender or grinder

Use a blender (shown in Figure 6-1) or grinder (see Figure 6-2) to reduce plant material (dry or fresh) to the smallest particle size possible — this increases the surface area of the herb that's exposed to the solvent during the extraction process. This blending/grinding process gives a more complete extraction and doesn't waste herb material. In the case of expensive herbs like ginseng, you want to get as complete an extraction as possible, so blending and grinding ginseng is particularly important.

- A good blender is one of the most important tools of the home herb product maker. While any high-quality blender will do, try to find one with a very high speed and strong motor. A Vita-Mix has an extra strong motor, which is reversible to help disentangle herb roots and stems that may get caught in the blade. The heavy-duty motor also gives a more complete breakdown of the plant material.
- A small seed grinder or coffee grinder (available in many kitchen shops) is handy for finely powdering small quantities of dry seeds, root slices, and leaves. A small grinder usually yields a finer particle size than a blender, but it can only process a small amount of herbs.
- Any food processor can be useful for shredding fresh roots, seeds, and leafy material.

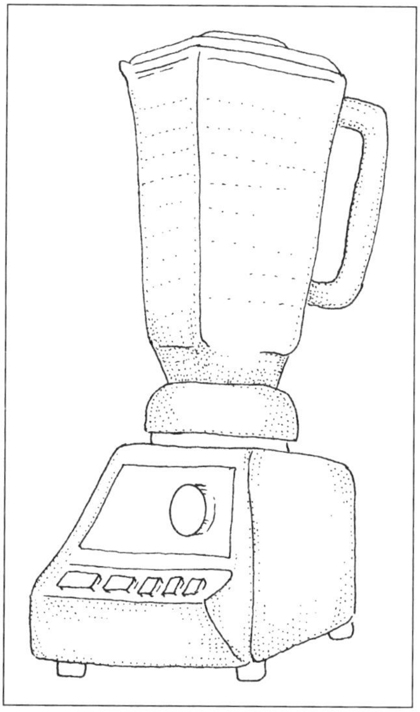

Figure 6-1: A blender is useful for making tinctures, infused oils, and creams.

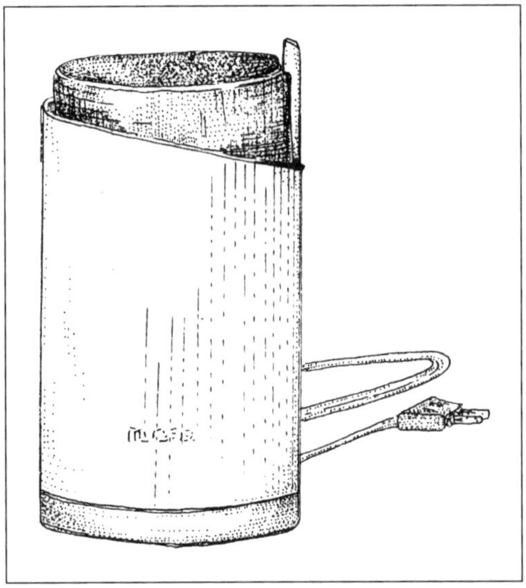

Figure 6-2: Using a grinder lets you get the most out of your herbs when making herbal products.

Pots and pans

A pot or pan is an important extraction tool for simmering roots, barks, and flowers. Remember that making an extract at home is as simple as steeping a tea bag in a cup of hot water for 20 minutes. You may want to use different kinds of pots and pans for making different kinds of herbal products.

- A quality stainless steel pot works nicely for making herbal products. Use one that has a heat-dispersing handle.
- Pyrex glass is my favorite material in which to cook herbs and herb oils.
- Coffee pots that are made of good quality heat-resistant glass are excellent for making tea, because you can see the process of extraction and the color of the tea. I judge the strength of the tea by its dark rich color.
- A double boiler, shown in Figure 6-3, is also useful for melting wax and other ingredients, while not overheating or scorching them.
- You may want to use a crock pot to make herbal oils. They're especially useful for keeping an oil warm when you're making an herbal oil, thereby increasing the extraction rate and concentration of the herbs in the final oil. Try to find a crock pot that allows the temperature to be set to about 100°.

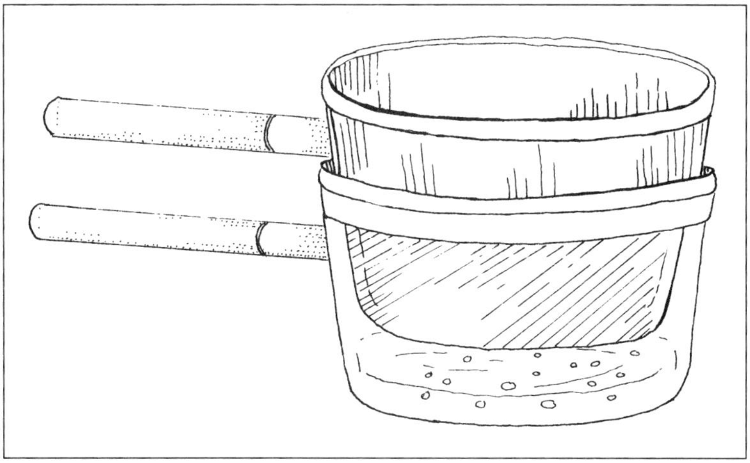

Figure 6-3: A double boiler maintains the desired heat level when making infused oils and salves.

Jars and containers

You can find a wide variety of jars and containers from suppliers listed in Appendix C. Think about obtaining the following types:

- Purchase a few one- or two-quart canning jars for extraction and for storing herbs. The rubber seal keeps oxygen out, preserving the freshness of the herbs.

  Some stores sell one-gallon jars for larger extraction batches.

- For tinctures, use one-, two-, or four-ounce Boston amber round bottles with droppers (available from pharmacies and herb shops). See Figure 6-4.

  A *tincture* is a concentrated liquid solution made by soaking herb powders in an alcohol and water blend, then filtering out the liquid. Put a teaspoon of the tincture in a cup of warm water to make an instant tea — even when you're on the move and away from your kitchen.

- Buy some one-ounce salve jars or tins for salves and creams.

  See Appendix C for sources of tins and bottles by mail. You can also find one- or two-ounce dropper bottles at your local pharmacy or herb shop.

You can make labels for your products by hand, on your printer at home, or by visiting a local printing shop. Labels for your laser or ink-jet printer are available in an amazing variety of shapes and sizes from an office supply store or paper-goods catalog.

Consider a food dehydrator

A food dehydrator is a good investment for the home herb product maker. Here's why:

- You can use it to dry flowers, leaves, root slices, and other herb parts quickly and preserve valuable active plant chemicals and color.
- You can make potent extracts — dried and powdered teas — with the aid of a good food dehydrator.
- You can dry kitchen spices, such as oregano and basil.

Appendix C has addresses for ordering food dehydrators by mail.

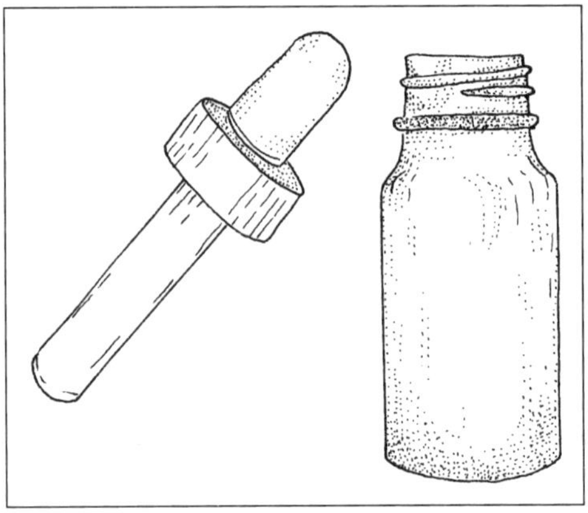

Figure 6-4: Boston amber rounds are convenient for storing liquid herbal products.

Miscellaneous tools

Here is a shopping list of other useful items that you may need to make herb products.

- **Measuring spoons:** You can buy a set that includes 1/4 teaspoon, 1/2 teaspoon, and 1 teaspoon. You can use these smaller measures to add potent essential oils to your salves, creams, cough syrups, or other preparations.
- **Mortar and pestle:** A mortar and pestle is a traditional device to grind small quantities of herbs to a coarse or fine powder by hand. Reducing herbs to a powder speeds up the extraction process (the process of removing the active chemicals from plants).

- **Muslin, linen, or cheesecloth:** You can use these fine-meshed cloths to filter tinctures or oils, seperating the spent herbs (that have all medicinal chemicals removed) from the finished oil or tincture.
- **Funnel:** A funnel is helpful for pouring finished oils or tinctures into small-mouthed bottles, such as a one-ounce dropper bottle.
- **Scale:** A weighing scale (in grams or ounces) is essential if you want to keep track of exactly how much herb you used to make a batch of tincture or oil. Knowing the weight enables you to make your next batch stronger or weaker by adding more or less herbs to the same amount of liquid oil or alcohol/water blend. I recommend keeping good records by writing these amounts in a small notebook.
- **Candy thermometer:** A candy thermometer helps you know just when to turn the heat off from a batch of herbal candy (like horehound candy for coughs) and pour it into the molds. If you pour the liquid candy too early, before all the water is removed, your finished candy will be sticky.
- **Candy molds.** Candy molds are available from some kitchen shops. You can buy them in different shapes. I like the plain, round ones because candies of that shape are easy to wrap with a little waxed paper and put into a small box to carry in your pocket or purse.

Stocking Your Pantry

To make herbal products like tinctures, salves, or creams, you need oils, alcohol, glycerin, vinegar, and wax to create an extract, and then, perhaps, to thicken the extract. Be sure to stock these items.

Oils

For making herbal oils, salves, and creams, buy good-quality oils that won't go rancid quickly. Try to avoid polyunsaturated oils (canola, sunflower, and safflower oils) because they're sensitive to heat and light and degrade rapidly. Store your oils in the refrigerator to avoid rancidity.

- **Sweet almond oil:** A light oil, less greasy than olive oil and one of my favorites for making medicated oils. Almond oil is especially soothing and helps relieve dryness and itching.
- **Apricot kernel oil:** A light oil more delicate than almond and often more expensive. Apricot kernel oil is blended with almond or other oils at about 10 to 50 percent of the total to lighten it up. The oil is excellent to use if you have sensitive skin.

- **Avocado oil:** A heavy, long-lasting oil for the skin. Avocado oil contains vitamins for the skin and adds a rich, dark green color to salves, creams, and other products.
- **Carrot oil:** A light oil that slows aging of the skin.
- **Castor oil:** Castor oil is pressed from the castor bean and processed to remove toxic substances in the bean. Commercially-available castor oil is commonly used as a laxative by the teaspoonful. Castor is a heavy oil, but one that is highly therapeutic in its own right. The psychic healer Edgar Cayce popularized its use for the treatment of cysts, tumors, and growths. The oil contains toxic protein-like compounds called *lectins,* which when applied to the skin, are absorbed and stimulate a local immune response to help break down a tumor or cyst. Use up to 20 percent in an oil blend.
- **Cocoa butter:** Obtained from the cocoa bean, this butter is used in lotion, cream, lip balm, and soap. Cocoa butter contains highly saturated fatty acids, so it's heavy and resists rancidity. Cocoa butter smells of chocolate, which may be a good thing if your partner is a chocolate freak. If the smell becomes overwhelming, use no more than 15 to 20 percent in your product.
- **Coconut oil:** This oil from the tropics is semi-solid at room temperature. Use coconut oil to thicken your creams and other skin products and to give them body. Coconut oil is one of the most stable oils and doesn't easily go rancid in your products.
- **Grapeseed oil:** An almost colorless, vitamin-rich oil that is easily absorbed. The oil is made from the seeds of the fruit. Grapeseed oil has a good texture that makes it ideal for massage oils, but it can't be cold-pressed, so all commercial grapeseed oil is solvent-extracted with industrial solvents like hexane. For this reason, I recommend skipping this oil.
- **Olive oil:** The finest all-around oil for making medicated oils. What could be more natural than the oil of olive, requiring only crushing the olives to release the nutritious and heart-friendly yellow-green oil? Many other oils require solvent extraction or heating during extraction, even when the product says *expeller-pressed* or *cold-pressed.* Olive oil stays fresh longer than other oils and is excellent for people with naturally dry skin.

  Olive oil is a heavy oil and sometimes has a decided scent of olives. If the scent and oily feel are pleasant to you, fine — but it may make you feel like a walking salad.

- **Jojoba oil:** A wax that's traditionally used as a hair restorer, jojoba oil is also an excellent moisturizer for dry skin. Jojoba oil is usually diluted by half with other oils for massage oils.
- **Palm kernel oil:** Add palm oil to products to give them a thick, creamy feeling and protect your skin. The oil is heavy, containing mostly saturated fatty acids and a good quantity of vitamin A, which is a natural skin protector and cancer fighter.

Choose cold-pressed organic oils whenever they're available. I try to use organic oils instead of commercial oils, which are made with harsh solvents that extract the oil from the seed mash.

Grain alcohol

Grain alcohol is absolutely the best solvent and delivery system to carry an herb's active constituents into the bloodstream. The proportion of alcohol to water is often adjusted in order to selectively pull out the constituents desired.

For instance, resins like bee propolis and the active constituents of milk thistle are only alcohol-soluble. Using a solvent with a high percentage of pure ethanol or grain alcohol yields the best extraction.

The active steroid-like compounds in ginseng are mostly water-soluble, so I choose a solvent that contains a fairly low percentage of alcohol (45-50 percent alcohol to 50-55 percent water).

For home use, tinctures and elixirs can be made with 100 proof vodka, which is the most widely available.

Vodka is the most effective distilled liquor for making tinctures or alcoholic herbal extracts. Be aware that 100 proof vodka actually contains a little less than 50 percent ethanol by volume, and 80 proof vodka, a little less than 40 percent.

Other kinds of alcoholic beverages such as rum and brandy are not ideal because they already contain coloring pigments, flavoring compounds, sugars, and other components. Without as many "binding sites" on the alcohol, the water molecules have to pull and hold active constituents from the herbal material. Vodka, on the other hand, is probably the purest and most effective. Even better is pure grain alcohol, distilled from corn. Pure grain alcohol is 190 proof, or a little less than 95 percent pure alcohol. The reason it's not 100 percent pure is because absolutely pure alcohol always pulls some moisture from the air, and the solution stabilizes at 95 percent. See Appendix C for suppliers.

Glycerin

Good-quality glycerin from vegetable sources is widely available in natural-foods stores and pharmacies. Glycerin adds body and a little sweetness to herbal preparations such as cough syrups and elixirs. It's often added to creams and helps bring oils and tinctures together in a smooth, easy-to-apply blend. For those who like taking a liquid herbal product, but don't want alcohol, glycerin can dissolve certain plant constituents and act as a reasonably good preservative. Many flavored herbal glycerites are available in natural-foods stores and herb stores, especially for children. These products are helpful for parents who want a good-tasting, liquid preparation that's easy to disguise in juice. In these products, flavorful essential oils like orange or cinnamon are often added to the glycerin and herb blends.

On the downside, glycerin isn't as good a solvent as alcohol — you get more activity in a one ounce echinacea alcohol-based tincture than in a one ounce echinacea glycerite. And glycerin isn't as good a preservative as alcohol, so glycerites have to contain at least 75 percent glycerin, which can render the taste sickly-sweet after repeated doses. Further, glycerin can be drying and irritating to the mucous membranes when used undiluted — as can alcoholic preparations. Finally, glycerin isn't as effective a carrier of the active herbal constituents into the body as alcohol. All in all, I recommend glycerites only for children or for people who can't take any alcohol.

Beeswax and other wax

Beeswax is used to harden salves and creams and turn them into a suitable consistency. You can buy beeswax at your local hobby shop or natural-foods store. Some grocery stores also carry beeswax.

- Look for beeswax that's pure and free from chips of paint, dirt, rocks, and dead insect parts. (Hives may be painted with lead-based paint.)
- Use wax that's a light amber color and has the delightful fragrance of honey with a slightly gluey smell.
- Look in the Yellow Pages of your phone book under beekeepers for sources of good beeswax.
- Prepackaged wax can be found in herb shops, natural-foods stores, and even craft shops. See Appendix C for mail-order sources.

Essential oils

An appealing smell can be achieved through the use of *essential oils,* which are extracts of essential oil-containing plants. You can buy oils of herbs to add an inviting smell to your herbal body products; for example, the citrus family members (orange, lemon, and grapefruit), mints (peppermint and spearmint), wintergreen, and lavender. See Chapter 3 for the lowdown on essential oils.

Miscellaneous

Other items you may need for making herbal products include the following:

- **Honey** is soothing to the throat and is a common ingredient in herbal cough syrups and throat lozenges.
- **Brown rice syrup** (available in natural-foods stores) is used in the same ways as honey and is less sweet with more complex sugars. Brown rice syrup is a good choice if you have diabetes or other blood sugar imbalance.
- **Ascorbic acid** (vitamin C powder) acts as a mild preservative for herbal creams.
- **Borax** is a natural substance (commonly used for washing clothes) that you can use to help the oily and watery ingredients mix together. It makes your herbal creams creamy.

Making Products for Internal Use

This section gives you numerous recipes that include teas, a tincture, a cough syrup, and an elixir.

Making teas

Blending an herbal tea is a pleasant, healthy ritual that encourages you to slow down a little and smell the herbs — no capsule or tablet can do that! I encourage my patients to drink invigorating teas such as rosemary or green tea instead of coffee to slow down even more. This section shows you how to prepare different herbal teas.

Infusions

Infusions are a simple way of preparing tea from leaves and flowers. To make an infusion, do the following:

1. **Pour boiling water over the herb and let steep, covered, for 10 to15 minutes.**

   Use 1 teaspoon herb per cup of water.

2. **Pour the tea through a strainer into a teacup.**

   You can also store your herb tea in the refrigerator for two to three days.

Herbs commonly used for infusions include peppermint, chamomile, lemon balm, raspberry leaf, and red clover.

An Infusion of Calmness

This combination of herbs is formulated to infuse a feeling of calmness throughout your body and spirit. Drink a cup several times a day or just before bed.

Preparation time: *20 minutes*

Yield: *4 cups*

1 quart boiling water

3 teaspoons linden flower

3 teaspoons chamomile herb

3 teaspoons eleuthero root

3 teaspoons passion flower

3 teaspoons orange peel

1/2 teaspoon stevia herb

1 Pour the boiling water over the herbs, roots, flowers, and peels and cover the pan.

2 Let the brew steep for 15 minutes.

3 Strain the mixture.

Elderflower Tea

Elderflower tea makes a good-tasting beverage with gentle cleansing power. Drink a cup or two several times a day to assist your body in getting rid of toxic waste products when you are going through a healing crisis (see Chapter 2) or any time you want an easy, yet efficient cleanse of your system.

Preparation time: *20 minutes*

Yield: *1 quart*

4 tablespoons dried elderflower

1 quart water

1 In a covered pan, steep the elderflower in freshly-boiled water for 15 minutes. Strain the mixture.

2 Store what you don't use in the refrigerator.

Vary It! Try adding a teaspoon of stevia (often referred to as "the sweet herb") to every 4 tablespoons of elderflowers for extra sweetness.

HERB TALK

Decoctions

A *decoction* is a method of extracting the heavier and denser parts of plants like roots, barks, and twigs. To make a decoction, do the following:

1. **Add 1 tablespoon of an herb or herb mixture (coarsely chopped or ground) to each cup of boiling water and simmer.**

   Thin barks like willow bark need only 15 or 20 minutes of gentle simmering. Thicker chunks of ginseng root need 1 hour of simmering to extract all the active constituents.

2. **Let the mixture step for 15 minutes or so, until it's cool enough to handle.**

3. **Pour the mixture through a strainer and add the herb residue to your compost pile.**

Herbs that are generally made as a decoction include licorice, yellow dock, dandelion root, and ginseng root.

REMEMBER

Decoctions are a time-honored way of using tonic herbs. Tonic herbs and herb formulas support and nourish your body systems. In China, decoctions of the tonic herb dong quai are used as a base to make vegetable chicken soups. The vegetables, grains, and chicken take on the medicinal qualities of the herb. By eating the soup, you get all the benefits of the food *and* the medicinal effects of the dong quai, such as building the blood, increasing energy levels, and strengthening the uterus. Take tonic teas for three to nine months to receive the full effects. Take the herbs daily for maximum benefits. Don't use tonic herbs during an acute infection. Begin again after the main part of the infection is over to bolster your immune system.

Immune Vitali-Tea

This time-honored decoction can be used daily, even for six to nine months, to strengthen your natural defenses against colds, flu, and other diseases. Drink 1 cup, morning and evening.

Preparation time: *1½ hours*

Yield: *1 quart*

3 to 4 sticks astragalus root

1 tablespoon ligustrum

3 to 4 roots codonopsis (about 4-5" long)

1 tablespoon burdock root

1 teaspoon licorice

5 cups water

1 Simmer all of the herbal ingredients in the water for 30 to 60 minutes.

2 Turn off the heat and let the tea steep for an additional 15 minutes.

3 Strain and pour into a quart jar for storage in the refrigerator.

HERB TALK

Light decoctions

For lighter barks and hard leaves or to remove heavier compounds from leaves and flowers, make a *light decoction* by doing the following:

1. **Place the herbs in water and simmer on the lowest heat possible, covered, for 10 to 15 minutes.**

   Use 2 tablespoons of the herb for each cup of water.

2. **Turn off the heat and let the mixture steep for an additional 10 to 15 minutes.**

3. **Strain the entire mixture and drink. Store whatever is left over in the refrigerator — it keeps for up to three days.**

Pass-on-Gas Tea

This delicious tea is a favorite with many of my patients for preventing gas after meals, as well as helping to ease gas pains and abdominal discomfort. Drink 1/2 to 1 cup of the tea after meals to help relieve that feeling of fullness.

Preparation time: *25 minutes*

Yield: *3 cups*

4 cups water

1 teaspoon cumin seed

1 teaspoon fennel seed

1 teaspoon caraway seed

1 teaspoon orange peel

1/2 teaspoon licorice root

1 Bring the water to a boil and add the herbs. Simmer, covered, in the water, for 10 minutes.

2 Remove from the heat and steep the mixture for another 10 to 15 minutes.

3 Strain the mixture. Drink immediately or store for later use.

Vary It! After you turn the heat off, add 2 teaspoons of peppermint leaf.

Understanding the art of tincture-making

HERB TALK

Tinctures are made by grinding up dry or fresh herbs in a solvent of alcohol and water or glycerin. Tinctures have several advantages over other types of herbal products — their medicinal properties are easily absorbed by the body, they have a long shelf life (up to three years), they act quickly on your body, and they're easy to use — they can be carried in one-ounce bottles in the pocket. The usual process for making a tincture is as follows:

1. **Place the herbs in a blender and add the solvent.**

   A tincture is made with 5 parts solvent liquid volume to 1 part herb by dry weight, which is notated (1:5).

   See the "Stocking Your Pantry" section for tips on choosing a solvent.

2. **Blend at high speed until smooth.**

3. **Place the mixture in a warm area, but out of direct sunlight.**
4. **Shake daily for at least two weeks.**
5. **Squeeze any liquid out through a linen cloth or press it out with a hydraulic press, such as a cider press.**
6. **Filter the remaining mixture, if desired.**
7. **Compost or discard the spent herb (the *marc*).**

You can add more dry herb to the solvent to make a stronger tincture. Keep adding the herb to the liquid and blend. After soaking, the herb settles out. Keep at least $^{1}/_{2}$ inch of pure solvent over the herb. If the herb sticks up out of the solvent at any time, your tincture may ferment and produce an off-flavor.

One teaspoonful (about 5 droppersful) of a tincture has approximately the same potency as one strong cup of tea. The average adult dose of most tinctures is about 1 to 3 droppersful, 2 to 3 times daily, for health maintenance and about twice that (4 to 6 droppersful, 4 to 5 times daily) for a therapeutic dose (when you are treating a specific medical condition). Adjust the dose for children, according to age and size. See Chapter 4 for children's doses.

Store tinctures in amber bottles to minimize the adverse effects of sunlight on their important medicinal components. They can keep their potency for up to three years if you store them in a cool place away from heat and light.

Echinacea Leaf and Flower Tincture

This widely-used tincture helps strengthen the body's natural defenses. Use it to prevent and help heal colds, flu, respiratory ailments, urinary tract infections, and other types of infections.

Preparation time: *10 minutes*

Yield: *6 ounces*

$1^{1}/_{2}$ ounces dried echinacea leaves (and flowers if available)

4 ounces grain alcohol (or 100-proof vodka)

4 ounces distilled water

1 Combine the echinacea, alcohol, and water in a blender.

2 Blend for about 1 to 2 minutes or until smooth.

3 Pour into a quart canning jar or other suitable container.

(continued)

(continued)

4 Shake the blend vigorously for 1 minute, every day for two weeks. Be sure to keep the mixture out of sunlight, but in a warm place.

5 Press or squeeze the blend through a piece of linen or other fine cloth.

6 Transfer the finished tincture to an amber dropper bottle. Keep away from heat and light; refrigeration isn't necessary.

Vary It! If you prefer a stronger echinacea tincture with more of a bite, add echinacea root to the leaves and flowers. Use the roots only for the most potent tincture. In my experience, the leaves and flowers are potent enough for most situations.

The best herbs to make into tinctures

Over the years, I've seen manufacturers and herb users choose a few herbs over and over again in tincture form. These following herbs are usually more potent in tincture form than in teas.

- **Orange peel, stevia, and licorice.** Great flavoring herbs to add to any of your tinctures. Orange tincture eases digestive discomforts, helps relieve gas pains, and has a mildly calming effect. Stevia helps you manage an out-of-control sweet tooth. Licorice soothes your stomach and digestive tract.
- **Ginkgo.** Used to improve memory, improve mental function, and increase circulation to your legs.
- **Milk thistle.** Made from the seeds, milk thistle tincture has a protective and rebuilding effect on your liver.
- **Valerian.** Probably the most popular sleeping and relaxing herb.
- **Kava.** Helps to relax your muscles and improve sleep.
- **American ginseng.** Counteracts stress and helps support adrenal function.
- **Goldenseal/barberry.** Goldenseal is popular for easing infections of the sinuses, bladder, intestines, and respiratory tract. Goldenseal is endangered in some states because of overharvesting. For this reason, I recommend using only 10 to 20 percent goldenseal along with 80 or 90 percent barberry root, Oregon grape root, or coptis root (a Chinese herb). All of these herbs have the same active principles as goldenseal.
- **Ginger.** This hot, spicy tincture helps to ease an upset stomach and promotes good digestion.
- **Dong quai.** One of the most popular herbs of all time, dong quai has a general strengthening effect on your energy and helps build healthy blood. For women, dong quai has a building effect on the uterus.
- **St. John's wort.** A popular herb for lifting your mood and helping to ease mild to moderate depression.

HERB TALK

Do fresh or dry herbs make a more potent tincture?

"Fresh herbs versus dry" is a debate that rages on among herbalists. Some herbalists contend that a number of herbs are more potent when tinctured fresh. This has been disproven by laboratory tests — most herbs make a more potent extract when extracted or tinctured *freshly dried.* This means that the plants are harvested at the peak of perfection (in full flower, in the fall for roots, and so on), and then carefully dried in the shade. If these herbs are tinctured within two to three weeks of drying and are kept away from heat and light, they can be called freshly dried.

You can find exceptions, however — sensitive herbs (chickweed, gotu kola, cleavers, and the roots of *Echinacea angustifolia*) are best when tinctured fresh, not freshly dried. For tincturing fresh, undried herbs, add the plant material to the solvent and blend well until you have only about 1/2 to1 inch of clear liquid over the settled solid material.

Making herbal cough syrup

Herbal cough syrups are sweet and thick and contain concentrates of herbs that help soothe inflamed tissues, calm your cough, help fight infection, and increase the elimination of thick, clogging mucus. You can buy a number of herbal cough syrups from your local herb store or pharmacy, but you can't find one that's as effective as the following classic Horehound Hack-Free Cough Syrup.

Horehound Hack-Free Cough Syrup

Ever had a hacking cough that kept you up at night? This classic horehound recipe is similar to ones that are available commercially. While I've tried several commercial syrups that contain horehound, sage, and wild cherry bark, I find that they don't work nearly as well as this formula — the commercial products just don't have enough horehound or sage in them to do the job.

Preparation time: *1 1/2 hours*

Yield: *2 1/2 cups*

(continued)

Besides adding hot to your pot and scorch to your borscht, cayenne is one of the most widely used herbal remedies. Its long list of uses can fill a small book.

- Cayenne powder arrests bleeding, decongests the lungs, and improves digestion.
- Sprinkle a pinch of cayenne powder on a cut to quickly stop the bleeding. Cayenne's antibacterial effect helps prevent infections.
- Cayenne, in tincture or powder form, invigorates the blood and facilitates the removal of toxins in the body and improves circulation.
- Make a paste by stirring a teaspoon of cayenne into a tablespoon of olive oil or other cooking oil. Rub a little on cold sores, sore joints, or sore muscles.
- Add 1/2 teaspoon of cayenne to 1/2 cup of vodka, let the mixture macerate (moisten) for a week or so, then filter and bottle. Rub this cayenne tincture on sore muscles or joints.

  A teaspoon of the cayenne tincture added to a cup of warm water makes a great gargle for sore throats and mucus congestion, but remember — it's hot.
- Use cayenne liberally when you have a cold or any sinus problems, such as hay fever, because it reduces immune reactivity, dries up mucus, opens nasal passages, and stimulates good immune function.
- Preparations of cayenne that contain a guaranteed amount of capsaicin (its primary active ingredient) block the pain response.
- You can apply a cayenne cream externally for shingles and the pain of arthritis.
- Make cayenne oil by soaking 1/2 cup of cayenne powder in 1 cup of oil for ten days to two weeks. Strain the oil and bottle for use. Rub the oil onto sore muscles and joints to increase circulation and reduce pain. Try using cayenne oil for stir-frying vegetables to crank up the temperature.
- Add a tablespoon of olive oil to make a liniment, which has long staying power on the skin. Cayenne liniment is great for rubbing on a sore back (when you're spending too much time bending over a hot stove).

TIP

Remember that cayenne causes burning and itching when it gets in the eyes. Although getting cayenne in the eyes isn't dangerous — people used to use it to help heal eye problems — it burns like blazes for ten or fifteen minutes. If you notice a burning sensation in your stomach after ingesting a strong dose of cayenne, don't worry — this is normal. If the burning makes you uncomfortable, reduce the dose next time.

Celery (Apium graveolens)

The seeds of this familiar vegetable are used medicinally to treat arthritis, mild nervousness, and water retention. Adding celery seeds to potato salad is a must, and they add a good flavor when making potato soups.

DOSAGE GUIDE

Celery seed tea has a slight cleansing and detoxifying effect on the body. Gently simmer a teaspoon of celery seeds in 1 cup of water for 15 minutes. Drink 1 cup daily.

Celery Seed Nerve Tonic

Celery seed is celebrated as a nerve restorative and relaxer. Take 1 teaspoon of this tonic in a little water or tea, twice daily as needed.

Preparation time: *5 minutes*

Yield: *1 1/2 cups*

2 tablespoons gotu kola tincture (tinctured fresh)

2 tablespoons wild oat seed tincture (tinctured fresh or in the milky stage)

1 cup vodka

3 tablespoons celery seed

1 Blend the tinctures and vodka together and add the celery seeds.

2 Store in a dark place for two weeks, shaking daily.

3 Strain and bottle for use.

Chives (Allium schoenoprasum)

Chives are in the same family as garlic and onions and are useful as an appetite stimulant. Sprinkle chives liberally on your food when you have a cold.

Chive Butter

You can use herbal butters as you would cream cheese — on crackers or bread, stuffed into celery sticks, or as a dip with carrots, cauliflower, jícama, or bell peppers. This one uses chives and parsley as its major ingredients.

Preparation time: *5 minutes*

Yield: *1/2 cup*

1 tablespoon finely chopped chives

1 tablespoon finely chopped parsley

1/2 teaspoon finely chopped rosemary

1/2 cup softened butter

1 Mash chives, parsley, and rosemary into the softened butter.

2 Cover and let stand in the refrigerator 2 hours before using.

Vary It! Substitute 1/2 cup of olive oil for the butter and/or add 2 cloves minced garlic for a healthy-heart alternative.

Cinnamon (Cinnamomum spp.)

Cinnamon powder is effective when taken in capsules for a wide variety of illnesses — colds, coughs, nausea, vomiting, diarrhea, and sluggish or delayed periods. But why take it in capsule form when cinnamon tastes so delicious? (You may remember chewing on delicious cinnamon oil-soaked toothpicks and cinnamon sticks — or having a warm cup of spicy apple cider as a kid.)

- Cinnamon toast or a cup of warming cinnamon tea tastes delicious and alleviates indigestion, nausea, or diarrhea.
- As a circulatory stimulant, use cinnamon for colds and chills.

- Try adding a few drops of the oil to a cup of almond oil or other vegetable oil as a liniment for use on sore muscles.
- Simmer 3 to 4 cinnamon sticks in 2 cups of water to make a tea.
- Add a teaspoon of the powder to a cup of hot water for a quick dose of this healing herb.

Medicated Cinnamon Sauce with Apples

This sauce is a good example of what Hippocrates said nearly two thousand years ago — "Let your food be your medicine, and your medicine your food." Try this recipe for colds, mucus congestion, an upset stomach, a sick feeling with nausea or vomiting, or for slowing down the flow of loose stools.

Preparation time: *$1^{1}/_{2}$ hours*

Yield: *3 cups*

5 cinnamon sticks or 2 tablespoons of cinnamon powder

4 cups of water

5 organic apples, washed, cored, and sliced into wedges

1 Simmer the cinnamon sticks or powder in a pan of water, covered, over low heat.

2 Turn off the heat and let the tea steep for a half-hour. Strain the tea and compost the herbs.

3 Add the apples.

4 Simmer over low heat until the slices are tender, in a covered pot, about 30 to 40 minutes. Let the mixture cool.

5 Place the mixture in a blender and blend until smooth. Pour into a canning jar and store in the refrigerator for later use. If you can't wait to sample the sauce, try a cup right away while it's still warm. Use the sauce on desserts or eat it plain with a little cow's milk, soy milk, rice milk, or almond milk.

Clove (*Syzygium aromaticum*)

I always keep a vial of clove oil in my medicine chest in case of a toothache. For a good pain reliever, rub a small amount of the oil on the tooth area (or while you're in the kitchen, place a whole clove on the spot). Cloves have antiseptic as well as pain-relieving properties — sprinkle clove powder on wounds to avoid infection.

A tea made from cloves settles an upset stomach and warms the body. Lightly simmer 3 to 5 cloves in 1 cup water for 15 minutes.

Coriander (*Coriandrum sativum*)

Coriander has a long history of use in herbalism for relieving indigestion. This herb has a cooling effect on the body and is a common ingredient in Indian and Mexican spice blends to aid the digestion of hot, spicy foods. Coriander is one of the best spices for preventing and assisting the body to get rid of intestinal worms. The tea works well for easing intestinal spasms.

The leaves of the coriander plant give you *cilantro* — a must for salsa. Try also adding coriander seeds to your salsas, to increase the healing properties (and flavor).

Plant coriander seeds in your garden, and soon you'll have an ample supply of delicious cilantro for salsa and salads.

To make a tea, put 2 teaspoons of coriander seed in 1 cup water and simmer gently for 15 minutes.

Coriander seeds are often included in recipes for the Indian spiced tea, chai — the "Cardamom" section in this chapter has a chai recipe.

Dill (*Anethum graveolens*)

Brew dill seeds (the same ones that flavor pickles) into a tea to relieve indigestion, heartburn, and flatulence and to stimulate the flow of breast milk. Dill seed tea is made by lightly simmering 2 teaspoons of seed in 1 cup of water for 15 minutes. Pickle cravings are famous in the early stages of pregnancy, but drinking dill seed tea after the child's birth helps promote mother's milk. Chew the seeds to freshen the breath.

Fennel (*Foeniculum vulgare*)

Try drinking a sweet-tasting tea made from fennel seeds to relieve gas, stomachache, and colic. This tea is safe for children, and they generally like the taste. Nursing mothers wishing to increase their supply of breast milk do well with fennel seed tea. The dose is 2 to 3 cups daily made by gently simmering 1 teaspoon of seeds in 1 cup water. You can also use the tea as a soothing eyewash.

Three Seed Tea

Three seed tea is a pleasant tasting, soothing tea that helps alleviate constipation, upset stomach, gas, and coughs and serves as a mild blood cleanser as well.

Preparation time: *20 minutes*

Yield: *3 cups*

1 teaspoon fennel seeds

1 teaspoon flaxseeds

1 teaspoon fenugreek seeds

3 cups water

1 Gently simmer fennel, flaxseeds, and fenugreek in the water for 15 minutes.

2 Strain and drink.

Fenugreek (*Trigonella foenum-graecum*)

Powdered fenugreek seeds are commonly used in Indian cooking to stimulate the appetite and improve digestion and assimilation. Studies show that fenugreek decreases serum cholesterol levels and helps stabilize blood sugar levels. The herb is also beneficial for lung congestion and facilitates the expulsion of mucus.

Drinking a tea or using the seeds in cooking on a regular basis helps prevent atherosclerosis — plaque formation in the arteries. To make a tea, simmer 2 tablespoons of fenugreek seeds in 2 cups water and drink 1 cup, 2 or 3 times daily.

A nice spice blend to keep by your stove and sprinkle on salads, fish, rice, and vegetable dishes includes fenugreek seeds combined in equal parts with fennel, cumin, and coriander seeds. You can purchase these herbs in powder form, but they taste especially great when you blend them up coarsely with a blender or grinder just before serving.

Doing some spring cleaning? Try a few cups of the Cleansing Polaritea, which contains fenugreek seeds.

Cleansing Polaritea

I learned about this tea at the Polarity Institute where I studied years ago. The tea helps remove gas from the system, gently stimulates liver function, and increases bile flow. I recommend it to many of my patients and keep the blend in ready-to-use packages. I always enjoy two cups of Cleansing Polaritea each day during a fast or following a liver flush. Try this tea and see whether it doesn't become one of your favorite blends. Drink 2 cups after a liver flush (see the following recipe) or anytime for promoting good digestion, good regularity, cleansing the liver and digestion, or improving fat digestion.

Preparation time: *40 minutes*

Yield: *4 cups*

1 tablespoon flaxseed

1 tablespoon fennel seed

1 tablespoon fenugreek seed

1 tablespoon burdock root

1/2 tablespoon licorice

4 cups water

1 heaping tablespoon peppermint

1 Add flaxseed, fennel seed, fenugreek seed, burdock root, and licorice to the water. Simmer, covered, for 15 minutes.

2 Turn off the heat and add the peppermint.

3 Let the brew steep for 15 minutes.

4 Strain, compost the herbs, and bottle for use.

Liver Flush

This liver flush is a great citrusy drink to help increase bile and cleanse and regulate your liver. I do a liver flush every spring and fall, as thousands of others do each year.

Preparation time: *10 minutes*

Yield: *1/2 cup*

Juice of 1 medium freshly squeezed grapefruit

Juice of 1/2 to 1 freshly squeezed lemon, depending on taste

1 tablespoon of fresh ginger

1 teaspoon to 1 tablespoon olive oil

2 cloves garlic, pressed

1 Put the grapefruit and lemon juices in a blender.

2 Make ginger juice by grating or slicing the fresh ginger and pressing the juice out in a garlic press.

3 Add the ginger juice, olive oil, and garlic. Blend until creamy.

Drink the liver flush first thing in the morning before breakfast — don't eat for at least an hour or two. Follow the flush with 2 cups of the Cleansing Polaritea.

Garlic (Allium sativum)

HERB TALK

People use garlic to prevent or treat an amazing array of ailments, including colds and flu, heart disease, high blood pressure, high cholesterol, cancer, worms, earache, and vaginal infections. This long-revered, well-proven herb is available in oil form (in capsules known as *perles*) and in powder form (in capsules), both guaranteed to not turn you into a social outcast.

My favorite way to use garlic, though, is in its fresh state — the more the better. Add a few crushed cloves of garlic to guacamole, a stir-fry, and sauces or roast whole bulbs as a delicious way to maintain good health. To deodorize your breath after eating fresh garlic, put a drop of peppermint oil on your tongue or chew fresh parsley. Or choose friends who like garlic as much as you do and add "garlic lover" to the top of your list of preferred traits when you choose a marriage partner.

Use garlic externally for infections. For ear infections, try dripping a few drops of the oil directly into the ear two or three times daily. Place freshly squeezed garlic on insect bites or stings. Swab athlete's foot with garlic oil, which also has antifungal properties.

Garlic Cough Syrup

The mucus-cutting, antibacterial, and expectorant action of the garlic often helps eliminate coughs. Take 1 teaspoon to 1 tablespoon at a time for coughs, colds, and mucus congestion. Kids like it, too. If they balk at taking a dose of the syrup, try adding several drops of orange or cinnamon oil to the blend.

Preparation time: *10 minutes*

Yield: *1 cup*

1 cup honey

5 to 10 cloves garlic

Juice from 1 medium lemon

1 tablespoon sage leaf

1 tablespoon lemon peel, fresh or dried

1. Pour the honey into a blender.
2. Add the garlic cloves, lemon juice, sage leaf, and lemon peel.
3. Blend on high speed until smooth.
4. Let the blend steep for several days away from heat.
5. Squeeze out the liquid. Filter and bottle it for use up to one week. If you plan on storing it longer, keep in the refrigerator.

Garlic, applied externally, can cause redness and skin irritation and even produce burns in people with sensitive skin.

Ginger (Zingiber officinalis)

Freshly grated ginger in sautéed vegetables or a tofu scramble imparts an exotic, spicy flavor to your food and improves your digestion as well. Ginger is a well-known remedy for motion sickness, used by sailors and astronauts alike, and is also used for tummy aches, nausea, and morning sickness. Make fresh ginger into a tea, take the powder in capsules, or even nibble on pieces of sliced candied ginger or pickled ginger.

For minor burns, immediately immerse the affected area in cool water or put ice on it for a few minutes. This often takes away most of the pain. Then put a fresh slice of ginger over the burned area and wrap with a bandage. Fresh ginger juice is even more effective for easing the pain of burns and to promote healing. Put three or four slices of fresh ginger into your garlic press and squeeze out the juice onto the pad of an adhesive bandage. Place the ginger juice pad over the burn.

Due to its antiviral properties, ginger is effective for relieving symptoms of colds and coughs. Drink 2 or 3 cups of the strong tea throughout the day. To make this tea effective for colds, make it spicy enough to induce sweating. This popular herb is also a circulatory stimulant, and drinking warm cups of the tea causes you to sweat and release toxins through your pores. I find that taking a warm bath with ginger tea added, at the onset of a cold, greatly speeds the healing process.

Candied Ginger

Candied ginger is a time-honored favorite for easing the unpleasant feeling of an upset stomach or nausea. Promote complete digestion or help reduce cold symptoms with a slice or two of candied ginger.

Preparation time: *45 minutes*

Yield: *1 cup*

5 tablespoons raw sugar

1 cup warm water

1 cup ginger, peeled and sliced into 1/4 inch slices

1. Dissolve the sugar in the water.
2. Place the sliced ginger into a small saucepan and add the sugar water.
3. Simmer until the slices are tender, about 40 minutes. Strain out the water.
4. Dry the slices in a food dehydrator (or in a glass pan in the oven turned to 200° until the slices are mostly dry to the touch, approximately 4 to 5 hours). Stop the drying process before the slices are fully dry, so that they are a little chewy.

Vary It! If you want to avoid using sugar, try simmering the slices in sweet pineapple juice or honey, instead. Be aware that slices cooked in honey are stickier than the sugar-cooked slices. To help dry out the outside of the slices, roll them in granulated raw sugar, cinnamon powder, or ginger powder.

Horseradish (*Armoracia rusticans*)

Some aficionados say that they have a religious experience after a big taste of horseradish. Known as *wasabi* in Japan, this green paste made with dried horseradish is the supreme kitchen remedy for plugged sinuses. The spicy preparation has strong antibacterial properties and helps prevent or subdue a sinus or other upper respiratory tract infection. Holding 1/2 to 1 teaspoon of this hot and spicy remedy in your mouth for a few seconds makes breathing easier. Horseradish is good for colds, flu, and respiratory infections. Cook with horseradish by adding it to soups and salad dressings and using it as a condiment. You can buy horseradish fresh in most markets, in jars as prepared horseradish, or in packets in powdered form.

Kudzu (*Pueraria lobata*)

This starchy root is an ancient Chinese medicine for colds and for its health-strengthening properties. You can buy the powder in grocery stores and natural food stores. Try substituting kudzu powder for flour to thicken sauces, stews, pudding, and gravy and add the healing benefits of this herb to your meals. The root powder may help you recover from an illness when used regularly as a tonic in your cooking.

- Add a teaspoon of the kudzu powder to a cup of hot water to make a drink to ease diarrhea and an upset stomach.
- Modern research shows that kudzu is one of nature's highest sources of *phytoestrogens,* mild plant estrogens that help create and restore hormone balance in your body. These natural, estrogen-like compounds may help prevent cancer and heart disease when used regularly.
- If you have to drive after dinner and are tempted to have that second glass of wine, try a cup of kudzu instead. Modern science shows the herb helps ease the craving for alcohol. And for those times when you may have had too much to drink the night before, try a cup or two of kudzu tea to help ease your hangover.

  For an energizing tea, stir 1 teaspoon kudzu root into 1 cup cool water. Add 1/2 teaspoon fresh grated ginger root and a few drops of tamari. Stir while heating. Drink 1 cup daily.

Lemon (*Citrus limon*)

For colds, fever, and sore throats, squeeze the juice of a lemon into 2 cups of warm water, add a little honey to taste, and sip it throughout the day. Use this tart-tasting remedy for liver congestion and obesity. Lemon peel is high in *flavonoids,* which benefit your blood vessels.

Marjoram (Origanum majorana)

This popular aromatic spice is soothing to the digestion and is beneficial for colds, fever, headache, and menstrual cramps. Use marjoram tea for coughs and sinus infections as a steam inhalant — place a towel over a bowl of the hot, steamy tea.

To make a tea, steep 2 tablespoons of the dried herb in 2 cups water, and drink 1 cup, 2 to 3 times daily.

Mustard (Sinapis alba)

Mustard seeds are traditionally used externally in the form of a plaster to stimulate circulation and treat rheumatism, sprains, and bronchitis. To make a plaster, add 1 tablespoon mustard powder to 4 tablespoons flour, and add sufficient water to make a paste. Place the paste on the affected area for 15 to 30 minutes, taking care not to blister your skin.

Watch out when using the mustard plaster. It can cause deep, slow-healing burns when left on too long. Don't use the plaster if you may fall asleep and closely supervise children when they use it.

To break up lung congestion, prepare a mustard foot bath by adding 1/2 cup mustard powder to 1 gallon of hot water and soaking your feet for 15 to 30 minutes.

Black mustard seeds (the Latin name is *Brassica nigra*) are commonly used in Indian cooking and have healing properties similar to the yellow ones. The seeds promote strong and complete digestion when used in cooking.

Nutmeg (Myristica fragrans)

Nutmeg is a delightfully aromatic herb that's used as a digestive remedy for indigestion, nausea, and diarrhea. Nutmeg powder is also commonly sprinkled on the tops of warm drinks and used in baking.

Onion (Allium cepa)

Onions, like garlic, have antiviral and blood-sugar balancing properties, as well as asthma prevention abilities. Eating onions regularly is a good general disease-preventive measure. When you have a cold, increase your intake of onions with a nice, warming onion soup or by liberally sprinkling onion powder or flakes on your food. If you're concerned about having onion breath, chew some fresh parsley or put a drop of peppermint oil on your tongue after you eat onions.

Onion Cough Poultice

For heavy chest congestion, coughs, or bronchitis, an onion poultice provides relief. Even young children happily submit to one as long as you read them a story while the poultice is doing its job.

Preparation time: *15 minutes*

Yield: *1 poultice*

2 tablespoons olive oil

1 large onion, coarsely chopped

3 tablespoons flaxseed

1 Heat the olive oil in a frying pan over medium heat.

2 Add the chopped onion and the flaxseed.

3 Cook until the onions are translucent, about 10 minutes.

4 Wrap the mixture in cheesecloth and apply very warm (but not too hot) to the chest.

5 Cover the cloth with a hot water bottle and a towel. Leave on for a half-hour.

Parsley (Petroselinum crispum)

Eating fresh parsley stimulates the appetite and encourages optimum digestion. The bitter and slightly spicy leaves are high in iron and Vitamin C content, helping to build the blood and protect the bones.

DOSAGE GUIDE

Fresh parsley tea helps rid the body of uric acid and is therefore beneficial for arthritis and gout. The herb is a good diuretic and is useful for relieving water retention. It has blood-moving properties and was traditionally used for suppressed menstruation. To make a tea, steep 2 or 3 tablespoons in 1 or 2 cups of boiled water to taste.

Parsley on the plate — the culinary holdover

Parsley is a holdover from the days when people actually ate herbs with meals for their health-promoting benefits. I often watch as friends and acquaintances push their parsley aside during restaurant meals. I'm only too happy to eat their parsley as well as my own, but as a health educator, I can't help but remind them that the parsley is on the plate for a reason. Your digestion often suffers and is unable to do its job optimally because your digestive tract was designed to absorb lots of wild bitter greens (like parsley) and roots along with richer foods. Today, people don't eat nearly as many bitter greens as their ancestors did.

Pepper, black (*Piper nigrum*)

Black pepper is one of the few healing spices found in American cuisine. Originally from India, black pepper is a favorite spice and healing herb all over the world. Black pepper is sometimes included as an ingredient in the spicy Indian drink chai (see the recipe in the section "Cardamom," earlier in this chapter). Black pepper increases the flow of hydrochloric acid and digestive enzymes, making digestion, especially of protein foods, more complete.

Rosemary (*Rosmarinus officinalis*)

Commonly found in spice racks, this herb is easy to grow and is valuable for both culinary and medicinal purposes. Rosemary has a beneficial effect on the circulatory and nervous systems and is used to alleviate headaches, aid indigestion, and increase energy. Rosemary is a fantastic antioxidant, helping to protect your cells and tissues from free radical damage. Some researchers say that regular use of antioxidants helps slow the aging process. Rosemary extracts are also added to oils and commercially processed foods to help prevent rancidity.

REMEMBER

Try adding a sprig or two of dried rosemary to your cooking oils to help extend their shelf life, add a refreshing aroma, and give an interesting flavor to salads and stir-fried vegetables.

DOSAGE GUIDE

Make a tea of rosemary by steeping 2 tablespoons of the leaves in 2 cups water for 15 minutes. Use the tea as a cleansing rinse for your hair and scalp after shampooing.

Sage (Salvia officinalis)

When slaving over a hot stove has you sweating and the aroma you smell is more than the spices, try a dash of sage leaf powder under your arms, not on the stew. Sage has great drying and deodorizing properties and is used in many commercial underarm deodorant products from Europe. A cup or two of a strong infusion, taken daily (internally), helps reduce body odor, especially when you use it regularly. Soak a cloth with a little tea and wipe under the arms while you're at it. You can also use sage tea, made by steeping a teaspoon of the herb in boiled water for ten minutes, as a wash for gum problems and mouth sores, as a gargle for sore throats and laryngitis, and as a drink that helps dry up mother's milk.

Thyme (Thymus vulgaris)

HERB TALK

Thyme, a favorite kitchen spice is also a famous respiratory remedy. The herb extract is a common ingredient in cough syrups and helps relieve spasms and clear congestion in the bronchial area. Thyme contains a strong antibacterial constituent, known as *thymol,* commonly found in mouthwashes, lozenges, and liniments.

Thyme Home Cleaner and Deodorizer

Try making this natural antibacterial and deodorizing spray. It has mild antibacterial effects and a refreshing, herbal scent.

Preparation time: *5 minutes*

Yield: *3 ounces*

1 ounce thyme tincture

2 ounces water

30 drops essential oils (try thyme, rosemary, lemon, or lavender, or a blend)

1. Add the thyme tincture to the water and shake well.
2. Add the essential oils and shake again.
3. Pour the mixture into a small spray bottle.

Turmeric (*Curcuma longa*)

The bright golden color you see in powders and curried vegetable dishes comes from the use of the popular East Indian herb, turmeric. Its yellow pigment, known as *curcumin,* not only causes strong anti-inflammatory activity — making it useful for arthritis, tendinitis, and swelling — but makes a fabulous Easter egg dye as well.

Turmeric lends itself particularly well to healing dishes like stir-fried vegetables, tofu scrambles, and Chinese noodle soups. Sprinkle the powder onto foods or pack it into empty gelatin capsules and take it as a supplement. Whole fresh roots are available from stores for cooking. You can also slice and simmer the roots to make a tea. Use one teaspoon per cup and simmer for 15 to 20 minutes. For therapeutic doses, turmeric is available as a standardized extract — you can find it in health food stores.

Curry Cure

Although a lot of people think that curry powder comes from a curry plant, it doesn't — the powder is actually an enticing blend of spices used in cooking vegetables, grains, and legumes. You can buy these herbs powdered and combine them to make a simple curry powder and then add the mixture when making curries. Start with 1 to 2 tablespoons of the mixture and then adjust according to your individual taste.

Preparation time: *5 minutes*

Yield: *1/2 cup*

7 teaspoons turmeric powder

5 teaspoons cumin powder

3 1/2 teaspoons fenugreek powder

3 teaspoons coriander powder

1 teaspoon ginger powder

1 teaspoon cinnamon powder

1/2 teaspoon mustard powder

1/4 teaspoon cayenne powder

1/2 teaspoon clove powder

1 Combine all ingredients and stir them together.

2 Store in a spice jar and use as needed.

A Kitchen Prescriber

In Table 7-1, you can look up common symptoms or conditions and pick out a common kitchen herbal remedy to try. This table is the key to your kitchen herbal first aid kit.

Table 7-1 Kitchen Cures for Common Ailments

Ailment	*Kitchen Remedy*
Acne, pimples	Basil
Arthritis	Cayenne, bay, celery seed, cinnamon
Bleeding	Cayenne
Breast milk (to promote)	Anise, fennel
Breath freshener	Anise, basil, cardamom, cinnamon, dill, fennel
Burn	Ginger
Cold	Anise, cinnamon, garlic, ginger, horseradish, kudzu, lemon juice, marjoram
Constipation	Fennel seed
Cough	Anise, cinnamon, fennel, garlic, ginger, marjoram, onion, thyme
Cut	Basil
Dandruff	Bay leaf
Deodorant	Sage
Diarrhea	Cinnamon, kudzu, nutmeg
Gas	Anise, caraway, cardamom, fennel
Hay fever	Cayenne
Headache	Basil, bay, marjoram, rosemary
Indigestion	Basil, caraway, cardamom, cinnamon, coriander, dill, nutmeg, rosemary
Nausea	Basil, cardamom, cinnamon, ginger, nutmeg
Runny nose	Cayenne, sage
Shingles	Cayenne
Sinus problems	Horseradish
Sore joints, rheumatism	Bay, cayenne, cinnamon, mustard
Toothache	Clove
Upset stomach	Cardamom, cinnamon, cloves, fennel, ginger, kudzu

Part III

The Part of Tens

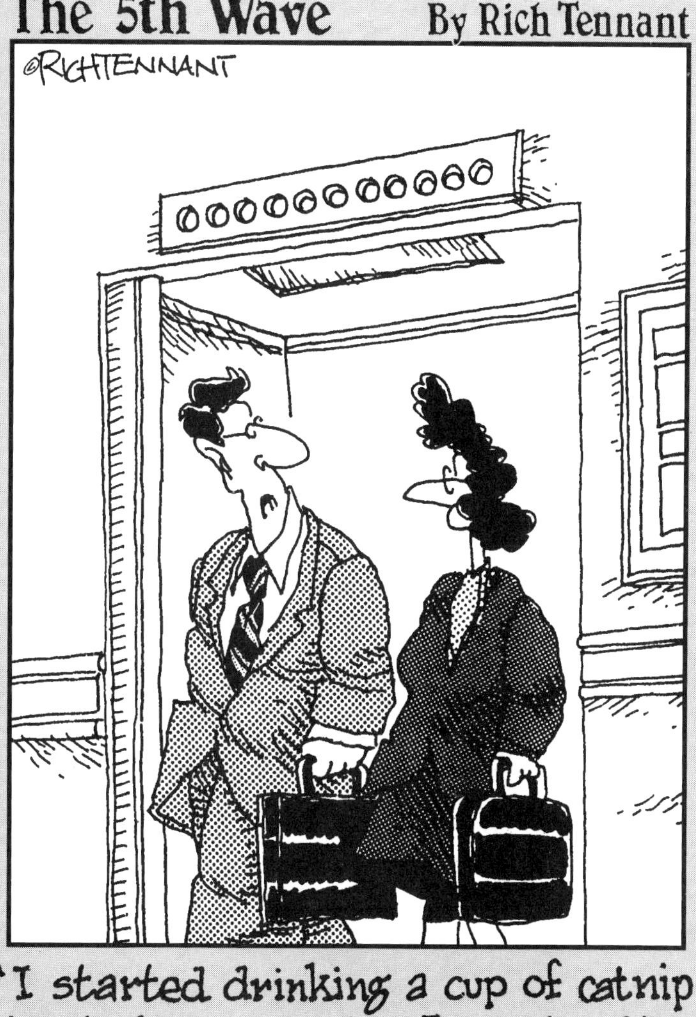
The 5th Wave
By Rich Tennant
©RICHTENNANT

"I started drinking a cup of catnip tea to help me relax. It works fine, except I keep wanting to curl up on someone's lap and take a nap."

In this part . . .

In this part, I sort out the many health benefits you can reap by using herbs on a regular basis. I also tell you how to use the top ten herbs that will keep you feeling great into your 90s. Finally, in this part, you can find recipes for herbal tea blends that are so delicious, you may even decide to give up coffee!

Chapter 8

Ten Reasons to Use Herbs Every Day

In This Chapter

- Creating more energy, greater health, and better mental clarity
- Preventing disease and promoting longevity
- Saving money and protecting the environment
- Empowering yourself and taking responsibility for your health

Taking herbs every day can help your body in so many ways — from building a stronger immune system to giving you more energy, from heightening your senses to helping you think more clearly. In this chapter, I share my ten best reasons for taking herbs.

Better Digestion

Many herbalists believe that your digestion is one of the most important health assets you have. Health and vitality start in the digestive area in the belly, the place the ancients called the *hara*. Your digestion supports your energy, strength, and muscle tone; helps you think clearly; and detoxifies your tissues. When your digestive fires are weak, you can't completely digest your food — residues end up circulating in your blood and irritating your immune system, potentially leading to symptoms of allergies, arthritis, and other degenerative diseases.

Support your digestion with the following herbs and helpful hints:

- Take bitters or *bitter tonics* — bitter-tasting herbs that can stimulate production of all your digestive enzymes — before meals, daily. My favorite bitter herbs are gentian root, centaury herb, angelica root, orange peel, and wormwood tea.

Try taking a teaspoon of a ready-made bitter tonic, mixed in a little water, before meals. Use the bitters for a few months to get full benefits. You may be surprised at how energized you feel with this simple, traditional way of increasing your body's natural storehouse of energy.

- Use warming herbs during the winter or anytime that you feel chilly and can't digest well. Ginger and a little red ginseng are a great combination. You can find several commercial products containing the Chinese herbs atractylodes and astragalus, which are also beneficial for digestion. Use them daily with meals.
- Try the following healthy habits:
  - Relax when you eat. Leave unpleasant talk and thoughts for later — don't worry, they'll still be there when you want to find them again! Focus instead on pleasant and relaxing companions and conversation.
  - Don't eat too fast — chew each bite thoroughly.
  - Try to eat meals that are tasty, zesty, colorful, and simple.
  - Don't forget to eat parsley, a bitter stimulant to get your digestion going before the meal.
  - Use as little oil in cooking as possible. According to the latest studies, cooked oil is the single most common cause of heart disease — *and* it coats your food and slows down digestion. If you do cook with oil, use it sparingly and use olive oil only. We *do* need a variety of oils in our diet for optimum health, but the best way to get them is through eating the whole foods that contain the oils naturally, like seeds, nuts, beans, and avocados.

A Stronger Immune System

If you have more than two or three colds or bouts with the flu every year, or if you're prone to getting other kinds of infections like vaginal yeast infections or bladder infections, you can strengthen your immune system with *immune tonics.* Maintaining a healthy immune system helps you avoid the common cold and other infections, as well as cancer and other degenerative diseases.

I recommend using an herbal blend with two or more reliable immune boosters like astragalus, ligustrum, codonopsis, reishi, shiitake, nettle herb, or maitake. You can find these herbal tonics in capsules or tablets, by themselves or in combinations. (See the *Herb Guide* in the green pages near the back of this book for the proper doses.) Try cooking with herbs by making a strong tea, then adding grains, beans, a little meat (if you choose), and lots of vegetables.

Look for products that contain extracts, not just herb powders, because herb powders are much weaker. Take 2 to 3 of the tablets or capsules, or $^{1}/_{2}$ to 1 teaspoon of a liquid tincture in a little water, 2 to 3 times daily.

Reduced Risk of Heart Disease and Cancer

Heart disease is still the leading cause of death in men and women in nearly all developed countries. Right behind heart disease is cancer. One out of three North Americans eventually develops some form of cancer in their lifetimes.

The following are heart- and cardiovascular-protective herbs, along with herbs to boost your immune system (which can help you avoid cancer in the first place).

- Use heart protectors like garlic and turmeric in your daily diet, or at least several times a week.
- Take herbs that strengthen your heart (like hawthorn, ginkgo, and motherwort) every day for years at a time. Heart tonics increase circulation and help increase blood flow to your heart and tissues.
- Immune-boosters that can help your body avoid the formation of cancer cells and can help remove them from your body include astragalus, ligustrum, and the immune-boosting mushrooms shiitake, reishi, and maitake. Use these protectants daily in extract form in capsules and tablets, or as a tea, daily or at least several months of the year.

More Energy

Nearly everyone wants more energy. I teach classes on human energy and energy management, and I often ask members of the audience, "How many of you have all the energy you would like to have to accomplish everything you want in life?" Guess what — out of one hundred people, maybe one or two people raise their hands, even in a college audience of 18-year-olds!

You probably already use herbal energy products — coffee, tea, and the kola nut — that provide the caffeine boost in many cola drinks. But caffeine doesn't actually give you energy; in fact, it robs your system of it. When you use caffeine on a regular basis, it can disrupt your sleep and make you feel nervous and jumpy.

Here are my suggestions for herbal products that can give you deeper, more lasting energy:

- **Bitter tonics.** Much of your daily energy comes from your digestion. When you have a powerful digestive system, you're able to access the energy that's inherent in the food you eat, locked up in the form of sugars, carbohydrates, proteins, fats, enzymes, and other nutrients. See the section "Better Digestion" (earlier in this chapter) for more details. You can find many ready-made products on store shelves or make your own.
- **Natural herbal energy boosters without caffeine.** Energy herbs are effective in maximizing your energy potential by helping your body use energy more efficiently. I see great results in patients who use one of the energy-promoting ginseng herbs — American ginseng, red Chinese or Korean ginseng (if you're over 40), and eleuthero (Siberian ginseng), which is especially good when you're under stress.

  Don't use red ginseng if you're under 30, if you currently have high blood pressure, or if you have an active infection.
- **Natural relaxers.** Holding chronic tension in your body is a sure way to waste energy. My favorite muscle-relaxing herb is kava, and it doesn't make you feel drowsy. California poppy extract and calming teas (like linden, chamomile, and passion flower) also help you relax, which saves the energy your body has to use to keep your muscles tight.

  Help your body create more energy by practicing conscious and deep breathing down to your diaphragm into your belly every day. You can also release muscle tension and save energy by stretching or practicing yoga each day. Finally, avoid sugar like the plague — it actually robs your body of deep energy — stick to whole fresh fruit to satisfy your sweet tooth.

Enlivened Senses

Millions of city-dwellers live in a grey, concrete and asphalt world, devoid of colors, smells, or feelings. To counteract this environment, use herbal scents — rosemary, peppermint, cinnamon, ginger, lavender, orange flower, gardenia, and roses — to enrich your imagination, sensuality, sexuality, and creativity. Use the essential oils of these aromatic herbs daily by rubbing them, smelling them, and brewing them (see Chapter 3).

Even if you don't have a backyard garden, you can grow a number of scented plants in pots in your apartment or house. Your windowsill is a good place for lavender, rosemary, lemon balm, and miniature roses to flourish. If you do have a yard, try planting a scented garden for a nightly stroll (see Chapter 5). My wife and I have created a scented garden where our back lawn used to be — we planted apricot, rose, cinnamon, nutmeg, and coconut geraniums. We love to walk through our garden in the evening and smell lavender, thyme, lemon flower, lemon-scented eucalyptus, and all the other scented plants. I always feel refreshed and enlivened after my walk. Our small garden is truly heaven-scent.

Better Mental Clarity

I don't think anyone would argue that to be successful in the modern world, a good memory is a valuable asset. In today's information age of computers and high-tech industries, you need good mental clarity and memory, because jobs dealing with information are essentially mental and often highly complex. A good memory also helps you develop business and personal relationships by keeping names and other personal information accessible to you.

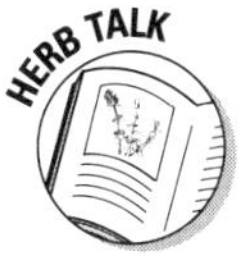

While you can never remember as much or think as quickly as the fastest high-capacity computers, daily use of herbs can help you maintain excellent memory and clarity. My favorite memory and mental clarity herbs include ginkgo (of course), gotu kola, rosemary, and lavender. These herbs work by increasing circulation, oxygen, sugar, and nutrients to the brain and by enhancing neurotransmitter activity and production, helping it to work more efficiently. (*Neurotransmitters* are the vital chemical messengers that make your brain and nervous system work.)

Control of Your Own Health Care

Herbal medicine is the people's medicine. Although you can buy sophisticated capsules and tablets that are standardized and processed to be extra potent, such as standardized ginkgo, you can also grow peppermint in an indoor pot and use it to make peppermint tea. Of course, when you grow your own, the quality and amount of what you're taking is unregulated — and this sometimes frightens people. I'm not sure that this is a bad thing, however. When medicine is completely controlled and regulated under a strict law the way pharmaceutical drugs are, you have less choice about your health care. And unregulated herbs right from your garden can be far, far safer than the most strictly regulated pharmaceutical drugs lined up in gleaming white bottles. In many cases, the herbs are just as effective.

Here's my suggestion for taking control of your own health care. The next time you have a cold or flu, resolve to handle it the herbal way:

- Take lots of echinacea, osha, peppermint, and elder flower as teas, as tinctures, or in powdered extract form in tablets and capsules.
- Try to curtail your normal activities and get as much rest as possible. By rest, I mean relaxing and allowing yourself to be pampered for a few days. Drink at least four cups of one of the herb teas listed above, as well as four to five glasses of water to which a few drops of lemon have been added.
- Don't eat too many heavy, greasy foods. Stay away from foods made from refined sugars — eat mainly fresh fruits, vegetables, and whole grains.
- Allow yourself to be nurtured by friends and family. You deserve it! (Don't forget that you always have an opportunity to pay your friends and family members back — sooner or later they will get sick, too.)
- Take a few days off of work — it will still be there when you get back.

Fewer Dangerous Drugs In Your System

A recent overview of 39 studies by researchers at the University of Toronto showed that pharmaceutical drugs are between the fourth and sixth leading cause of death in the United States, even when used as directed. The researchers cited 106,000 deaths in U.S. hospitals in 1994 as due to bad drug reactions. By using herbs, you can keep these drugs out of your body. What people tend to forget is that herbs have been around for several thousand years, and drugs have existed for only a few, or at most for sixty or seventy years. Your ancestors used herbs for hundreds of generations. Herbs can be powerful medicines.

However, no herbalist can tell you that herbs are completely safe under every condition. Yet in my thirty years of working with herbs nearly every day, I've seen very few problems. Poison control centers in the United States and Europe have few reports filed that involve the therapeutic use of herbs, despite their rapidly-growing popularity. Most poisonings from plants come from ornamental plants and houseplants.

To ensure your own safe use of herbs, remember the following:

- Review any side effects or safety tips about an herb before you start using it.
- Start with one-half of the recommended therapeutic dose for a few days (to check for individual sensitivity) and then increase to a full dose.

- If you experience any unpleasant symptoms after starting on an herb or herb formula, consult with your herbalist or supplement specialist in the herb shop where you bought the product. If necessary, call or write the manufacturer, because they're accountable for the purity and quality of the product.
- If a product states that it's "not for long-term use," limit your intake of the product for only a week or two, unless you're under the guidance of a qualified herbalist.

More Money

Herbs are many times more cost-effective than drugs or modern medical intervention, especially when you remember how effective herbs are for prevention. When you use immune tonics, stress-relieving herbs, digestive herbs, and calming herbs every day, you feel better and get sick less often. That's the best way to save money, because you're more productive and spend less money on drugs and visits to the doctor.

In my experience, well-formulated herbal products are a good value, providing what is arguably the best health insurance you can buy. Herbs work with your body's natural healing process and don't place excessive stress on your vital resources. With herbs you can often ease your symptoms and create a higher state of health in the process.

For getting rid of symptoms and easing common ailments, here are more ways to save money with herbal medicine.

- Grow your own herbs and harvest local weeds (like yellow dock) and local wild plants (like elder flower). Make your own teas, tinctures, and extracts and save big money. When you have more time than money, making your own products is the most cost-effective way to use herbs.
- If you don't have the time or confidence to grow and harvest your own herbs, buy bulk herbs — this way, you can still make your own teas and extracts. Teas are always the cheapest way to get a therapeutic dose of herbs because you do the work of making the teas yourself. On the other hand, you pay for the equipment and labor that a manufacturer uses to process extracts in tablets, capsules, or liquids. Remember that the manufacturer also has to pay for advertising and distribution of their products and they pass these costs on to you.
- When you're on a budget, avoid the most famous brand names (unless they also have a good price), but *do* buy by brand. Do your research by talking to your supplement salesperson, reading articles, and calling manufacturers to ask them details about their products. Buy your extract from a reputable company, but not necessarily from the one

that does the most advertising. Ask your herbalist or the buyer at your local herb shop whether they can recommend a good company that doesn't charge too much.

You actually get a better deal if you don't buy simply on price. When you buy on price alone, skipping from brand to brand to find the lowest price, you likely get what you pay for. Find a few quality brands that don't do an excessive amount of advertising and stick with them. I have been taking just a few brands for a number of years because I've been to their plants and am satisfied that they pay attention to quality.

- Choose a few herbs or herbal products, such as a digestive tonic that meets your needs, and stick with them. Take the herbs daily, at least twice a day, and take them faithfully. Don't skip around to different herbs erratically. I see remarkable results with people who choose a good formula (or two or three) and take it every day. Generally, you need to take the herbs for one to three months before you begin to see the full benefits.

A Sustainable Environment

Herbal medicine doesn't just help your body, it also helps the planet, animals and insects, trees and plants — in fact, all life on earth. Here are some specific environmental benefits you can feel good about.

- Herb cultivation, processing, and product manufacture are sustainable processes that support the health of the natural environment.
- Growing medicinal herbs, shrubs, and trees adds oxygen to the air and removes and helps break down waste products from the environment.
- Herbal medicine is life-affirming and seeks to understand the causes of disease and, more important, how to maintain a healthy mind, body, and spirit.
- Herbs often smell good and taste good; the flavors and aromas enhance the enjoyment and digestion of food.
- Your connection with healing plants is ancient. Through studying, growing, and taking herbs, you draw from a deep well of wisdom and healing power.

Chapter 9

Ten Top Power Herbs

In This Chapter

- Using time-honored herbs to keep you feeling young, healthy, and active
- Discovering herbs that wake you up and ones that help you calm down and sleep
- Finding out which herbs enhance communication and lift depression
- Using herbs daily to help prevent illness and promote longevity

From ancient pharaohs to today's film stars, humans have long depended on the power of healing herbs. Even the cast of *Star Trek: The Next Generation* used the immune-enhancing herb echinacea when colds and flu threatened to slow down the show's production schedule to below Warp 1.

In this chapter, I list the top ten power herbs to stock in your medicine chest. You can put the top ten of nature's time-tested medicines to work for you — keeping colds at bay, sharpening your memory, and increasing your energy. The herbs in this chapter can help you accomplish more during the day, feel more relaxed, and get a great night's sleep. The instructions you need to put them to work are all here!

Echinacea — Immune Support

Echinacea can stimulate the immune system, helping to quickly eliminate infections of all kinds. Scientific studies show that volunteers using echinacea overcome the unpleasant symptoms of colds and flu faster than people in a placebo group. Echinacea is a top-selling herb in the U.S. and Europe and has been featured on the evening news of major networks and in many other mainstream news stories. The taste is tingly and exotic; the benefits are hard to beat — you may find that echinacea becomes your constant winter companion. Echinacea liquid products also come in flavors and some are sweetened.

DOSAGE GUIDE

The liquid extract (also called a *tincture)* is often recommended by herbalists. Take $^1/_2$ to $^3/_4$ of a teaspoon (3 to 4 droppersful) of the liquid in a little water, 3 to 4 times daily, away from meals. It is best to take it at the first signs of a cold or flu, and not stop taking it for five to ten days to avoid getting sick entirely. Echinacea also speeds up elimination of wastes, so it doesn't suppress symptoms the way over-the-counter aspirin and decongestants can.

Discovering echinacea

As he traveled across Sioux country in the mid-19th century, a German doctor noticed that tribe members chewed on the root of a small prairie plant (the purple coneflower) when they had a cough or cold. As time went by, he discovered that the plant seemed to have almost miraculous healing powers — it caused respiratory and other infections to disappear quickly and never return. He began making his own proprietary medicine and was so excited about it he sent some off to prominent medical doctors in Cincinnati. At first they weren't impressed, yet twenty years later, it became the top-selling medicine in the U.S. It remained an official drug in the *United States Pharmacopeia* until the late 1930s.

Garlic — The Heart Protector

In the past, garlic protected people from vampires and werewolves. Today, however, garlic is known as a protector of another sort — against heart attack and stroke. Garlic epitomizes the modern quandary for regulatory agencies like the U.S. Food and Drug Administration (FDA) — is it a food or is it a medicine? The modern doctor can now say, "Eat two pieces of garlic bread and call me in the morning." If the FDA has its way, soon all garlic sold in stores will carry a label reading, "Take only as directed."

Modern science has thoroughly explored the chemistry and pharmacology of garlic and declares it a valuable aid to keep the heart and blood vessels healthy into old age. It can help keep the blood pressure in the normal range — even if you're late to work and stuck in rush hour traffic — and can lower cholesterol. Because heart disease and stroke are still the leading causes of death in developed countries, the daily use of garlic seems like a must. But not everybody likes the pungent flavor in their sauces and stir-fry, so products are available that have great benefits and a lot less of the smell.

Take 2 capsules or tablets of a good odor-controlled garlic, morning and night, with meals for full benefit. Odor-controlled capsules or tablets have a slight smell of garlic, but do not usually leave a garlic odor on your breath. Garlic is also known as the "poor-person's antibiotic." It lives up to its name to help the body fend off respiratory infections like bronchitis, pneumonia, colds, flu, and other infections of the urinary tract and digestive tract. Use the capsules or tablets 2 or 3 at a time, several times daily, along with echinacea.

Better to stay home?

Garlic is now and has been an important medicine in the East and West for over 5,000 years. The ancient Egyptian royalty were said to have given garlic to the workers building the pyramids to keep them from getting sick so that they could stay on the job. This may be less effective in our modern office environment.

Ginger — The Root of Good Digestion

If you've ever had a queasy feeling, ginger can help. Several clinical studies have favorably compared ginger extract with Dramamine and other over-the-counter preparations for easing nausea and stomach ailments. If traveling by boat, car, or plane makes your stomach jumpy, ginger is just the thing — it's quite soothing to the stomach and helps ease any digestive upset.

An herb of fame and fable in both ancient Egypt and China, its modern reputation is supported by science that says its digestive worth lies in its rich oils that warm and stimulate stomach and intestinal juices, encouraging complete digestion from top to bottom. Ginger is great for a congested liver, with notable protective and stimulating properties. For kids and grown-ups alike, ginger tea with a little lemon and honey is the perfect "tum-ease." Try adding 1/2 cup of ginger tea to 1 cup of plain sparkling water to make your own tummy-settling ginger ale. A cup after meals will help settle things down and increase the digestive fires, leading to more complete digestion, assimilation, and elimination. A few bites of either pickled or candied ginger work well, too.

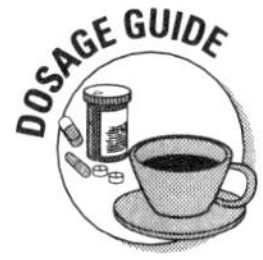

Ginger extract is available in liquid form, as well as in powder form made into capsules and tablets. Take 1 or 2 tablets or capsules, several times daily, around mealtimes. One-half teaspoon of the liquid extract in a little hot water makes an instant, quick-acting ginger tea anytime it's needed. A teaspoon in 1 cup of sparkling water makes an instant ginger ale, without the sugar.

Ginkgo — Super Brain Food

If you feel a major brain strain from work and all of the myriad of details you have to take care of, an extract of the leaves of the ancient ginkgo tree can help. Known for its healing powers for over 3,000 years, recent research has catapulted this herb to superstar status worldwide, from Macao to Moscow. A concentrated extract of the leaves is the top-selling pharmaceutical in Europe and is prescribed by doctors in both Europe and increasingly in the U.S.

Ginkgo is well documented to increase circulation to the brain, improve memory and alertness, and protect the heart. Take two capsules or tablets containing a standardized extract in the morning around breakfast time and one in the evening with dinner.

You should notice a distinct difference within one to two weeks — if you just remember to take it!

Ginseng — The Energy Herb

Everyone wants more energy. After all, who doesn't want to be able to work hard all day, accomplish more, and still have the energy for your evenings and weekends? For increasing energy and protecting human health, ginseng has taken on a healing and protective aura of magical proportions — it has been in use for over 5,000 years!

- In China, ginseng is a cultural treasure and used by the young and old alike.
- The official botanical name *panax* means "panacea."
- Today ginseng is a worldwide phenomenon. It is taken daily by millions and — as humans tend to do — overused by thousands (see dosage guides later in this list).
- Sales are skyrocketing in the U.S., and it is now one of the top-selling herbs sold in natural food stores, drugstores, and supermarkets everywhere. TV host Larry King wants us to believe he can't get through his monster week without it.
- Look for red Korean or red Chinese ginseng to warm up your hormones and get your juices flowing again! Red ginsengs support energy, sex drive, and powerful digestion.

  Take standardized extracts in capsule or tablet form, 1 in the morning and 1 each evening, preferably before meals. Use it on and off for several weeks or months as needed.
- If you "do" stress, whether by choice or by circumstance, American ginseng products can help protect and soothe jangled nerves and regulate hormones. This is the ginseng for cooling out and promoting good sleep and rejuvenation. American ginseng is fine for any age, unlike red ginsengs that should only be used by people over 40 or so.

  Use the powdered extract in capsules or tablet form, 2 to 3 in the morning and 1 to 2 in the evening, around mealtimes. Use it continuously for three to nine months for full effect.

- Eleuthero, or Siberian ginseng, is from a different plant group in the ginseng botanical family than American, Korean, or Chinese ginseng. Eleuthero is used to help you adapt to stress of any kind and to help you maintain balance in all your activities. This herb helps you go the distance, whether you run, play tennis, or engage in any sports activities. It's also great for travelers and for reducing the unpleasant side effects of jet lag.

  Take eleuthero continuously for three to nine months (or longer). Its effects get better as time goes on. Use 2 to 3 capsules or tablets containing an extract, morning and evening, around mealtimes.

All ginsengs have an enjoyable bittersweet taste and are world-renowned as rejuvenating teas. Try a cup of ginseng tea with a little stevia or licorice (or any of the sweet herbs) instead of that cup of cappuccino to get going in the morning. It doesn't go as well with whipped cream, but the boost may surprise you!

Kava — The King and Queen of Relaxation

How about a nice cup of morning kava to start the day? Or to end it for that matter? Kava has a memorable name *and* a memorable taste — though not completely pleasant, unless you're from Fiji, Vanuatu, or Hawaii, in which case you probably grew up with the herb all around you and acquired a taste for it. Now that the wonderful muscle-relaxing and mellowing-out qualities of the herb are known in Europe and the U.S., it is quickly becoming one of the most popular herbs in use.

If you feel stressed, nervous, tight, tense, or have trouble relaxing enough to get a refreshing night's sleep, this herb may be worth a try. The tea works wonders and can stimulate memorable, full-color dreams!

See Chapter 10 for a delicious Kava Kocktail. Products are available in capsule, tablet, or liquid extract form in many pharmacies and natural food stores. Happy dreams!

St. John's Wort — Mood Food

Unless you've been living in a cave, you've probably heard of St. John's wort. It's commonly prescribed by medical doctors throughout Europe as a safe, natural way to ease depression. It's been on TV, in newspapers, and in magazines such as *Newsweek* and *Time*. It was advertised on prime time TV during *Seinfeld*.

So what's so great about it? German medical researchers have shown the herb to be just as effective as commonly-prescribed pharmaceutical anti-depressants — *selective serotonin reuptake inhibitors* (SSRIs), such as Prozac and Zoloft — with few, if any, side effects. It can help millions of people who are depressed, unable to sleep at night, or feel anxious.

Over 20 modern clinical trials support the use of extracts of the herb for easing mild, moderate, and even some cases of severe depression. Some forms of insomnia and anxiety also benefit from St. John's wort.

To an herbalist, the usefulness of St. John's wort doesn't stop there. It is also widely recommended for use on the skin for healing and easing the pain of burns, cuts, scrapes, and bites. Internally, it is also effective as an antiviral to slow replication of the AIDS virus, help to heal stomach ulcers, and soothe nerve pains.

Most pharmacies, grocery stores, and natural food stores carry it in two forms — a liquid extract that should be a rich red color to be active, and in tablet or capsule form. Take $1/2$ to $3/4$ teaspoon of the liquid, morning and evening in a little water, away from mealtimes, or 2 capsules or tablets in the morning and 1 in the evening containing a standardized extract. It can take two to three weeks before you feel the effects, and up to two months before it becomes fully active.

What about St. John's wort for mood enhancement if you aren't depressed and can sleep just fine? A good friend, Dr. Paul Lee, who is normally quite cheerful, recently asked me to send him some. When I said, "Why do you need it Paul, are you depressed?" He replied, "No, I just want to see if it makes me feel better than I already do!"

Saw Palmetto — A Good Fate for the Prostate

As men get older, a strange thing happens — the prostate gland starts to grow. As it gets bigger, the little tube that conducts the urine out of the body that the prostate is wrapped around naturally gets smaller. This leads to a common problem in men over 40 or so — they have trouble going with the flow! Or it goes in little spurts and it takes too long. It can be painful. All-in-all, not very pleasant. Modern medicine wants to perform surgery, which can increase the flow, but can also lead to other major problems like no erections and dribbling after urinating. Time for a diaper? Not if you get hold of a special herb called saw palmetto.

The not-so-secret herbal marvel is an extract from the fruit of a scrubby palm that grows in northern Florida called saw palmetto. The herb has become so popular worldwide that cattle ranchers who were clearing thousands of acres of the trees to plant grass for their cows are now planting palms. They can actually make more money on berries than on beef!

Saw palmetto is available in soft-gel capsules nearly everywhere, even by mail-order. Purchase only brands that claim that they are "solvent-free," "hexane-free," or "supercritically-extracted." Take 2 capsules morning and evening. You should notice the full effects — which include less pain and irritation, more control, less frequent urgency, and more comfort — after three to six weeks.

Many herbalists also feel that the regular use of saw palmetto can improve the health of the prostate gland. For women, regular use can help prevent urinary tract infections and improve the health of the entire genito-urinary tract.

Valerian — To Sleep, To Sleep, Perchance to Dream

For over 1,000 years, the spicy and (to some) smelly root of valerian has been part of the ambiance of many herb shops. Valerian is known as the sleep-promoting and relaxing herb — studies show that it works on the brain and spinal cord, activating some of the same receptor sites as common pharmaceutical drugs, notably the benzodiazepines Xanax and Valium. These drugs are widely prescribed — especially in the elderly — for anxiety, nervousness, and insomnia. Unfortunately benzodiazepines can also lead to addiction, memory loss, and even worse mental and emotional symptoms than they are designed to treat.

Valerian has none of these side effects and coupled with a natural program of relaxation and good diet, can be as (or more) effective. Liquid extracts or tinctures made from the fresh roots and rhizomes (underground parts) are calming and relaxing and can be taken daily as needed. Actual clinical trials show that valerian can help users fall asleep faster and have a deeper, more refreshing night's sleep.

Using $^1/_2$ to $^3/_4$ of a cup of tea before bedtime is often effective, as is $^1/_2$ to $^3/_4$ teaspoon of the liquid extract in a little water. You can also blend valerian with other relaxing herbs such as passion flower, California poppy, hops, and linden flower.

Vitex — The Hormone Helper

Two thousand five hundred years ago, the father of natural medicine, Hippocrates, discovered that small berries of a shrubby plant native to Greece and the Mediterranean were an effective remedy to regulate the women's monthly cycle and to help new mothers produce an ample supply of breast milk. In the 1950s, German researchers looked into the matter and found that an extract could stimulate the hypothalamus gland in the brain to tell the ovaries to produce more of a key hormone that regulates milk production and the menses — progesterone. Today, the herb vitex, also called chaste-berry, is the most popular natural medicine throughout Europe for helping to ease unwanted symptoms of premenstrual syndrome, as well as those symptoms that may occur during menopause.

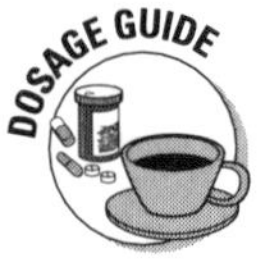

Use 1/2 teaspoon (3 droppersful) of the liquid extract in a little water, first thing in the morning. This simple remedy can help ease such symptoms as mood swings, irritability, sugar cravings, acne, excessive menstrual bleeding, and irregular cycles associated with PMS. During menopause, the remedy can be used for several months to a year, or longer under the guidance of your herbalist, to make the journey more pleasant, reducing such symptoms as hot flashes, vaginal dryness, mild depression, and other mood swings.

Chapter 10

Ten Delicious Herbal Teas

In This Chapter

- Preparing healthy alternatives to black tea or coffee
- Making nutritious herbal teas for kids
- Enjoying herb teas for nervousness or indigestion

Recipes in This Chapter

- Chai
- Hibiscus Party Punch
- Calm Day Tea
- Summer Garden Tea
- Seven Flower Tea
- Kava Kocktail
- Herbal Cup of Coffee
- Children's Delight
- Herbal Root Beer

In this chapter, I provide recipes for my favorite herb teas. Using these simple recipes, you can make either hot or iced teas. Either way, you reap the benefit of these delicious, vitamin- and mineral-rich herbal beverages.

Chai

This spiced tea is a traditional drink throughout the Middle East and Far East. The flavors and ingredients vary and many recipes include black tea, which can add quite a bit of caffeine. This recipe is a decaffeinated version, specifically formulated to promote powerful digestion. If you prefer a caffeinated version, look for the variation at the end of this recipe. This tea can help settle an upset stomach and it makes your house smell great!

Preparation time: *25 minutes*

Yield*: 2 cups*

2 cups water

2 tablespoons freshly grated ginger

2 cinnamon sticks

3 to 4 whole peppercorns

8 to10 cardamom pods

1/2 cup milk (or substitute almond, rice, or soy milk)

1 pinch nutmeg powder

Honey to taste

1 In a medium saucepan, combine the water, ginger, cinnamon sticks, peppercorns, and cardamom pods.

2 Cover and simmer for 10 minutes over low heat.

3 Add the milk and simmer an additional 10 minutes.

4 Strain into mugs, sprinkle nutmeg powder on top, and sweeten with honey, if desired.

Vary It! If you want to add black tea to this blend, add it after you've simmered the herbs. Let it steep for three minutes, then strain, add milk, and sweeten, if desired.

Hibiscus Party Punch

This refreshing tea is great to serve cold at summer parties and to have on hand on hot days. This cooling blend can be made to look festive by adding fresh slices of lemons and oranges and a few sprigs of spearmint.

Preparation time: *1 hour*

Yield: *5 quarts*

1 gallon water

2 cups red clover

2 cups hibiscus

4 or 5 whole cloves

1/3 cup cinnamon sticks

1/2 cup honey

1 cup lemon juice

2 cup orange juice

1 cup apple juice

1 Bring the water to a boil and pour over the red clover, hibiscus, cloves, and cinnamon sticks. Steep for 20 minutes.

2 Add honey, lemon juice, orange juice, and apple juice. Refrigerate until chilled.

Vary It! This tea also turns out wonderfully when made as a sun tea. Put the herbs in room-temperature water and let them sit out in the sun from morning until mid-afternoon. Add the honey and juices; refrigerate. You can enhance the aesthetic appeal of this sun tea by adding a few calendula petal ice cubes. To make the flower ice cubes, pick the petals off of 3 or 4 calendula flowers, mix with water in a measuring cup, and pour the mixture into ice cube trays.

Calm Day Tea

Serve this delicious-smelling tea blend after lunch or dinner to promote digestion and relaxation.

Preparation time: *20 minutes*

Yield: *4 cups*

4 cups boiling water

1 teaspoon linden flower

1 teaspoon lemon balm

1 teaspoon orange peel

1/2 teaspoon chamomile

1/2 teaspoon lavender

1/2 teaspoon hops

Pour the boiling water over the other ingredients and let steep for 20 minutes. Strain and drink.

Summer Garden Tea

This tea is made up of a combination of herbs from the garden that can relax you and keep your immune system healthy. It's refreshing and tasty, iced or hot.

Preparation time: *20 minutes*

Yield: *4 cups*

5 cups water

1 teaspoon bee balm

1 teaspoon chamomile

1 teaspoon echinacea flowers and leaf

1 teaspoon lemon balm

1 teaspoon anise hyssop

1 teaspoon red clover blossoms

1 Bring the water to a boil.

2 Combine ingredients and cover with the boiling water. Steep for 20 minutes.

Vary It! This tea is also good made as a sun tea. Use the same proportions and instead of bringing the water to a boil and steeping the herbs, let the mixture sit in the sun for 5 or 6 hours.

Seven Flower Tea

You can make this fragrant tea with herbs from your garden or dried herbs that you buy. Seven Flower Tea cools you down on a warm summer's day, helping to keep you calm and soothe your digestion.

Preparation time: *20 minutes*

Yield: *6 cups*

1 quart boiling water

2 teaspoons chamomile flower

1 teaspoon linden flower

1 teaspoon calendula flower

1 teaspoon lavender flower

1 teaspoon honeysuckle flower

1/2 teaspoon passion flower

1/2 teaspoon orange flower or orange peel

1 Pour boiling water over the flowers.

2 Allow to steep for 20 minutes. Strain and enjoy.

Kava Kocktail

Kava is a traditional, relaxing, ceremonial herb from the South Pacific. Kava imparts a feeling of ease and help reduce muscle and mental tension. Try this easy recipe from Herbal Ed Smith using kava powder that's available in most natural food stores or herb shops.

Preparation time: *10 minutes*

Yield: *2 cups*

1 teaspoon kava powder

1 1/2 cups water

1 teaspoon lecithin liquid or granules

2 tablespoons pineapple juice (optional)

1 Simmer the kava powder in the water for 5 minutes, let cool.

2 Add 1 teaspoon of lecithin liquid or granules and 2 tablespoons of pineapple juice, blend in a blender for a few minutes on high speed.

3 Strain thoroughly and drink.

Herbal Cup of Coffee

If you'd like to stop drinking coffee to get a more healing sleep, but still keep your energy up, try this full-flavored morning herbal beverage. Unlike coffee, the herbs in this blend are healthy for your liver and help promote a relaxed state of heightened energy.

Preparation time: *10 minutes*

Yield: *3 cups*

2 teaspoons roasted chicory root

2 teaspoons roasted dandelion root

1 teaspoon fennel seed

1 teaspoon ginger root

2 teaspoons carob chunks (or powder)

2 cups water

Milk to taste

Honey to taste

1 Gently simmer the chicory, dandelion, fennel, ginger, and carob in the water for 10 minutes.

2 Strain and add milk and honey, if you like.

Vary It! If you want to ease off of caffeine gradually, add a pinch or two of bancha twigs to this tea. It complements the flavor of the blend and contains a very small amount of caffeine.

Children's Delight

This tea is an extremely healthful drink to give your kids as a substitute for fruit juice and soft drinks. The herbs in this blend help your children support their immune and digestive systems and build strong, pliable bones.

Preparation time: *35 minutes*

Yield: *5 cups*

1 teaspoon fennel

1/2 teaspoon cloves

1/4 teaspoon cinnamon bark chips

6 cups water

1 teaspoon peppermint

1 teaspoon chamomile

1/2 teaspoon red clover

1/2 teaspoon nettles

1/2 teaspoon oatstraw

1 teaspoon stevia herb

(continued)

(continued)

1 Simmer the fennel, cloves, and cinnamon in the water for 15 minutes.

2 Add the remaining ingredients. Remove from heat and allow the entire mixture to steep for 20 minutes.

3 Strain. Serve warm or refrigerate for iced tea.

Herbal Root Beer

Try this herbal alternative to commercial, sugary root beer. Not only do the herbs in this blend increase health and vitality, but they also have the popular root beer flavor.

Preparation time: *25 minutes*

Yield: *1 quart*

1 teaspoon sarsaparilla

1/2 teaspoon sassafras bark

1/4 teaspoon licorice

3 cups water

1 teaspoon wintergreen herb

1/4 teaspoon stevia or honey

1 cup mineral water

1 Simmer the sarsaparilla, sassafras, and licorice in the water for 10 minutes.

2 Remove from heat and add the wintergreen and stevia or honey. Allow to steep an additional 10 minutes.

3 Add the mineral water. Refrigerate the root beer.

Symptom Guide

The 5th Wave By Rich Tennant

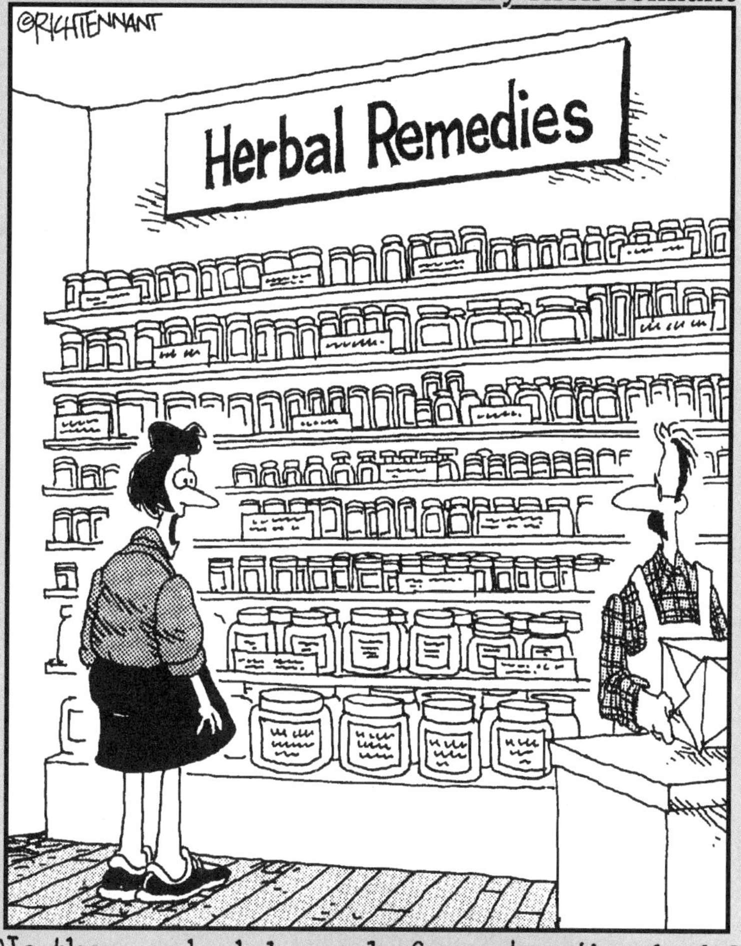

"Is there an herbal remedy for acute option shock?"

In this guide . . .

This *Symptom Guide* is a practical reference guide based on what I've learned from over thirty years of experience with herbs. In this guide, I put together my favorite herbal remedies and supportive programs that I've seen work and that are safe under most conditions. I organize the information under the following categories to help you find the remedies quickly.

Medical description: This category includes the modern medical understanding or definition of your symptom or condition.

Holistic understanding: Holistic concepts and viewpoints about your symptoms and ailments are the way many herbalists think about disease — this category explains disease in a holistic way that takes into account the influence of your environment, diet, and health habits.

Herbal remedies: In this category, I discuss today's most useful herbs as a natural way to care for most symptoms and ailments — the ones with the best track records of safety and effectiveness.

Herbal formulas: In this category, I recommend specific herbal formulas that you can easily make at home, using common kitchenware. Alternatively, you can find many of the commercially-prepared formulas in capsules, tablets, or liquids.

Healthy habits: Herbs are designed to work in a total program for health — when you eat a healthy diet and follow healthy habits like exercising and singing to help supercharge your cells with oxygen, the herbal remedies that you take work even better. In this category, I recommend specific healthy habits that can help ease symptoms and prevent disease in an enjoyable way.

Keep in mind that the information in this reference is not intended to substitute for expert medical advice or treatment; it is designed to help you make informed choices. Because each individual is unique, a professional health care provider must diagnose conditions and supervise treatments for each individual health problem. If you're under a doctor's care and receive advice that is contrary to the information provided in this reference, the doctor's advice should be followed, because it is based on your unique characteristics.

Abscess

Medical description: A bacterial infection surrounded by inflamed tissue where pus collects.

Holistic understanding: Often caused by an overheated system from stress, eating too much sugar or spicy and greasy foods, and buildup of toxic waste products in the blood and tissues.

Herbal remedies: Use cleansing herbs like the roots of echinacea, dandelion, burdock, and/or yellow dock to help remove excess heat and toxic waste products from the bowels and liver. Try using bowel cleansing herbs like yellow dock root and psyllium seed for a week, and repeat once a month for several months, especially if you have trouble with boils, acne, and other skin problems. Apply a flaxseed meal poultice to the abscess.

Herbal formulas: Make a decoction by simmering 1 tablespoon each of echinacea leaf or root, dandelion root, and Oregon grape root together with 1 teaspoon of licorice for each 2 cups of water for 30 minutes. Drink 1 cup of the tea, 2 or 3 times daily. If you prefer, mix 1 teaspoon each of the individual tinctures, (for licorice, 1/2 teaspoon), to 1 cup of water and drink 1/2 cup, 2 times daily.

Healthy habits: Increase your intake of fresh fruits, vegetables, and whole grains to speed recovery and prevent abscesses from forming. Avoid fatty foods, red meats, and spicy foods for a week or two.

Acne

Medical description: Inflammation of the sebaceous glands.

Holistic understanding: Acne is generally the result of hormonal imbalance or toxicity of the bowel or blood.

Herbal remedies: Use cleansing herbs like burdock root, yellow dock root, or echinacea root to help cleanse your blood and remove toxic waste products from your liver. Use bowel-cleansing herbs like yellow dock root and psyllium seed for a week, and repeat once a month for several months, especially if you have trouble with boils, acne, and other skin problems. Take evening primrose oil in capsules. Apply tea tree oil externally.

Herbal formulas: Make a decoction by simmering 1 tablespoon each of Oregon grape root, yellow dock root, burdock root, and red clover flowers for each 2 cups of water for 30 minutes. Drink 1 cup of the tea, 2 or 3 times daily. If you prefer, mix 1 teaspoon each of the individual tinctures in 1 cup of water and drink 1/2 cup, 2 times daily.

Healthy habits: During a breakout, eat mainly fresh fruits and vegetables, and add a six-ounce glass of cleansing vegetable juice with equal parts of cucumber, carrot, and celery, with a little parsley. Identify and drastically reduce all forms of refined sugar and fried foods in your diet — this includes honey. Alternate hot and cold water compresses over pimples once or twice a day to open the pores, cleanse them, and increase circulation to remove wastes.

Anemia

Medical description: A deficiency of hemoglobin or red blood cells in the blood or in the total blood volume.

Holistic understanding: Anemia is related to the holistic concept of blood deficiency and is a symptom of various metabolic and bodily disorders. Anemia is thought to be related to weak digestion.

Herbal remedies: Take herbs to build the blood, such as dong quai root or nettle leaf. Also take digestive stimulants, such as gentian root and artichoke leaf, which are available in bitters formulas in natural food stores. Consider taking yellow dock, which increases the body's assimilation of iron.

Herbal formulas: Combine 1 teaspoon each yellow dock root and nettle leaves and 1/2 teaspoon dandelion root and dong quai with 4 cups water. Bring herbs and water to a boil, and simmer the mixture for 20 minutes. Drink 2 cups daily with meals. If you prefer, mix 1 teaspoon each of the individual tinctures in 1 cup of water and drink 1/2 cup, 2 times daily.

Healthy habits: Increase your intake of iron rich foods, such as the sea vegetables wakame and nori, and eat blood-building beets, beans, and green leafy vegetables (including chard, kale, collard greens, and beet greens). Wild greens, including dandelion leaves, lamb's quarters, nettles, and yellow dock leaves, have a particularly high iron content. Note that certain foods inhibit iron absorption — these include bran, tea, coffee, eggs, and milk. Also try adding liquid chlorophyll to your bath.

Angina Pectoris

Medical description: Commonly called *angina,* this condition is a feeling of suffocating pain in the chest caused by narrowing of coronary arteries. Consult your doctor and/or herbalist if you experience this condition.

Holistic understanding: Problems with the heart are generally lifestyle diseases, which can be prevented by eliminating risk factors, such as smoking, eating a high-fat diet, and being too sedentary. A recent study pointed to intake of cooked fats, refined sugar, and lack of exercise as the most important factors that cause heart problems.

Herbal remedies: Take hawthorn flowers and leaves and ginkgo leaves to dilate your coronary arteries and bring more blood to the heart muscle. This can help prevent heart muscle damage. Garlic and flaxseed oil can help keep the blood from thickening up and discourage clot formation. Take cactus flowers and motherwort herb to gently stimulate and steady the heart. Take herbal antioxidants daily to protect your heart and prevent heart disease in the first place — these include green tea, ginkgo, and grapeseed extract.

Herbal formulas: Combine 1 teaspoon each hawthorn flowers and leaves, motherwort leaf, and linden flowers in 4 cups water. Bring herbs and water to a boil, and simmer the mixture for 20 minutes. For extra strength, add 1 teaspoon of ginkgo leaf tincture. Drink 1 cup of the tea, 2 or 3 times daily. If you prefer, mix 1 teaspoon each of the individual tinctures in 1 cup of water and drink 1/2 cup, 2 times daily.

Healthy habits: Try one of the two diets that have long resulted in healthy hearts — a Mediterranean diet, which emphasizes grains, vegetables, fish, olive oil, and moderate fat intake with very low animal fats; and the Asian diet, with its emphasis on tofu, sea vegetables, aduki and mung beans, and rice. Add plenty of onions, cayenne, ginger, and garlic to your food. Fiber is also important, so add psyllium, flaxseed, and bran to your diet. Countless studies have shown the benefits of regular exercise on the heart. Try to exercise at least a half-hour daily and make it vigorous, if you can.

Anxiety

Medical description: A type of neurosis characterized by a feeling of apprehension. May also include insomnia, fear, and difficulty concentrating.

Holistic understanding: People experience mild anxiety during times of stress, such as when going through an illness, speaking in front of a group of people, or taking an exam. Other causes of anxiety include emotional stresses, major life transitions, habitual use of stimulants (such as coffee, tea, and other caffeinated beverages), and excessive intake of sugar.

Herbal remedies: Use calming and relaxing herbs such as California poppy root, valerian root, St. John's wort leaf and flowers, linden flowers, and/or passion flower herb to calm anxiety.

Herbal formulas: Combine 1 teaspoon each valerian root, California poppy herb and root, hawthorn leaves and flowers, and kava root in 4 cups water. Bring herbs and water to a boil, then simmer the mixture for 20 minutes. Drink 1 cup of the tea, 2 or 3 times daily. If you prefer, mix 1 teaspoon each of the individual tinctures in 1 cup of water and drink 1/2 cup, 2 times daily. Also try the Kava Kocktail in Chapter 10.

Healthy habits: Avoid stimulants such as coffee, tea, chocolate, and cola drinks. Incorporate daily relaxation methods such as deep breathing, meditation, visualization, stretching, and walking in the woods or by the ocean. During times of high stress and anxiousness in my life, I've found that strenuous activity helps burn off the tension, and it benefits my cardiovascular system as an extra bonus! Dancing is my favorite, but biking and skipping rope are also great.

Appetite (Poor)

Medical description: Also called anorexia, loss of appetite can result from stress, but see a doctor if the feeling persists, because it can result from a serious metabolic imbalance, disease of the liver, or other diseases, such as hepatitis.

Holistic understanding: Loss of appetite can be a symptom of a wide range of disorders, including food stagnation (when your food just sits on your stomach and won't digest), weak digestion, or mental or emotional turbulence.

Herbal remedies: To improve your appetite, combine digestive stimulants, such as ginger root and artichoke leaf, or bitters-containing formulas with relaxing herbs, such as hops strobiles and California poppy root. Three of the most effective herbs that combine bitter digestive-stimulating properties with calming effects are wild lettuce leaf, California poppy root, and hops strobiles.

Herbal formulas: Make a decoction by simmering 1 teaspoon each of angelica root, orange peel, and artichoke leaf and 1/2 teaspoon of gentian root in 2 cups of water for 30 minutes. Add wild lettuce leaf or California poppy root if your digestive problem is related to nervousness. Drink 1 cup of the tea, 2 times daily, 1/2 hour before meals. If you prefer, mix 1 teaspoon each of the individual tinctures in 1 cup of water and drink 1/2 cup, 2 times daily, before meals.

Healthy habits: Eat a diet made up of lightly steamed or cooked vegetables, well-cooked grains, and legumes. Eat raw vegetables and fruit during the warm times of the year. Try taking a good bitters formula 1/2 hour before meals — continue this for several months.

Arthritis

Medical description: Joint inflammation with pain, swelling, and stiffening of the surrounding tissues.

Holistic understanding: Arthritis occurs when excess heat accumulates in and around the joints. This pathogenic heat often occurs in people who eat a lot of red meat, sugar, and spicy foods, and drink stimulants such as coffee. Other causative factors include food allergy, poor dietary habits, and a sedentary lifestyle.

Herbal remedies: Take burdock root, celery seed, feverfew herb, nettles herb, devil's claw rhizome, black cohosh root, meadowsweet herb, and/or yucca root to lower inflammation and counteract pain. Some herbalists strongly promote the daily use of cayenne pepper in food and 2 capsules, 2 times daily to ease the symptoms of arthritis.

Herbal formulas: Make a decoction by simmering 1 teaspoon each of meadowsweet herb, licorice root, black cohosh root, and kava root in 2 cups of water for 30 minutes. Drink 1 cup of the tea, 2 to 3 times daily. If you prefer, mix 1 teaspoon each of the individual tinctures in 1 cup of water and drink 1/2 cup, 2 to 3 times daily.

Healthy habits: Avoid red meat, caffeine, sugar, fruit, and fruit juices. I've seen arthritis sufferers completely eliminate their symptoms by avoiding all foods in the nightshade family (including tomatoes, potatoes, eggplant, and peppers) for three months — if your symptoms aren't improved by then, avoiding nightshades probably won't work. Apply alternate hot and cold compresses to the affected areas. Get regular, moderate exercise, including walking, biking, or swimming, that doesn't place any additional stress on affected joints. I've seen regular acupuncture and moxibustion treatments help some of my patients.

Athlete's Foot

Medical description: A fungal infection of the skin of the feet, usually starting between toes three and four or four and five. The infection can spread to the toenails, if left untreated.

Holistic understanding: The dampness and heat accumulating between the toes creates an environment where various fungi proliferate. Maintaining a strong immune system helps tremendously in maintaining fungus-free feet.

Herbal remedies: Apply tea tree oil directly, 2 or 3 times daily, on infected areas. For cracking and peeling of the sole or other large areas of the feet, apply a tea tree cream several times daily. A good soothing calendula or chamomile cream can help relieve redness, itching, and irritation.

Herbal formulas: Apply a cream or salve with herbs like tea tree, calendula, echinacea, or bloodroot several times daily.

Healthy habits: Walking barefoot occasionally can help prevent athlete's foot.

Back Pain

Medical description: Pain that occurs in various parts of the back.

Holistic understanding: Back pain is due to stagnation of blood and vital energy in the area due to injury or from long periods of inactivity.

Herbal remedies: Apply a hot ginger poultice, 2 or 3 times daily. Rub on St. John's wort oil, a cayenne liniment, or one of the pain-relieving essential oil herbs like chamomile, rosemary, or camphor.

Herbal formulas: Blend together 1/2 teaspoon of the oils of wintergreen, cinnamon, and ginger in 1/2 cup of aloe gel and add a teaspoon of gum arabic. Shake well and apply to the painful area, 2 times daily. Reduce the dose if you experience redness or irritation of the skin.

Healthy habits: Apply alternate hot and cold compresses, or better yet, hot and cold ginger compresses. Regular exercise to strengthen the lower back is essential for eliminating long-standing pain. I have tremendous results with daily yoga and other gentle stretching exercises every morning. Be careful with a new stretching regime, because you can easily hurt yourself. Instead, start slowly and gradually increase the duration and range of stretching. If you aren't an experienced therapeutic stretcher, I recommend taking a class.

Bladder Infection

Medical description: Inflammation of the bladder usually associated with the bacteria *E. coli*. Consult your doctor and/

or your herbalist if you have prolonged or recurrent bladder infections, because these conditions can lead to kidney problems.

Holistic understanding: Bladder infections are often caused by improper hygiene around the sex organs. Try using tea tree oil soap when you shower to cleanse the pelvic area and help disrupt the bacteria. Other possible causes are the use of vaginal sprays and perfumes, bubble baths, scented toilet tissue, and soaking in jacuzzis or hot tubs that use chlorinated water.

Herbal remedies: Try using one herb from each of the following categories of beneficial urinary tract herbs: soothing herbs such as marshmallow root, plantain leaf, or corn silk; antiseptic herbs such as usnea lichen, uva ursi leaf, or pipsissewa leaf; gentle diuretic herbs such as dandelion leaf, parsley root, cleavers herb, or horsetail herb; and a urinary tract sedative herb such as kava root. A simple, yet highly effective, remedy is half marshmallow root and half plantain leaf as a tea, tincture, or in capsules.

Herbal formulas: Make a decoction by simmering 1 teaspoon each marshmallow root and echinacea root and 1/2 teaspoon of Oregon grape root for each 2 cups of water for 30 minutes. Drink 1 cup of the tea, 2 to 3 times daily. If you prefer, mix 1 teaspoon each of the individual tinctures in 1 cup of water and drink 1/2 cup, 2 to 3 times daily. For extra potency, add 1/2 teaspoon of tincture of usnea to your tea or tincture blend.

Healthy habits: Eat plenty of rice and beans and include soothing foods such as barley, flaxseed, and okra. Eat foods at room temperature or warmer and avoid hot, spicy foods, cold foods and drinks, processed sugars, and caffeine. Drink unsweetened cranberry juice or take cranberry juice powder in capsules to help reduce the infection. You can try alternate hot and cold sitz baths, in which you sit in just enough water to cover your pelvic region, to help bring blood to the area and get rid of the infection.

Bleeding

Medical description: The escape of the blood from the vessels after a cut or other injury. Consult your doctor if you have internal bleeding — for example, if you notice blood in your urine or stools.

Holistic understanding: None.

Herbal remedies: Herbs that stop bleeding from cuts, wounds, and scrapes are called *styptics.* The best styptics include yarrow leaf, wild geranium root, oak bark or oak twig tea, blackberry root, horsetail herb, and calendula flowers. Apply these herbs fresh and juicy, after chewing or grinding them up, or sprinkle the dry powders directly on the bleeding wound. After the bleeding stops, apply a good healing preparation to the wounded area. I suggest calendula and plantain creams or salves.

Herbal formulas: Thoroughly grind into a powder, equal parts of the dry herbs yarrow leaf, calendula petals, and echinacea leaf, and keep the powder in a small vial or jar available in your medicine chest, kitchen cabinet, back pack, or purse. Sprinkle the powder right onto the bleeding area to quickly stop the bleeding and help prevent infection of everything from shaving nicks to scratches.

Healthy habits: None.

Burn

Medical description: Tissue damage caused by heat, fire, or radiation. For severe burns, seek medical attention.

Holistic understanding: None.

Herbal remedies: Apply calendula cream, St. John's wort oil, lavender oil, or a cool ginger compress to the affected area. If you have access to fresh comfrey or plantain, crush or grind the herbs with a little water until a creamy liquid is produced, and spread some onto a small piece of cloth or bandage. Fasten in place and change several times daily as the herbs dry out.

Herbal formulas: Purchase creams containing herbs such as calendula flowers, plantain leaf, and St. John's wort oil. Apply throughout the day.

Healthy habits: Apply cold water for 5 or 10 minutes as soon as possible, and then the herbs. See a doctor if you have a serious burn.

Carpal Tunnel Syndrome

Medical description: A compression of the median nerve in the wrist as it enters the palm of the hand that causes pain, numbness, and weakness.

Holistic understanding: This condition is caused by repetitious movement, such as typing, working a cash register, or hammering. Carpal tunnel syndrome is often caused or aggravated by adrenal or immune weakness, which can lead to an autoimmune condition.

Herbal remedies: Apply St. John's wort oil, wintergreen essential oil, or cayenne cream externally for pain relief, daily. You can use St. John's wort leaf and flower, butcher's broom herb, skullcap leaves and flowers, California poppy root, and/or wild oats internally to soothe affected nerves, reduce inflammation, and restore flexibility.

Herbal formulas: To reduce pain and inflammation, apply a combination of St. John's wort oil with the essential oils of wintergreen and rosemary oil. (Don't use wintergreen internally, though!) Add 3 drops of each of the essential oils to 4 ounces St. John's wort oil and apply externally, as needed.

Healthy habits: Eat enough good-quality protein. I recommend fish and organic chicken or turkey, along with beans, seeds, nuts, and nutritional yeast. Use sugar sparingly.

Cholesterol (High)

Medical description: An excessive amount of the fatty sterol cholesterol that's in the blood and most tissues of the body. You're at an increased risk of dying from cardiovascular disease when your total cholesterol is above about 180 mg/dl, or your high-density cholesterol (HDL) is below 35 mg/dl.

Holistic understanding: High cholesterol is often the result of stress and a regular consumption of meat and dairy products, sugar, and oily foods.

Herbal remedies: You can add garlic, artichoke leaf, shiitake mushroom, guggul oleoresin, fenugreek seed, and devil's claw rhizome to your foods or take them as teas or supplements to help lower cholesterol.

Herbal formulas: Combine 1 teaspoon each guggul oleoresin, reishi mushroom, shiitake mushroom, artichoke leaf, ginger rhizome, and fenugreek seed in 4 cups water. Bring herbs and water to a boil, then simmer the mixture for 20 minutes. Drink 1 cup of the tea 2 or 3 times daily. If you prefer, mix 1 teaspoon each of the individual tinctures in 1 cup of water and drink $^{1}/_{2}$ cup, 2 times daily.

Healthy habits: Eat a diet of about seventy percent cooked grains, beans and legumes, and steamed vegetables. Increase your intake of raw fruits and vegetables during warm months. Try to keep the consumption of dairy products, sugar, coffee, and alcohol at a minimum. Eat artichokes regularly to help normalize your cholesterol levels. You may be able to lower your total cholesterol and increase your HDL cholesterol by exercising regularly several times a week.

Cold

Medical description: An acute viral infection of the upper respiratory tract with inflammation of the mucous membranes of the nose and throat, sore throat, runny nose, and sinus congestion.

Holistic understanding: Herbalists consider the common cold a blessing in disguise. During a bout of the ailment, your body increases its elimination of waste products through the skin and by mucus discharge, and your immune system is activated and exercised. The fatigue you often feel during a bout of the common cold is telling you to rest and replenish stores of vital energy. I recommend assisting nature and avoiding the use of antihistamines, aspirin, and other over-the-counter medications that only suppress your symptoms and go against what your body is trying to do to create better health.

Herbal remedies: Herbs are the best way to work with nature, while accelerating the healing process and easing symptoms. Use echinacea root and leaf to stimulate your immune system, eyebright herb to decongest, elder and yarrow flowers to help increase sweating and elimination, yerba santa leaf and osha root to stimulate your respiratory tract and help remove mucus, elder flowers to remove heat from your body, and lemon balm herb and wild indigo root to help manage the effects of the virus.

Herbal formulas: Combine 1 tablespoon each echinacea leaf and/or root and ginger rhizome in 4 cups water. Bring herbs and water to a boil, then simmer the mixture for 20 minutes. Drink 1 cup of the tea, 3 or 4 times daily. If you prefer, mix 1 teaspoon each of the individual tinctures in 1 cup of water and drink $^1/_2$ cup, 3 or 4 times daily.

Healthy habits: Try to eat warming foods when you have a cold. Spice up your diet with garlic, onions, cayenne, and ginger to help rid your body of toxins by increasing sweating. Take a hot bath with ginger tea added at the onset of a cold to help reduce unpleasant symptoms. Do an essential oil steam by adding about 6 drops of eucalyptus oil to a bowl of steaming water, covering your head with a towel, and inhaling the steam.

Cold Sore

Medical description: Small blisters (also called fever blisters) caused by the *Herpes simplex* virus.

Holistic understanding: Stress and overheating your system with stimulants like coffee and sugar can contribute to an outbreak of blisters.

Herbal remedies: Soak a cotton ball with lemon balm decoction or apply a small amount of lemon balm cream or lavender essential oil directly to the sores to fight the virus. Use calendula flowers, echinacea root and/or leaf, or St. John's wort leaf and flower cream or oil in the same way. Take yellow dock root and/or Oregon grape root internally along with St. John's wort flower and leaf, lemon balm herb, and echinacea leaf and root to clear internal heat, counteract the virus, and enhance your immunity.

Herbal formulas: Make a decoction by simmering 1 tablespoon each of calendula flowers, lemon balm herb, and echinacea leaf for each 4 cups of water. Drink 1 cup of the tea, 2 or 3 times daily.

Healthy habits: Increase your intake of lysine-containing foods such as turkey, chicken, fish, cottage cheese, ricotta cheese, wheat germ, yogurt, and sauerkraut. Avoid chocolate, peanuts, other nuts and seeds, and sour foods like citrus fruits and pineapple during the breakout.

Colitis

Medical description: Inflammation of the colon, often accompanied by diarrhea, constipation, and cramping.

Holistic understanding: Colitis is generally an autoimmune disorder related to food allergies, poor eating habits, and stress.

Herbal remedies: Use anti-inflammatory herbs, such as licorice root, marshmallow root, or chamomile flowers; anti-allergenic herbs, such as nettle herb, ginkgo leaf, or dong quai root; and heat-clearing herbs for the bowels, such as yellow dock root or cascara bark. Drink 4 to 6 ounces of aloe vera juice, 2 times daily, to soothe and heal the colon. Homeopathic belladonna is often helpful. Follow the instructions on the label.

Herbal formulas: Simmer 1 tablespoon each of plantain leaf, marshmallow root, and yellow dock root for every 2 cups of water. Bring herbs and water to a boil, then simmer the mixture for 20 minutes. Add 1 tablespoon of chamomile flowers and steep for 20 minutes. Drink 1 cup of the tea, 2 or 3 times daily. If you prefer, mix 1 teaspoon each of the individual tinctures in 1 cup of water and drink 1/2 cup, 2 times daily. The tea is more effective.

Healthy habits: Do gentle stretching exercises and avoid fried foods, spicy foods, and dairy products. Self-massage of the abdominal area for 5 or 10 minutes daily helps to keep the area loose.

Conjunctivitis

Medical description: Inflammation of the mucous membrane around the inner surface of the eyelid and part of the eye surface. This ailment is highly contagious. Pay careful attention to hygiene to avoid passing it on to others.

Holistic understanding: The eye is associated with the liver in Traditional Chinese Medicine. Herbalists believe that when your liver is overheated from alcohol, drugs, sugar, and stress, your eyes are much more likely to become inflamed or infected.

Herbal remedies: Take echinacea root to stimulate your immune response and eyebright herb to reduce inflammation around the eye. Apply well-strained goldenseal root and eyebright tea as a wash to lower inflammation. Try grating a raw potato and applying the pulp as a poultice to soothe the affected area. Liver cooling herbs, such as dandelion root, Oregon grape root, and gentian root, are a must, especially if you indulge in alcohol or recreational drugs, or take any pharmaceutical drugs like antibiotics.

Herbal formulas: Make a light decoction by simmering 1/2 teaspoon of goldenseal powder with 1 tablespoon each of eyebright herb and echinacea leaf and then steeping the mixture for minutes. Let the tea cool, filter it well, and wash the eye, several times daily. Soak a small cotton pad in the tea and tape over the eye for 1 or 2 hours.

Healthy habits: Follow a cooling, cleansing diet emphasizing fruits and vegetables and avoiding sugar for at least a week.

Constipation

Medical description: Infrequent or difficult bowel movements.

Holistic understanding: A low-fiber diet, stress, overeating, and eating foods that are over-cooked can all contribute to constipation.

Herbal remedies: To tone your bowels, take bulk laxatives such as psyllium seed or husk twice daily for a week. Try drinking a tablespoon of flaxseed meal ground up and added to a cup of warm water. Follow any mucilage-containing seeds like flax or psyllium with at least two glasses of water or herb tea. For bowels that are *really* stuck, try an herbal laxative like cascara bark, buckthorn bark, aloe resin, or senna leaves for one week only.

Herbal formulas: The most successful long-term bowel toning formula that doesn't lead to habituation is a blend of cascara bark, yellow dock root, and burdock. Simmer 1/2 teaspoon each cascara bark and licorice root and 1 teaspoon each burdock root and yellow dock root in 2 cups of water. Drink 1/2 cup a day, preferably before bedtime. For difficult constipation that doesn't respond to this remedy, try taking the tea morning and evening. Tinctures of these herbs are also effective. Take 1 teaspoon of each in a little water, and drink 1/2 cup, in the evening, or morning and evening.

Healthy habits: Eat plenty of fruits and vegetables and avoid processed foods. Avoid eating flour products like pasta, bread, or baked goods more than once or twice a week for a treat. Drink a glass of prune juice, once or twice a day. Exercising is a good preventive to constipation. You may find that taking the time to *let it flow* is all it takes to get regular.

Cough

Medical description: A violent exhalation that expels irritant particles in the airways. For chronic coughs and coughs continuing longer than two months, consult with your doctor and/or herbalist.

Holistic understanding: Coughing is a protective mechanism that rids the body of mucus and waste products in the bronchial area during an infection.

Herbal remedies: To soothe the cough and remove congested matter, try yerba santa leaf, yerba mansa root, and grindelia tops. For dry coughs, use demulcent soothing herbs like marshmallow root, flaxseed, mullein leaf, and Irish moss to soothe the throat. I find that herbal cough syrups containing loquat leaf, horehound leaf, and/or wild cherry bark are effective for calming a cough along with soothing and expectorant herbs.

Herbal formulas: For dry coughs, combine 1 tablespoon each licorice root, mullein leaf, and marshmallow root in 2 cups of water. Bring herbs and water to a boil, then simmer the mixture for 20 minutes. Drink 1 cup of the tea, 2 or 3 times daily. For wet coughs, combine grindelia flowers, yerba santa leaf, and wild cherry bark, and follow the same directions. Tinctures of the expectorant herbs work well, and you can take them alone, or add them to the soothing tea. Add 5 to 7 drops of bloodroot tincture for each cup of expectorant tea for extra potency. Don't exceed the recommended dose of bloodroot and don't take it undiluted because the herb is highly irritating.

Healthy habits: Eat soups and other cooked, warming foods. Add extra cayenne, ginger, garlic, and horseradish to your food.

Dandruff

Medical description: A scaly, itchy condition of the scalp caused by drying and flaking of dead skin.

Holistic understanding: Dandruff is often related to food allergies or a bowel imbalance. Eliminating milk and wheat from the diet may bring relief.

Herbal remedies: Add a few drops of tea tree oil to your shampoo. You can also massage 2 or 3 drops ginger oil into your scalp or make a ginger tea and use it as a rinse. Take evening primrose oil in capsules.

Herbal formulas: After shampooing, rinse your hair with a mixture of 1/4 cup vinegar and 3 cups rosemary tea, working it in well and leaving it on for 5 minutes to increase circulation to the scalp.

Healthy habits: Add one or two tablespoons of flaxseed to your daily diet and avoid fried foods and sugar. If you have trouble digesting your food, take the bitter tonic formula as described under the "Fatigue" section.

Depression

Medical description: A mental state characterized by sadness and in extreme cases hopelessness and a loss of enjoyment in normal activities.

Holistic understanding: Depression is an imbalance due to a lack of vital energy, often as a result from prolonged stress, poor nutrition and overwork, and the resulting weakening of the adrenal, nervous, and digestive systems.

Herbal remedies: Take St. John's wort tincture or standardized extract, the most proven herbal antidepressant. I often add ginkgo leaf extract to increase brain energy and metabolism, and/or red Korean or red Chinese ginseng root to increase vital energy, especially if you're over 45 or so. Use essential oil of lavender as an inhalant daily to lift your spirits.

Herbal formulas: Combine 1 teaspoon each of the tinctures of St. John's wort leaf and flower, ginkgo leaf, rosemary leaf, lavender flowers, and 1/2 teaspoon of red ginseng tincture in 1 cup of water, and drink 1/2 cup, morning and evening, away from mealtimes.

Healthy habits: Include more vegetables, fruits, and whole grains in your diet. Decrease fat intake. Make sure you're getting enough high-quality protein from fish, daily beans like tofu, and nutritional yeast, because your nervous system runs on the amino acids that you get from protein. Regular exercise, fresh air, and deep breathing are good depression busters.

Diaper Rash

Medical description: A painful red and raw area of skin over the buttocks and under areas covered by a diaper.

Holistic understanding: The redness and irritation from exposure of tender skin to ammonia in urine.

Herbal remedies: Apply natural salves, creams, and body powders containing calendula flowers, plantain leaf, comfrey leaf and root, and chamomile flowers.

Herbal formulas: None.

Healthy habits: Thoroughly rinse diapers and allow the baby time without a diaper when weather and circumstances permit.

Diarrhea

Medical description: Frequent evacuation of loose, watery bowel movements. If food poisoning is the cause of your diarrhea, or if you have chronic diarrhea, consult your physician and/or herbalist.

Holistic understanding: This condition is sometimes caused by stress and buildup of dampness and heat (damp heat) in the intestines. Other causes include food poisoning, food allergies, drinking contaminated water, caffeine, or unripe fruits.

Herbal remedies: Use blackberry root tea, kudzu root tea, black walnut hull tincture, and/or psyllium husks to normalize your bowels.

Herbal formulas: Make a blackberry root decoction by simmering 2 tablespoons of the chopped herb for every 3 cups of water for 30 minutes. Add a tablespoon of chopped dry or fresh orange peel, and a teaspoon of chopped dry licorice root, and steep the brew for 15 minutes. Drink 1 cup, 3 times daily. If the diarrhea persists, add 1 tablespoon of chopped dry barberry root to the mixture and take it for another three or four days. A tablespoon of pectin powder in a glass of water often helps. If the diarrhea still persists, I recommend consulting with your herbalist.

An extremely effective ready-made Chinese herb formula, called Huang Lian Su, is sold in many herb shops. The pills contain pure berberine sulfate, an active compound from the Chinese herb coptis. I've used them extensively in my clinic. They're convenient and safe when used as directed. Take two of the small yellow pills twice daily for up to a week. Consult with your herbalist or Chinese medicine practitioner if you have any doubts.

Healthy habits: The recommended diet for this condition consists of applesauce (with the peel) with cinnamon, yogurt, toast, rice, and bananas. Take a few tablets of activated charcoal 2 times daily.

Digestion (Weak and Painful)

Medical description: The inability to completely digest your food, affecting assimilation of nutrients and elimination of wastes.

Holistic understanding: Stress and poor dietary habits, such as eating on the go, are often the causes of this condition. Symptoms include gas, bloating, abdominal pain, poor appetite, and diarrhea.

Herbal remedies: Long-term use of digestive bitter herbs, such as artichoke leaf and gentian root, and bitters formulas usually help your digestion to improve. Other helpful digestive herb teas include chamomile flowers, ginger rhizome, peppermint leaf, and hops strobiles.

Herbal formulas: Combine 1 teaspoon each gentian root, orange peel, and ginger rhizome, and 1/2 teaspoon of licorice root, and simmer in 2 cups of water for 5 minutes, then steeping for 15 minutes. Drink 1/2 to 1 cup of the tea, 2 times daily, before your big meals. If you prefer, mix 1 teaspoon each of the individual tinctures in 1 cup of water and drink 1/2 cup, 2 times daily, before meals.

Healthy habits: Avoid drinking cold liquids with meals. Add sauerkraut and yogurt to improve your digestion. Eat moderate portions of food during meals. Don't eat too late at night, and give yourself an hour or two after rising to get your blood and energy moving before eating. Avoid eating on the run. Also, try to be relaxed and thinking happy thoughts during your meal — heavy, argumentative, or depressing thoughts or conversation during meals doesn't help promote good digestion.

Earache and Ear Infections

Medical description: An ache or pain in the ear caused by inflammation or infection of the inner or outer ear. For severe or painful earaches, or for ones that last more than a few days, consult your doctor and/or herbalist.

Holistic understanding: This condition is often related to food allergies such as wheat or dairy.

Herbal remedies: Take 1/2 teaspoon of echinacea root tincture in a little water several times daily to help get rid of the infection. Use garlic-mullein oil directly in the ear to help reduce inflammation, discourage the infection, and reduce pain. Squeeze 3 or 4 drops of the oil, 1 time daily, right into the ear with the head tilted, so that the oil reaches the eardrum. Placing a few drops of aloe vera juice in the ear helps reduce inflammation and pain.

Herbal formulas: Simmer 1 teaspoon each of echinacea root, Roman chamomile flowers, and eyebright herb for each 2 cups of water, and drink 1 cup, 2 times daily.

Healthy habits: Eliminate dairy and wheat products from your diet during the infection. If the problem is ongoing, I recommend eliminating wheat and dairy products for one month on a trial basis. If you have a significant improvement, consider replacing dairy with almond, rice, soy, or oat milk, and wheat with other whole grains like rice and millet. Place hot compresses with a washcloth just behind the ear to help relieve pain.

Eczema

Medical description: Skin inflammation with redness and itching. Lesions form which ooze and then become crusted and scaly.

Holistic understanding: Eczema is often caused by food allergies, stress, or environmental toxins. Taking herbs that are beneficial to the liver and cleanse and detoxify the colon often gives improvement in this condition.

Herbal remedies: Take evening primrose oil in capsules, and follow the manufacturer's label directions. Try single herbs or formulas with a combination of herbs that help detoxify the liver and colon like dandelion root, burdock root, Oregon grape root, and yellow dock root. Herbalists also recommend blood cleansers like echinacea leaf and root, sarsaparilla root, and red clover flowers to reduce inflammation, cleanse the blood, and remove heat from the liver and intestines. I find that milk thistle extract in capsules or tablets (take 1 capsule or tablet, 2 or 3 times daily) is highly effective in many cases. Externally apply calendula ointment or cream, tincture of heartsease pansy, or a compress of chamomile tea to soothe your skin and reduce inflammation. Leave the compress on the affected area for fifteen minutes to a half hour at a time, once or twice a day. You can use a topical chamomile cream instead of the tea compress to save time, though the compress is sometimes more effective.

Herbal formulas: Simmer 1 teaspoon red clover flowers, red root, burdock root, and Oregon grape root in 4 cups of water. Bring to a boil, then simmer the mixture for 20 minutes, and then steep for 15 minutes. Drink 1 cup of the tea, 2 or 3 times daily before meals. If you prefer, mix 1 teaspoon each of the individual tinctures in 1 cup of water and drink 1/2 cup, 2 times daily.

Healthy habits: Follow a cleansing diet, emphasizing fresh fruits and vegetables and fruit juices for a few weeks. Avoid refined foods. Follow the cleansing diet with a building diet consisting of lightly-steamed vegetables, whole grains, and legumes.

Fatigue

Medical description: Mental or physical tiredness; no energy or enthusiasm to do anything. If the fatigue persists for more than a few days, or you wake up tired, you may have chronic fatigue.

Holistic understanding: Fatigue is often the result of continual illness, stress, overworking, worry, or periods of emotional upheaval.

Herbal remedies: Take ginger rhizome and eleuthero (Siberian ginseng) root internally to increase your energy and balance your digestive and hormonal systems. Herbs such as maté and green tea give you a temporary boost, but don't take them long-term, due to their caffeine content. Traditional medicine views fatigue as a common symptom of digestive weakness. Herbalists recommend taking digestive-strengthening herbs to increase the ability of your digestion to release energy from the food you eat. I use two basic digestive tonic formulas and then vary them for each patient. You can try the basic formulas to see if they help give you more natural deep energy, as they do with many of my patients. The first formula includes astragalus root, ginger rhizome, and red ginseng root. Take them as a tea, tincture, or extract in capsule or tablet form. The second formula is a *bitters* formula with one part each of ginger rhizome, cardamon seed, artichoke leaf, and 1/2 part of gentian root. These single herbs and formulas that contain them are widely available in liquid tincture form. Capsules and tablets don't work as well.

Herbal formulas: Combine 1 teaspoon each wild oats spikelets, damiana herb, ginseng root, and ginger rhizome in 3 cups water. Bring herbs and water to a boil, then simmer the mixture for 20 minutes. Drink 1 cup of the tea, 2 or 3 times daily before meals. If you prefer, mix 1 teaspoon each of the individual tinctures in 1 cup of water and drink 1/2 cup, 2 times daily.

Healthy habits: Even if you feel tired, try to at least take short walks in the fresh air, and practice deep breathing down in your belly as you walk. Walk at least 20 to 30 minutes daily if you can. Gradually work up to longer, more frequent exercise, including 20 minutes of aerobic activity every other day. Avoid processed foods and don't overeat. Eat plenty of greens, grains, legumes and lightly-steamed vegetables. Eat organic food that has lots of natural vitality and nutrients. Taking a bath with 3 or 4 drops of rosemary added is a good pick-me-up.

Fever

Medical description: A body temperature exceeding 98.6°. Consult your doctor and/or herbalist if your temperature exceeds 104°.

Holistic understanding: Fevers are a normal part of the immune system response to bacterial and viral infections. When you have an infection with a fever, work with nature by using diaphoretics rather than suppressing your body's best efforts to clear the infection by taking aspirin or acetaminophen.

Herbal remedies: Drink teas made from calendula flowers, chamomile flowers, elder flowers, yarrow herb, chrysanthemum flowers, lemon balm herb, white willow bark, meadowsweet herb, and feverfew herb, either singly or in combination, to move heat out of your body and increase elimination through your sweat and urine. Sponge your hands and feet with a cool washcloth soaked in a bowl of water with 2 or 3 drops of lavender oil.

Herbal formulas: Mix 1 tablespoon each of peppermint leaf, yarrow flowers, and elder flowers in 3 cups boiling water. Allow the mixture to steep 20 minutes. Drink 1 cup of the tea, 2 or 3 times daily. You can also blend the individual tinctures and add 1 teaspoon each to 3 cups of water. Drink 1 cup, 3 times daily.

Healthy habits: Drink plenty of liquid. Add lemon juice to water to make it a more appealing drink and cool down the fever.

Fibrocystic Breast

Medical description: Cysts and lumpiness in the breast — mostly benign. If you're uncertain about a lump that occurs in your breast, seek a diagnosis from a physician.

Holistic understanding: Breast lumps can occur from frequent use of coffee, sugar, and other refined or stimulating foods.

Herbal remedies: Use calendula flowers, burdock root, mullein leaf, nettle leaf, and/or cleavers herb to help cleanse and stimulate your lymphatic system. Apply a compress with a tea of any of the same herbs. Take evening primrose oil in capsules. Herbalists often view cysts as a result of accumulation and stagnation of dampness and phlegm in your tissues. Phlegm is sticky and persistent and is hard to get rid of when it builds up in your system. Try mucus-dissolving herbs for two or three months, either singly or in combination — the best ones include fennel seed, anise seed, licorice root, and bloodroot. Use bloodroot cautiously, only a few drops of the tincture for each dose, with 1/2 teaspoon of fennel tincture and 1/2 teaspoon of licorice for each cup of water.

Herbal formulas: Simmer 1 teaspoon each of echinacea root, mullein leaf, and red clover flowers for each 3 cups of water for 20 minutes. Add 1 teaspoon of fennel seed and steep for 15 minutes. Drink 1 cup of the tea, 2 or 3 times daily before meals. If you prefer, mix 1 teaspoon each of the individual tinctures in 1 cup of water and drink 1/2 cup, 2 times daily. You can make a clay pack by adding water to cosmetic clay to form a paste and then applying it to the affected area daily for 30 minutes. Cover with a towel and then a hot water bottle. Try applying a little castor oil over the cysts, morning and evening.

Healthy habits: Eat a low-fat, high-fiber diet, emphasizing whole grains and beans. Reduce caffeine intake, because it's a known risk factor.

Flu

Medical description: An acute viral infection of the upper respiratory tract or digestive tract with fever, chills, sore throat, nausea, diarrhea, abdominal pain, usually with lethargy.

Holistic understanding: According to holistic healing principles, a flu is often a *healing crisis,* during which toxic waste products are eliminated, and is part of a periodic process of the body to find a greater level of health. A flu or cold is often painful, but positive healing is taking place. The knowledge and acceptance that you're working with the natural processes of your body can often enhance your immune function and shorten the acute symptoms.

Herbal remedies: Use immune-enhancing and heat-relieving herbs such as echinacea root, eyebright herb, yarrow leaf, lemon balm herb, and elder flowers to eliminate the infection and remove heat from your body. When your deeper respiratory tract is infected and you have a fever with thick yellow mucus, add usnea lichen, goldenseal root, and thyme herb to clear the infection and help expel mucus from your lungs.

Herbal formulas: Simmer 1 teaspoon each of echinacea root, Oregon grape root, elder flowers, with 1/2 teaspoon of yerba mansa root in 3 cups of water for 15 minutes. Add 1 teaspoon of thyme herb and steep for 15 minutes. Drink 1 cup of the tea, 2 or 3 times daily before meals. If you prefer, mix 1 teaspoon each of the individual tinctures in 1 cup of water and drink 1/2 cup, 2 times daily. Use thyme herb in the tea version only. To encourage elimination through sweating, drink a tea of equal parts peppermint leaf, yarrow flowers, and elder flowers.

Healthy habits: Eat lightly and add plenty of cayenne, garlic, and ginger to your food. Drink lemon water throughout the day. Give yourself permission to get plenty of rest and recharge your vital energy.

Gas

Medical description: The presence of air or gas in the intestines that can lead to a feeling of fullness and pain.

Holistic understanding: Flatulence is caused by overeating, incomplete digestion, inadequately cooked beans, and poor food combining. Eating sugar with meat is an especially gas-promoting combination.

Herbal remedies: Make teas from the seeds of anise, caraway, fennel, and/or dill. You can also take peppermint leaf, lavender flowers, ginger root, and/or wild yam root. Try carrying a small vial of peppermint oil in your purse or pocket if you're traveling or eating out. Add 2 or 3 drops of the oil to a cup of hot water or peppermint tea and drink immediately after eating.

Herbal formulas: Mix 1 teaspoon peppermint leaf, 1/2 teaspoon ginger root, 1/2 teaspoon fennel seed, and 1/4 teaspoon cardamom seeds, and licorice root. Bring herbs and water to a boil, simmer the mixture for 5 minutes, and then let the blend steep for 10 minutes. Drink 1 cup of the tea, as needed.

Healthy habits: Don't mix protein with fruit and avoid cold drinks and coffee and tea with meals.

Gum Problem (Periodontal Disease)

Medical description: Gum inflammation and bleeding.

Holistic understanding: Gum problems are often the result of poor hygiene and dietary habits.

Herbal remedies: You can use bloodroot, available in many toothpastes and mouthwashes or as a diluted tincture, to protect your teeth and gums against bacteria. Other useful herbs include myrrh gum to tighten gums and echinacea root to help your body resist bacteria.

Herbal formulas: I use a tincture formula containing echinacea root, myrrh gum, ginger root, with a little bloodroot and peppermint oil as a preventive measure against gum disease and plaque. Similar commercial formulas are available in herb shops and natural food stores. Apply 1 or 2 drops of these tinctured herbs on top of your toothpaste and brush regularly.

Healthy habits: Keep sweet treats to a minimum and try to at least rinse, if not brush, your mouth after every meal. Floss and brush thoroughly with an herbal rinse at the end of each day.

Hangover

Medical description: Unpleasant physical symptoms like headache, nausea, and vomiting resulting from excessive use of alcohol.

Holistic understanding: The toxic effects of alcohol (and other chemical by-products that your body creates from alcohol) affect your entire body.

Herbal remedies: Take ginseng root in tincture, tea, or capsule form to regulate your digestion and balance your energy. Always take 2 tablets or capsules of milk thistle extract twice daily when you're drinking. Liver cooling and detoxifying herbs can assist your body in geting rid of toxins. I recommend dandelion leaf and root, yellow dock root, and chicory root and about half the amount of gentian root.

Herbal formulas: Simmer 1 tablespoon each of dandelion root, dandelion leaf, and a teaspoon of ginger rhizome per 3 cups of water for 20 minutes. Drink 1 cup of the cool tea, several times a day. Add 1 tablespoon of the Chinese herb kudzu when it's available.

Healthy habits: After drinking alcohol, drink as much pure water as possible to help clear the bloodstream. I recommend 2 eight-ounce glasses of pure water, with a little lemon added, for each drink that you've had.

Hay Fever

Medical description: An acute allergic condition of the mucous membranes of the upper respiratory tract and eyes with inflammation and symptoms of runny nose, itchy eyes, and sneezing.

Holistic understanding: Adrenal, immune, and digestive system weakness are often at the heart of hay fever.

Herbal remedies: Use nettle leaf and ginkgo leaf to calm your immune system and help prevent overreaction to pollen. Add eyebright herb, Mormon tea, and/or horseradish root to dry up excess secretions and keep your sinuses open. Add eleuthero (Siberian ginseng) root if you commonly experience fatigue. Take evening primrose oil in capsules to reduce inflammation. In severe cases, try also taking a good respiratory tract formula with herbs such as yerba santa leaf, grindelia flowers, marshmallow root, and usnea lichen. Do an essential oil steam with eucalyptus or peppermint once or twice daily by adding about 6 drops of eucalyptus or peppermint oil to a bowl of steaming water, covering your head with a towel, and inhaling the steam.

Herbal formulas: Mix 1 teaspoon each nettle leaf, eyebright herb, Oregon grape root, cleavers herb, and yarrow flowers in 4 cups water. Bring herbs and water to a boil, then steep the mixture for 20 minutes. Drink 1 cup of the tea, 2 or 3 times daily before meals. If you prefer, mix 1 teaspoon each of the individual tinctures in 1 cup of water and drink $^1/_2$ cup, 2 times daily.

Healthy habits: Add 1 or 2 tablespoons of flaxseed to the diet daily, and eat plenty of cayenne, ginger, garlic, onions, and horseradish. Choose high-quality whole foods, such as grains, legumes, and vegetables, including steamed greens. Get plenty of rest and avoid stressful situations to help keep your immune system strong.

Headache

Medical description: A pain felt in the head.

Holistic understanding: Headaches are often a sign of stress and tension with chronically tight neck and shoulder muscles or a liver imbalance.

Herbal remedies: Take pain-relieving herbs like valerian root, Roman chamomile flowers, Jamaican dogwood, or meadowsweet herb, and/or beneficial circulatory herbs like ginger root and ginkgo leaf. You can apply peppermint or lavender essential oil compresses to the forehead, using 2 drops essential oil in 1 cup water.

Herbal formulas: Mix 1 teaspoon each wood betony leaves and flowers, ginger root, feverfew herb, passion flower herb, and periwinkle leaf (if available) for each 3 cups of water. Bring herbs and water to a boil, then steep the mixture for 20 minutes. Drink 1 cup of the tea, 2 or 3 times daily, before meals. If you prefer, mix 1 teaspoon each of the individual tinctures in 1 cup of water and drink 1/2 cup, 2 times daily. Feverfew is the best herb for preventing migraines. I've seen patients get results when nothing else would work, but remember to take it every day for at least four months to see whether or not it works for you. Take 1 capsule of the powdered herb or extract, or 1 dropperful of the liquid tincture, 2 times daily.

Use liver regulating and cooling herbs for chronic headaches or temple headaches. I get good results with the herbs boldo leaf, artichoke leaf, and dandelion root, either singly or in combination.

Healthy habits: Take hot foot baths and practice deep breathing. Exercising regularly can help prevent tension headaches. Massage of the neck, shoulders, and the area at the back of your skull often provides relief.

Heartburn

Medical description: A burning pain behind the breastbone, associated with a spasm or irritation of the lower end of the esophagus or upper stomach.

Holistic understanding: This condition is often the result of stress, eating highly spiced food, or eating rich foods like greasy sauces and casseroles.

Herbal remedies: Use soothing herbs such as marshmallow root, licorice root, ginger root, peppermint leaf, and/or chamomile flowers. Herbs to relax your intestinal tract include chamomile flowers and wild yam root.

Herbal formulas: Simmer 1 teaspoon each of marshmallow root, licorice root, and wild yam root for every 2 cups of water. Turn off heat, add 1 teaspoon of peppermint leaf, then steep for 15 minutes. Drink 1 cup of the tea, 2 or 3 times daily, before meals. If you prefer, mix 1 teaspoon each of the individual tinctures in 1 cup of water and drink 1/2 cup, 2 times daily.

Healthy habits: Avoid high protein foods and overly spicy foods and emphasize grains and steamed vegetables. Try not to eat when you're emotionally upset or in a hurry. Eat slowly and chew your food well.

Hemorrhoids

Medical description: Enlarged veins in the wall of the anus, sometimes with pain and bleeding.

Holistic understanding: Hemorrhoids are often caused by excessive sitting or standing, lack of exercise, dry feces, and straining when constipated.

Herbal remedies: Take horse chestnut extract in capsule or tablet form. Follow instructions on the package. Add 1 teaspoon of stone root tincture in 1 cup of water, and drink 1/2 cup, 2 times daily. Apply a witch hazel liniment or horse chestnut ointment externally to the area to help strengthen the veins. Use soothing, anti-inflammatory, and bowel-softening herbs, such as marshmallow root, flaxseed, and chamomile flowers as teas. If your feces are dry or hard, drink 1/2 cup of aloe juice, 2 times daily, or take bowel tonic herbs like yellow dock root or cascara bark for short periods.

Herbal formulas: Simmer 1 teaspoon each of stone root, wild yam root, and witch hazel leaf for each 2 cups of water for 20 minutes. Add 1/2 cup of aloe juice, and drink 1 cup of the mixture, 2 or 3 times daily before meals. If you prefer, mix 1 teaspoon each of the individual tinctures in 1 cup of water or 1/2 cup of aloe juice, and drink 1/2 cup, 2 times daily.

Healthy habits: Increase your intake of water, yogurt, and fiber, including psyllium seeds, and get plenty of exercise. Add three capsules a day of a good acidophilus supplement, which supports the health and balance of your intestinal flora, found in many natural food stores and even supermarkets. Take 2 capsules in the morning and 1 in the evening, with meals.

Hepatitis

Medical description: An inflammatory condition of the liver associated with viral infection, toxic substances, or an autoimmune condition. If you have hepatitis, you must consult with your doctor and/or herbalist.

Holistic understanding: Hepatitis is inflammation of the liver due to a virus. You can overheat your liver and create an internal environment where a virus can flourish by indulging in strong emotions (like anger) and consuming substances that are irritating or toxic to your liver (like alcohol).

Herbal remedies: Take the liver protecting herbs milk thistle seed and schisandra berry, the anti-inflammatory herbs turmeric root and St. John's wort leaf and flower (also an anti-viral), the immune enhancing shiitake mushroom, and/or the bile-moving herb artichoke leaf.

Herbal formulas: Mix 1 teaspoon each of dandelion root, artichoke leaf, Oregon grape root, 1/2 teaspoon turmeric and ginger rhizomes, and 1/2 teaspoon gentian root in 4 cups water. Bring herbs and water to a boil, then simmer the mixture for 20 minutes. Drink 1 cup of the tea, 2 or 3 times daily before meals. If you prefer, mix 1 teaspoon each of the individual tinctures in 1 cup of water and drink 1/2 cup, 2 times daily.

Healthy habits: Avoid any foods, drinks, or other substances that can irritate or overheat your liver. This includes alcohol; recreational or pharmaceutical drugs; and fried, spicy, or heavy foods. Focus on greens, grains, and legumes. Incorporate juiced vegetables, such as carrot, celery, cabbage, and parsley, into your diet.

Herpes (Genital)

Medical description: Infection with several types of herpes viruses. The virus may be latent in nerve centers for many years with no symptoms, or it may produce small painful sores on the genitals or mouth from time to time.

Holistic understanding: Herpes is related to damp heat in Traditional Chinese Medicine. A weakened immune system and continual exposure to stress can bring on the herpes sores.

Herbal remedies: Herbs to clear damp heat from the bowels can help prevent breakouts. I recommend cooling herbs like yellow dock root, Oregon grape root, the Chinese herb coptis, or dandelion root. You can also take immune strengthening herbs like shiitake and reishi mushrooms as a tea, or as an extract in capsules or tablets, or the immune stimulant echinacea for ten days during an outbreak. Anti-viral herbs to discourage the virus from staying active include lemon balm herb, garlic, and St. John's wort leaf and flower.

Herbal formulas: Make a decoction of lemon balm herb by simmering 1 tablespoon for every cup of water for 30 minutes. Let the brew steep for 15 minutes and drink 1 cup, several times daily. You can also apply a lemon balm cream externally right on the sores to speed healing.

Healthy habits: See suggestions under the "Cold Sore" section.

High Blood Pressure

Medical description: Mild hypertension or high blood pressure is a systolic pressure over 140 mm/hg, and a diastolic pressure over 90 mm/hg. If you have high blood pressure, consult with your doctor and/or herbalist.

Holistic understanding: Blood pressure is affected by stress, diet, and heredity. Blood pressure tends to go up as people age and is influenced by salt intake.

Herbal remedies: Use beneficial cardiovascular herbs, such as shepherd's purse herb, alfalfa leaf, garlic, and hawthorn leaves and flowers and relaxing herbs, such as passion flower herb and California poppy root.

Herbal formulas: Make an infusion by steeping 1 tablespoon each of hawthorn leaves and flowers and shepherd's purse herb and a teaspoon of celery seed and yarrow herb in 3 cups of water. Drink 1/2 to 1 cup of the tea, 2 or 3 times daily before meals. If you prefer, mix 1 teaspoon each of the individual tinctures in 1 cup of water and drink 1/2 cup, 2 times daily.

Healthy habits: Relaxation is an ingredient in lowering your blood pressure. Try meditation, stretching, walking, or yoga. Use coffee, black tea, and salt in moderation. Reduce your salt intake drastically. I recommend a salt-free vegetable salt substitute or a sea vegetable seasoning (like nori flakes) that do have a little salt, but also contain many other minerals.

Hot Flashes

Medical description: Feelings of heat in the body, especially in the face and neck, followed by sweating, generally associated with changing levels of sex hormones during menopause.

Holistic understanding: Hot flashes (feminine power surges) are possibly the result of the body attempting to normalize hormone balance.

Herbal remedies: Use hormone-regulating herbs such as vitex berries, dong quai root, black cohosh root, or ginseng root and evening primrose oil.

Herbal formulas: Simmer 1 teaspoon each of linden leaf, red raspberry leaf, and black cohosh root in 3 cups water for 15 minutes, and remove from the heat. Add 1 teaspoon of lemon balm and 1 teaspoon of yarrow herb and flowers and steep for 15 minutes. Drink 1 cup of the tea, 2 or 3 times daily, before meals. If you prefer, mix 1 teaspoon each of the individual tinctures in 1 cup of water and drink 1/2 cup, 2 times daily.

Healthy habits: Follow a low-fat, high-fiber diet, with plenty of flaxseed oil and the omega-3 fatty acids found in trout, salmon, and mackerel. Include ample phytoestrogen-containing foods, such as soybeans, tofu, black beans, red kidney beans, black-eyed peas, azuki beans, and red lentils. Red clover extracts are available in tablet form standardized to phytoestrogens. Many women who exercise at least 3 or 4 hours per week don't experience hot flashes at all.

Infection

Medical description: Invasion of the body by pathogens, such as viruses or bacteria. If you have a particularly severe or prolonged infection, consult with your doctor or herbalist.

Holistic understanding: Acute infections are often the result of poor hygiene, weakened immunity, or exposure to bacteria or fungus.

Herbal remedies: Take immune-strengthening, antibacterial herbs such as echinacea root and usnea lichen, the antivirals osha root and garlic, and the antiseptic and immune-activating herb yerba mansa root. You can also use infection-fighting essential oils of lavender, cedar, lemon, sage, or thyme in baths or massage oils.

Herbal formulas: Mix 1 teaspoon each of American ginseng root, echinacea root, and wild indigo root in 4 cups water. Bring herbs and water to a boil, simmer for 10 minutes, then steep the mixture for 20 minutes. Drink 1 cup of the tea, 2 or 3 times daily before meals. If you prefer, mix 1 teaspoon each of the individual tinctures in 1 cup of water and drink 1/2 cup, 2 times daily.

Healthy habits: Adopt a cleansing diet emphasizing fresh fruits and vegetables and freshly-squeezed juices. Eat 1 clove of raw garlic twice daily with meals, preferably juiced in carrot-parsley juice to cut the odor. You can also use an odor-controlled garlic product that contains some of garlic's main antibiotic compound, allicin, but don't use an aged product.

Indigestion

Medical description: Pain or discomfort in the abdomen after eating.

Holistic understanding: Eating while stressed or in a hurry, improper food combining, and overeating all contribute to poor or painful digestion.

Herbal remedies: Take gentian root, dandelion root, and artichoke leaf in tincture form to move the bile and increase digestion. Also use the digestion-enhancing herbs ginger rhizome, peppermint leaf, and chamomile flowers in tea form. Sprinkle cayenne powder on your food or take it in capsules.

Herbal formulas: Mix 1 teaspoon each of artichoke leaf, orange peel, hops strobiles, gentian root, and angelica root in 3 cups water. Bring herbs and water to a boil, then simmer the mixture for 20 minutes. Drink 1 cup of the tea, 2 or 3 times daily, before meals. If you prefer, mix 1 teaspoon each of the individual tinctures in 1 cup of water and drink 1/2 cup, 2 times daily.

Healthy habits: Eat papaya and pineapple, which both aid digestion. Try to eat slowly, without distractions, and refrain from drinking cold beverages at mealtime. Eat small, frequent meals.

Insomnia

Medical description: The inability to fall asleep or to remain asleep.

Holistic understanding: Insomnia is caused by a wide variety of factors including genetics, emotional difficulty, and physical imbalances.

Herbal remedies: Take herbs to relax you and strengthen your nerves such as St. John's wort leaf and flower, valerian root, California poppy root, kava root, passion flower herb, and/or reishi mushroom. Try adding a few drops of lavender oil to a foot bath or regular bath before bedtime.

Herbal formulas: Mix 1 teaspoon each of valerian root, kava root, linden flowers, chamomile flowers, and catnip leaf in 4 cups water. Bring herbs and water to a boil, then simmer the mixture for 20 minutes. Drink 1 cup of the tea, 2 or 3 times daily before meals. If you prefer, mix 1 teaspoon each of the individual tinctures in 1 cup of water and drink 1/2 cup, 2 times daily.

Healthy habits: Massage therapy, meditation, and regular exercise are often helpful when dealing with sleep problems. Add plenty of tryptophan-rich foods, such as spirulina (a popular blue-green algae supplement), yeast, legumes, nuts, yogurt, and grains to your diet. I find that mineral supplements with at least 800 mg of calcium and 600 mg of magnesium, taken daily, help calm some of my patients and improve their sleep quality.

Irritable Bowel Syndrome

Medical description: A condition involving recurrent abdominal pain with constipation and/or diarrhea.

Holistic understanding: This condition is often associated with food allergies and may be the result of chronic irritation from eating too much processed food, meat, and sugar.

Herbal remedies: Use soothing, anti-inflammatory herbs such as chamomile flowers, marshmallow root, plantain leaf, licorice root, wild yam root, and flaxseed. Take peppermint oil in enteric-coated capsules. Homeopathic belladonna tablets are sometimes effective.

Herbal formulas: Mix 1 teaspoon each of marshmallow root, wild yam root, and 1/2 teaspoon of licorice root in 4 cups water. Bring herbs and water to a boil, then simmer the mixture for 20 minutes. Add one tablespoon of peppermint leaf and let the brew steep for 15 minutes. Drink 1 cup of the tea, 2 or 3 times daily, before meals. If you prefer, mix 1 teaspoon each of the individual tinctures in 1 cup of water and drink 1/2 cup, 2 times daily.

Healthy habits: Avoid alcohol, tobacco, caffeine, dairy, and eggs.

Jet Lag

Medical description: Jet leg is a set of symptoms that occur after a plane flight, especially longer flights where more than a three-hour time change occurs. Symptoms include a feeling of pressure in the head, fatigue, dizziness, depression, and nausea. The changes are related to the disruption and readjustment of hormone levels and biorhythms.

Holistic understanding: I find that you usually suffer more from jet lag if you have a weak adrenal or digestive system.

Herbal remedies: Take herbs which help you adapt to stress, such as eleuthero (Siberian ginseng) root, reishi mushroom, and shisandra berries. I travel a lot, and I find if I take eleuthero a few days before, during, and after flying, I rarely experience unpleasant symptoms. If you're constantly traveling, or if you have serious jet lag, take St. John's wort leaf and flower continuously for a few weeks before a major trip and for a week or two after.

Herbal formulas: Mix 1 teaspoon each of eleuthero (Siberian ginseng) root, shisandra berries, echinacea root, and wild oats spikelets in 4 cups water. Bring herbs and water to a boil, then simmer the mixture for 20 minutes. Drink 1 cup of the tea, 2 or 3 times daily, before meals. If you prefer, mix 1 teaspoon each of the individual tinctures in 1 cup of water and drink 1/2 cup, 2 times daily.

Healthy habits: Fast or eat lightly during long trips and drink plenty of water. Try to get aerobic exercise just before and just after a trip.

Laryngitis

Medical description: Inflammation of the larynx with symptoms of hoarseness and sore throat.

Holistic understanding: Laryngitis is commonly associated with stress and tension, as well as throat strain or infection.

Herbal remedies: Drinking warm cups of one or more of the following soothing teas may help you get your voice back more quickly: licorice root, marshmallow root, plantain leaf and/or sage leaf, with lemon juice added. If you like it hot, try gargling with a pinch of cayenne powder mixed with water. Try a steam inhalation with water and vinegar, or you can do an essential oil steam by adding about 6 drops of sandalwood or lavender oil to a bowl of steaming water, covering your head with a towel, and inhaling.

Herbal formulas: You can purchase throat sprays containing herbs like echinacea root, sage leaf, and marshmallow root to help heal laryngitis.

Healthy habits: Try to rest your voice during the healing process.

Leg Cramp

Medical description: Painful tightening or contractions of the leg muscles.

Holistic understanding: Leg cramps occur when you have improper circulation to the legs, as a result of inactivity, vascular disease such as atherosclerosis, and venous spasms of the legs caused by smoking.

Herbal remedies: You can improve your circulation and prevent leg cramps by drinking teas made from kava, hawthorn leaves and flowers, motherwort herb, ginkgo leaf, ginger rhizome, prickly ash bark, and/or cayenne fruits. Horse chestnut is a modern and effective treatment. Use it for several months to see if you respond to the herb. You can also rub a small amount of horse chestnut cream onto the areas that cramp. If you have troublesome leg cramps that occur often, see your herbalist about trying a preparation of Peruvian bark.

Herbal formulas: Mix 1 teaspoon each of hawthorn leaves and flowers, motherwort herb, and ginger rhizome in 4 cups water. Bring herbs and water to a boil, then simmer the mixture for 20 minutes. Drink 1 cup of the tea, 2 or 3 times daily, before meals. If you prefer, mix 1 teaspoon each of the individual tinctures in 1 cup of water and drink 1/2 cup, 2 times daily.

Healthy habits: Add the magnesium-rich herbs oatstraw, Irish moss, licorice root, kelp, and nettles to your diet. For persistent leg cramps, add magnesium and vitamin E supplements to your diet. Take 400 to 500 mg of magnesium, twice daily, and 400 IU to 800 IU of vitamin E per day.

Lice (Head and Pubic)

Medical description: A small wingless parasitic insect that lives in your pubic or head hair, biting and sucking blood for nourishment. Itching can be severe in people who react to the bites.

Holistic understanding: Lice thrive in overcrowded, unclean environments, but kids can easily transmit them anywhere during social interaction.

Herbal remedies: Make a strong tea with quassia bark, rosemary leaves, or horsetail herb and wash the affected areas with it. You can also add 20 drops essential oil of tea tree and 20 of rosemary oil to 2 ounces almond, apricot, or other vegetable oil. Apply it to the hair and massage into the scalp. Leave on for 1 hour and shampoo it out. Don't let any oil get into your eyes.

Herbal formulas: Add 1 tablespoon each of quassia bark, rosemary leaf, and horsetail herb tincture to 1/2 cup of water and 1/2 cup vinegar and rinse your scalp or pubic area with it, several times daily.

Healthy habits: Frequently wash your bedding, clothes, and combs, and avoid contact with others who are infected.

Lymph Gland (Swollen)

Medical description: Inflammation and swelling of the lymph nodes, most commonly those in the neck, under the arms, and groin area.

Holistic understanding: Swollen lymph glands are often the result of an infection. When lymph node swelling goes on a long time, suspect a viral infection and immune weakness.

Herbal remedies: Try using herbs that have a cleansing effect on the lymphatic system, such as red root, echinacea root, wild indigo root, ocotillo bark, mullein leaf, and/or cleavers herb. Figwort root is a specific and effective remedy for lymphatic swelling in the neck. It is available as a Chinese herb or western herb in tincture form and as a bulk herb. Don't take figwort if you're taking heart medications like digoxin.

Herbal formulas: Mix 1 teaspoon each of red root, red clover flowers, burdock root, echinacea root, and figwort root (if it's available) in 4 cups water. Bring herbs and water to a boil, then simmer the mixture for 20 minutes. Drink 1 cup of the tea, 2 or 3 times daily, before meals. If you prefer, mix 1 teaspoon each of the individual tinctures in 1 cup of water and drink 1/2 cup, 2 times daily. Ask your herbalist about poke root tincture. Poke is toxic unless used carefully, but it's a potent lymphatic stimulant.

Healthy habits: Apply alternate hot and cold compresses to your swollen glands. Pour 5 or 6 drops of castor oil in your palm and rub the oil into the skin over the swollen lymph node, several times daily.

Menopause

Medical description: Cessation of menstruation when the ovaries cease releasing eggs and producing estrogen.

Holistic understanding: Your body naturally shifts to a less stimulating estrogen called estrone, usually during your late forties and early fifties. If you're in good emotional and physical health, this transition is often smooth and symptom-free. After a few years, you may start losing bone density and experience vaginal dryness and a thinning of the vaginal wall, as well as a weakening of the bladder. After ten years, you're more prone to dying of a heart attack or stroke than before menopause when you received protection from your strong circulating estrogen. Hot flashes and night sweats may be a problem for women going through menopause.

Herbal remedies: Take the hormone-regulating herbs vitex berries, black cohosh root, red ginseng root, and dong quai root. I've seen great results with a combination of vitex and black cohosh for relieving hot flashes, sugar cravings, depression, and other unpleasant symptoms that often occur during menopause. If you feel depressed, add St. John's wort leaf and flower to the mixture. Exciting new evidence indicates that regular use of phytoestrogens can help protect your bones and cardiovascular system while reducing hot flashes and other symptoms that sometimes occur. Phytoestrogens are found naturally in flaxseed meal and oil, all beans, including soybeans and soy products, and other members of the pea family like red clover and kudzu root. Ready-made products are available in capsule, tablet, and powder form.

Herbal formulas: Mix 1 teaspoon each of black cohosh root, vitex berries, ginseng root, kudzu root, dong quai root, and motherwort herb in 4 cups of water. Bring herbs and water to a boil, then simmer the mixture for 20 minutes. Drink 1/2 to 1 cup of the tea, 2 or 3 times daily, before meals. If you prefer, mix 1 teaspoon each of the individual tinctures in 1 cup of water and drink 1/2 cup, 2 times daily.

Healthy habits: Follow a high-fiber, low-fat diet with emphasis on phytoestrogen-containing foods, such as soybeans, tofu, black beans, red kidney beans, black-eyed peas, azuki beans, and red lentils. Eat at least 2 teaspoons flaxseed daily, or take high-lignan flaxseed oil by the teaspoon or in capsules daily. Use the following essential oils in bath or massage oils: lemon, clary sage, jasmine, and lavender. Get plenty of exercise to help keep this period of your life symptom-free. Don't forget that you can get better protection from heart disease with a healthy diet, exercise, and stress-reduction than from estrogen.

Menstrual Cramps

Medical description: Cramping of the uterine muscle, often during menses.

Holistic understanding: Menstrual pain is sometimes aggravated by tension, insufficient exercise, poor dietary habits, nervous tension, tight muscles, and the use of stimulants.

Herbal remedies: Use cramp bark, valerian root, and kava root to ease menstrual cramps. Massage your abdomen and lower back with a massage oil containing lavender, marjoram, and chamomile essential oils in a base of St. John's wort oil.

Herbal formulas: Try this powerful blend of relaxing and pain-relieving herbs. Mix 1 teaspoon each of cramp bark, motherwort herb, valerian root, kava root, and skullcap leaves and flowers in 4 cups water. Bring herbs and water to a boil, then simmer for 20 minutes. Add 1 tablespoon of chamomile flowers and let the tea steep for another 20 minutes. Drink 1 cup of the tea, 2 or 3 times daily before meals. If you prefer, mix 1 teaspoon each of the individual tinctures in 1 cup of water and drink $^1/_2$ cup, 2 times daily.

Healthy habits: Increase your intake of spinach, beans, millet, green leafy vegetables, and seeds (especially flaxseed) and nuts. Avoid fried foods, alcohol, meat, and dairy products. Get plenty of exercise and sunshine and try to take time for relaxation around the time of your period.

Memory (Poor)

Medical description: Memory generally declines with age, often accompanied by loss of alertness and awareness.

Holistic understanding: Poor memory often occurs in the elderly as the brain is progressively starved for blood, oxygen, and nutrients as the blood vessels are clogged and hardened from a poor diet, stress, and stimulants. The vessels decline, and the brain doesn't receive adequate oxygen. Poor memory sometimes results from inadequate exercising of the brain. As you get older, keep stimulating and challenging your mind, for example, by taking a new course of study every five or ten years.

Herbal remedies: Drink ginkgo leaf and rosemary leaf teas and take cayenne powder in capsules to increase circulation to your brain. You may also want to use the brain tonic, gotu kola herb.

Herbal formulas: Mix 1 teaspoon each of ginkgo leaf, gotu kola herb, ginseng root, wild oats herb, and nettle leaf in 4 cups water. Bring herbs and water to a boil, then steep the mixture for 20 minutes. Drink 1 cup of the tea, 2 or 3 times daily, before meals. If you prefer, mix 1 teaspoon each of the individual tinctures in 1 cup of water and drink $^1/_2$ cup, 2 times daily.

Healthy habits: Follow a cardiovascular health program, do deep breathing, and avoid excessive worry. Rest the mind with regular meditation breaks. Habitual stress can wreak havoc with your memory. Reduce stress with meditation, yoga stretching, and regular exercise.

Migraine

Medical description: Severe, recurring headaches which often affect only one side of the head.

Holistic understanding: Although this condition can have a genetic component, it's often related to food allergies, immune weakness, and chronic stress or tension.

Herbal remedies: Feverfew herb, skullcap herb, ginkgo leaf, and ginger rhizome all have good track records for migraines by reducing inflammation, increasing circulation to the brain, and relieving pain. I've seen patients get great results with feverfew herb. The key is to stick with feverfew daily for several months. Feverfew works slowly, and you can't count it out as being effective for you unless you take the herb for at least three to five months in my experience. It's effective in capsule, tablet, or liquid tincture form. You can even grow the plant in your garden and eat 2 leaves every day, if you like bitter and spicy herbs.

Herbal formulas: Mix 1 teaspoon each of feverfew herb, periwinkle herb, ginger rhizome, and skullcap herb in 4 cups water. Bring herbs and water to a boil, then steep the mixture for 20 minutes. Drink 1 cup of the tea, 2 or 3 times daily, before meals. If you prefer, mix 1 teaspoon each of the individual tinctures in 1 cup of water and drink 1/2 cup, 2 times daily.

Healthy habits: Try stretching and massage therapy to keep blood flowing evenly into your head. Check for sensitivity to the following foods known to trigger migraines: ripened cheeses, sausage, onions, pickles, cured meats, red wine, sour cream, nuts, chocolate, coffee, and tea.

Morning Sickness

Medical description: Nausea and vomiting that often occur during the first 3 months of pregnancy.

Holistic understanding: Morning sickness is generally the result of the hormonal changes taking place in the body. Some researchers feel that morning sickness is the body's natural way to protect the baby by removing toxic chemicals from the body with regular purging. I find that mothers who prepare for pregnancy by following a regular program of cleansing and fasting for six months or so have much less morning sickness.

Herbal remedies: Prepare nausea-preventing tea infusions like ginger rhizome, lavender flowers, peppermint leaf, peach leaf, and/or wild yam root. In Chinese medicine the herb perilla, taken as a tea, is used for morning sickness. Ginger is the most important remedy for morning sickness and is valuable and effective for many mothers. Use fresh ginger rhizome infusion right from the store — dried ginger is not recommended for use during pregnancy in Traditional Chinese Medicine.

Herbal formulas: Mix 1 teaspoon each fresh ginger rhizome, wild yam root, orange peel, and lavender flowers in 4 cups water. Simmer the herbs for a few minutes, then steep the mixture for 20 minutes. Drink 1 cup of the tea, 2 or 3 times daily, before meals. If you prefer, mix 1 teaspoon each of the individual tinctures in 1 cup of water and drink 1/2 cup, 2 times daily.

Healthy habits: Eat dry toast or crackers first thing in the morning and eat small, frequent meals during the day. Keep oils to a minimum.

Motion Sickness

Medical Description. Feeling of nausea, sometimes accompanied by vomiting, caused by movement during car, boat, or air travel.

Holistic understanding: None.

Herbal remedies: Try taking ginger capsules 1/2 hour before departure and then every 2 or 3 hours as needed. This herb has been shown in clinical trials to be more effective than Dramamine to reduce the tendency of nausea, vomiting, and dizziness. You can also try eating crystallized ginger or drinking ginger ale — not the kind with ginger flavoring and sugar — but the high quality kind with real ginger available in natural-foods stores.

Herbal formulas: Simmer 1 tablespoon of dried ginger rhizome for every cup of water for 10 minutes. Add 1 teaspoon of lavender flowers, and let the mixture steep for 10 minutes. Drink 1/2 cup to 1 cup, several times daily.

Healthy habits: Try to slow your breathing. You may also apply cool compresses to your forehead. The best pressure point for preventing and reducing nausea from motion sickness is called P6 in Chinese medicine. The point is located two finger-widths above the wrist (toward your elbow) on the inside of your wrist between the two tendons. Press hard for a minute or two as needed.

Muscle Ache

Medical description: Soreness in the muscles.

Holistic understanding: Aching muscles are often the result of exercise, injury, muscular tension, and blood stagnation caused by sedentary habits.

Herbal remedies: Apply arnica cream or oil or horse chestnut cream to your aching muscles, and take arnica internally as well in homeopathic form only. Drink teas or take tinctures made from black cohosh root, a known muscle relaxant, and St. John's wort flowers and leaves, an excellent anti-inflammatory and pain-relieving herb. Kava root is one of the best muscle relaxants, and it helps you let go of tension and enjoy your body again. Kava root is available in tincture form or in capsules and tablets.

Herbal formulas: Simmer 1 teaspoon each of kava root and passion flower herb in 4 cups water. Add 1 teaspoon of linden flowers, chamomile flowers, and lemon balm herb, and let the brew steep for 15 minutes. Drink 1 cup of the tea, 2 or 3 times daily, before meals. If you prefer, mix 1 teaspoon each of the individual tinctures in 1 cup of water and drink $^1/_2$ cup, 2 times daily.

Healthy habits: For muscle soreness due to injury or stretching, apply cold compresses to the affected area for the first day, then do several rounds of alternate hot and cold ones (3 minutes hot, 1 minute cold). Use ginger compresses for 15 minutes at a time for muscular soreness.

Nausea

Medical description: Nausea is the feeling of being on the verge of vomiting. For prolonged nausea, seek the advice of your doctor or herbalist.

Holistic understanding: Nausea may be related to a variety of disorders, including infections, emotional stress, metabolic disorders, or from eating bad food or too much food.

Herbal remedies: Drink teas made from the stomach-settling herbs like lavender flowers, ginger rhizome, peppermint leaf, wild yam root, and/or cinnamon bark. Inhale a whiff of essential oils of peppermint, lavender, chamomile, or rose to help settle your stomach.

Herbal formulas: Take 1 capsule each of these herb powders: cinnamon, ginger, cayenne, and goldenseal. The anti-nausea Chinese medicine, called Curing Pills, is available in many herb shops and natural food stores.

Healthy habits: If you're prone to nausea after eating, reduce your food intake, and eat small, frequent meals. Eat only when you're hungry, and especially when you're relaxed and not stressed or distracted. I'm a big advocate of daily self-massage of the abdominal area. Lie flat on your back with a pillow under your knees, and gently but firmly massage your entire abdomen using small circular movements with your finger tips. Practice breathing deeply into your belly during the process. I've noticed that many of my patients are unaware of tension they store for years in the abdomen. When this tension is released, a major improvement occurs in energy and in the ease of digestion.

Osteoporosis

Medical description: A loss of bony tissue resulting in brittle bones, and eventually fractures.

Holistic understanding: Although heredity is a factor, you can decrease the risks of osteoporosis in later life through proper diet and adequate exercise, especially when you're young, but also all through your life. At any age, you can improve your diet and exercise patterns to improve bone strength.

Herbal remedies: Herbal sources of calcium include parsley leaf, dandelion greens, and watercress leaves. You may want to include other mineral-rich herbs like nettles, alfalfa, and horsetail in your herbal program.

Herbal formulas: Mix 1 teaspoon each horsetail herb, oat straw, nettles herb, parsley leaf, and dandelion leaf in 4 cups water. Bring herbs and water to a boil, then steep the mixture for 20 minutes. Drink 1 cup of the tea, 2 or 3 times daily, before meals. If you prefer, mix 1 teaspoon each of the individual tinctures in 1 cup of water and drink $^1/_2$ cup, 2 times daily.

Healthy habits: Exercise is the single most important preventive measure against osteoporosis. Include weight-bearing or isometric exercises in your regime. Eat plenty of high-calcium foods, such as collard and turnip greens, yogurt, dried figs, spinach, kale, broccoli, and tofu. Regular use of sea vegetables like wakame, nori, and kelp is essential because these foods are the highest vegetable source of calcium, magnesium, and all the other elements you need to build strong bones. Besides calcium, you need magnesium, silica, and vitamin D to build the strongest bones. You may want to take a supplement with these nutrients for extra protection, especially if you're not eating an excellent diet. I recommend that you be moderate with coffee, refined sugar, and soft drinks, which rob your bones of minerals and strength, especially if you have weak bones.

PMS

Medical description: PMS comprises many symptoms, such as depression, irritability, and water retention, which occur in the few days before the onset of menstruation. These symptoms must come and go in relationship to your menstrual cycle for a doctor to give that medical diagnosis.

Holistic understanding: A number of interconnected factors, including diet, hormones, stressors, and physical and mental health, play a role in PMS.

Herbal remedies: To help you with PMS symptoms, take vitex berries for four to six months to regulate your hormones. Continue indefinitely if you find it helpful. Dandelion root is another important herb, because it helps the liver remove excess estrogen. If you're also feeling tense and irritable, take liver-balancing herbs like boldo leaf or burdock root and calming herbs like chamomile flowers, valerian rhizome, skullcap herb, and kava root.

Herbal formulas: Mix 1 teaspoon each vitex berries, dandelion root, burdock root, lavender flowers, and prickly ash bark in 4 cups water. Bring to a boil, then steep the mixture for 20 minutes. Drink 1 cup of the tea, 2 or 3 times daily, before meals. If you prefer, mix 1 teaspoon each of the individual tinctures in 1 cup of water and drink $^1/_2$ cup, 2 times daily.

Healthy habits: Reduce your intake of salt, refined sugar products, coffee, and chocolate for at least 10 days before menstruation. Add 1 tablespoon flaxseed to your diet daily. I've often seen a big reduction in symptoms of PMS in my patients with regular practice of relaxation methods, including yoga, meditation, deep breathing, and aerobic exercise.

Pneumonia

Medical description: A bacterial or viral lung infection in which the air sacs fill up with exudate and pus. If you have a fever and severe respiratory symptoms, including a deep cough with yellow mucus, you may have pneumonia. Consult with your doctor or herbalist.

Holistic understanding: Pneumonia is usually caused by a number of different viruses or bacteria and often follows an upper respiratory tract infection. A condition of damp heat in the body, as well as a weakened immune system, increase your risk of developing pneumonia.

Herbal remedies: Try antibacterial herbs, like echinacea root, wild indigo root, osha root, goldenseal root, and usnea lichen, and soothing herbs such as marshmallow. Do a steam inhalation with eucalyptus oil.

Herbal formulas: Mix 1 teaspoon each echinacea root, osha root, goldenseal root, and 1/2 teaspoon of licorice root in 4 cups water. Bring herbs and water to a boil, then steep the mixture for 20 minutes. Drink 1 cup of the tea, 2 or 3 times daily, before meals. If you prefer, mix 1 teaspoon each of the individual tinctures in 1 cup of water and drink 1/2 cup, 2 times daily.

Healthy habits: Drink watery soups containing lots of onions and garlic. Eats a few cloves of fresh garlic each day. You may also want to apply onion externally in the form of a poultice. To make an onion poultice, sauté 1 large chopped onion and 3 tablespoons flaxseed in 2 tablespoons olive oil until onions are translucent. Wrap the mixture in cheesecloth and apply to the chest while warm. Cover with a hot water bottle and a towel. Leave on for 20 to 30 minutes. Rest and reduced stress are extremely helpful.

Poison Oak and Poison Ivy

Medical description: A red, hot, itchy rash caused by contact with poison oak or poison ivy leaves.

Holistic understanding: In Chinese medicine, poison oak or ivy rash is considered to relate to blood toxins and blood heat, so cooling and detoxifying herbs are used to treat this condition.

Herbal remedies: Take echinacea root, red clover flowers, or grindelia flowers tincture internally to cleanse the blood and reduce inflammation. Externally, apply the fresh juice of the astringent herbs jewelweed leaf or mugwort leaf or lotions made from these herbs, or grindelia tincture which stops the spreading of poison oak. Cooling and detoxifying herbs include dandelion root and Oregon grape root. Use them liberally as a tea or in tincture form during the rash. I find elder flower tea infusion, 3 or 4 cups a day, is excellent for helping to clear a poison oak or ivy rash.

Herbal formulas: For an external formula, dissolve 1/2 teaspoon salt in 1/2 cup water and add cosmetic clay until the mixture is creamy. Stir in 25 drops peppermint oil and apply to the affected area. For a quick lotion that I've found effective for reducing the heat and itching of the rash, add 1 teaspoon of salt and 1 teaspoon of peppermint oil to a bottle of calamine lotion and shake well before applying to the rash, 1 or 2 times daily.

Healthy habits: You can assist the body in its efforts to eliminate the heat and toxins from the poison oak or ivy by eating lightly for four or five days. Drink an eight-ounce glass of celery, cucumber, and parsley juice with a little apple or carrot every day. Drink lots of water with lemon juice.

Prostate Imbalance

Medical description: Benign prostatic hyperplasia (BPH) is the diagnosis given to this common condition of men over 50, with symptoms of nocturnal urination and restricted flow due to an enlarged prostate gland. The condition may be related to a reduction or change in metabolism in the hormone testosterone and in health habits.

Holistic understanding: Prostate imbalances are often caused by over consumption of red meat and sugar and excessive sitting.

Herbal remedies: Use saw palmetto berries, nettle root, and kava root to reduce prostate swelling and pain, improve urine flow, and increase blood circulation to the prostate. Saw palmetto is amazingly effective for some men. Start with 3 capsules or tablets a day of the hexane-free or *supercritical CO2* extract, and increase to 5 or even 6 a day if that doesn't work after two months or so.

Herbal formulas: Simmer 1 teaspoon each nettle root and herb, dandelion leaf, goldenrod herb, and 1/2 teaspoon of licorice root for each cup of water and drink 1/2 cup, 2 times daily.

Healthy habits: Include lots of vegetables, fruits, nuts, seeds, grains, and legumes in your diet. Eat plenty of zinc-containing foods, such as unroasted sesame butter, wheat germ, wheat bran, and pumpkin seeds. Avoid sugar, foods that are high in fat, and excessive sitting. Practice Kegel exercises, which are regular contraction and relaxation of the perineum, the area between your anus and the bottom of your scrotum. About 100 to 200 contractions a day is often the magic number.

Psoriasis

Medical description: A chronic skin disease with scaly white patches and inflammation.

Holistic understanding: Many herbalists contend that this chronic skin disease is related to digestive and liver imbalances.

Herbal remedies: Try liver-regulating herbs, such as burdock root, dandelion root, and the liver protector milk thistle seed; heat-clearing herbs, such as cleavers herb and elder flowers; blood purifiers, such as red clover flowers and sarsaparilla root; and immune tonics, such as reishi mushroom, ligustrum berries, and shiitake mushroom.

Herbal formulas: Simmer 1 teaspoon each of burdock root, dandelion root, red clover flowers, sarsaparilla root, and 1/2 teaspoon of ginger in 4 cups of water for 15 minutes and let steep for 15 minutes. Drink 1 cup of the tea, 2 or 3 times daily, before meals. If you prefer, mix 1 teaspoon each of the individual tinctures in 1 cup of water and drink 1/2 cup, 2 times daily.

Healthy habits: Follow a cleansing diet emphasizing fruits, vegetables, and juices for a few weeks. Avoid refined foods. Follow with a diet of steamed vegetables, whole grains, and legumes. Ocean swimming (not pool swimming) is recommended where possible, as well as an exercise program and fresh air.

Sciatica

Medical description: Pain along the sciatic nerve that usually radiates down the back of your leg.

Holistic understanding: Weakness of the bones and back muscles from excessive sitting and lack of exercise can lead to stagnation of blood, nutrients, and vital energy to the nerve roots of the lower back. This in turn can irritate the sciatic nerve and send a radiating pain down the leg. Injuries caused by strain from improper lifting can easily lead to a compressed disk that irritates the sciatic nerve.

Herbal remedies: Apply ginger rhizome compresses, wintergreen oil, St. John's wort oil, or horse chestnut cream externally to relieve pain and reduce inflammation. Try taking anti-inflammatory herbs, such as St. John's wort leaf and flower and Roman chamomile flowers, and pain-relieving herbs, such as California poppy flowering plant and valerian root internally.

Herbal formulas: Use a supplement daily containing one or more anti-inflammatory herbs like standardized turmeric extract, DGL (a special licorice extract), or bromelain, extracted from pineapple.

Healthy habits: Try daily walking, stretching, physical therapy, and hydrotherapy (the therapeutic application of hot and cold water) combined with a natural foods diet with high-quality protein. I've seen patients who had so much lower back and sciatic pain that they were willing to go for an operation, completely turn their pain around using this natural program. Through a total program of exercise, stretching, physical therapy, massage, diet, and herbal supplements, they were able to strengthen their back and relieve the pain. I don't recommend surgery except under the direst situations, because more often than not, this won't bring about permanent relief, and it does nothing to strengthen your back.

Shingles

Medical description: An acute inflammatory disease of the nerves caused by the virus *Herpes zoster,* accompanied by pain and burning, sometimes over large parts of the body.

Holistic understanding: Many causative factors lead to an attack of shingles, such as weakened immunity and emotional or physical stress.

Herbal remedies: Apply topical anti-inflammatories such as St. John's wort oil, lavender oil, or calendula oil. Try using flaxseed poultices or pain-relieving creams made from cayenne. Take oatmeal or barley baths to soothe the skin. Drink soothing teas, such as St. John's wort leaf and flower, lemon balm herb, passion flower herb, or skullcap herb. Apply a few drops of bergamot or basil essential oil diluted in St. John's wort oil directly to the affected areas. The use of a wild oat tincture is often recommended by herbalists.

Herbal formulas: Mix 1 teaspoon St. John's wort leaf and flower, calendula flowers, and lemon balm herb in 4 cups water. Bring herbs and water to a boil, then steep the mixture for 20 minutes. Drink 1 cup of the tea, 2 or 3 times daily, before meals. If you prefer, mix 1 teaspoon each of the individual tinctures in 1 cup of water and drink $^1/_2$ cup, 2 times daily. You can add 1 teaspoon of wild oat tincture to the blend.

Healthy habits: Reduce your intake of salt and high-protein foods and eat a whole-foods diet that emphasizes grains, legumes, and lightly-steamed vegetables. You may find relief from a concentrated preparation for external use that contains a natural ingredient from cayenne, called capsaicin, which is available as a prescription item.

Sinusitis

Medical description: Inflammation of the sinuses with labored breathing.

Holistic understanding: Accumulation of damp heat in your body, along with a weakened immune response, can increase your chances of having sinusitis.

Herbal remedies: Try a strong sinus-clearing herb like horseradish root, immune-supporting herbs like echinacea root and garlic, and heat-clearing herbs like goldenseal root or wild indigo root.

Herbal formulas: Simmer 1 teaspoon each of echinacea root and either goldenseal root or the Chinese herb coptis in 4 cups water. Bring herbs and water to a boil, then steep the mixture for 20 minutes. Drink 1 cup of the tea, 2 or 3 times daily, before meals. If you prefer, mix 1 teaspoon each of the individual tinctures in 1 cup of water and drink $^1/_2$ cup, 2 times daily. The Chinese herb formula called *Huang Lian Su* is effective for sinusitis when taken for 4 or 5 days, along with echinacea leaf and root tincture. The product is available in some herb shops or from your acupuncturist.

Healthy habits: Add plenty of onions, garlic, cayenne, and horseradish to your food to help clear your nasal passages. Grate horseradish and hold a small amount of it in your mouth. Even inhaling the fumes while grating horseradish helps relieve sinusitis symptoms. Avoid sugar and fried foods during the infection.

Smoking (to Stop)

Medical description: An addiction to the nicotine in tobacco from smoking or chewing the product is extremely difficult for most people to break.

Holistic understanding: To stop smoking, the most important step is to make the decision to quit. Cleansing the body through fasting and diet is a great help.

Herbal remedies: Herbalists often recommend lobelia, which has an alkaloid lobeline, similar to nicotine, to assist you in the process of stopping smoking. I don't recommend taking lobelia herb or tincture by itself unless you're under the advice of an herbalist. A number of other natural products to help you stop smoking are available at your local herb shop.

Herbal formulas: Adequate cleansing of the nicotine and other by-products that can continue to cause a craving for tobacco is essential for success in my experience. Simmer 1 teaspoon each of dandelion root, burdock root, sarsaparilla root, Oregon grape root, and 1/2 teaspoon of American calamus root in 4 cups of water for 10 minutes and steep for another 15 minutes. Drink 1 cup, several times daily. Take the cleansing formula with a natural smoking withdrawal formula.

Healthy habits: I've found from personal experience that a 5-day vegetable juice fast is one of the best ways to quit smoking. After a good cleanse and fast, the last thing your body craves is the potent toxin nicotine.

Sore Throat

Medical description: A sore throat is a common symptom that's often associated with viral or bacterial infections of the upper respiratory tract.

Holistic understanding: Weakening the throat from irritation caused by too much talking or breathing polluted air can increase your chances of developing a sore throat.

Herbal remedies: Gargle with any of the following herbs: myrrh gum tincture diluted in water, warm calendula flowers tea, Roman chamomile flowers tea, cool sage leaf tea, or ginger root tea. Do essential oil steams with peppermint, eucalyptus, or lavender by adding about 6 drops of the oil to a bowl of steaming water, covering your head with a towel, and inhaling the steam. Internally, take echinacea root and/or propolis resin tinctures several times a day. You can buy sore throat lozenges containing herbs such as slippery elm bark, licorice root, marshmallow root, echinacea root, and thyme leaves in natural food stores and herb shops.

Herbal formulas: My favorite sore throat remedy is a formula made with white sage leaves, lemon peel, and lemon juice. You can simmer the lemon peel in a covered pan for 5 minutes, then add the sage leaves and lemon juice and allow the mixture to steep for another 15 minutes.

Healthy habits: Eat soothing foods like barley soup, to which you have added infection fighters such as echinacea root, garlic, and cayenne.

Sprain

Medical description: The wrenching of a joint causing the rupture of ligaments and small blood vessels, accompanied by pain, and sometimes swelling and inflammation.

Holistic understanding: None.

Herbal remedies: Apply witch hazel liniment, horse chestnut cream, arnica oil or ointment (or tincture as a compress), or St. John's wort oil to the affected area. Internally, take calendula flowers and St. John's wort leaf and flower tincture and arnica in homeopathic tablets.

Herbal formulas: None.

Healthy habits: To prevent sprains from occurring try to incorporate gentle stretching into your daily exercise routine to increase flexibility of your joints, muscles, and ligaments.

Stress

Medical description: A factor that threatens the body's health, such as worry, disease, injury, or toxic chemicals.

Holistic understanding: When the adrenal glands are chronically stimulated by the body's reaction to stress, the long-term results are often immune, hormone, and digestive system depletion, as well as high blood pressure.

Herbal remedies: Popular anti-stress herbs include eleuthero (Siberian ginseng) root and licorice root. Use calmative herbs such as California poppy flowering plant, valerian root, hops strobiles, kava root, and passion flower herb on a regular basis.

Herbal formulas: Mix 1 teaspoon each valerian root, California poppy flowering plant, hawthorn flowers and leaves, and kava root in 4 cups water. Bring herbs and water to a boil, then steep the mixture for 20 minutes. Drink 1 cup of the tea, 2 or 3 times daily, before meals. If you prefer, mix 1 teaspoon each of the individual tinctures in 1 cup of water and drink $^{1}/_{2}$ cup, 2 times daily.

Healthy habits: Detaching from the daily pressure of life is the most important factor in stress reduction. You can do this with meditation, deep breathing, visualization, stretching, and spiritual practices. Follow a natural-foods diet with lightly steamed vegetables, grains, and legumes and a little meat if you desire. Increase your intake of raw vegetables and fruits in warmer months. Emphasize foods that nourish the adrenals such as aduki beans and yams.

Sunburn

Medical description: Skin damage from prolonged exposure to the sun.

Holistic understanding: Your skin is a sensitive organ and is easily damaged from strong or prolonged exposure to harsh sunlight.

Herbal remedies: Use any of the following herbs externally in oil or ointment form to reduce the pain and help speed healing of the skin: St. John's wort leaf and flower, chamomile flowers, and calendula flowers. Apply fresh aloe leaves if available. A few drops of lavender oil added to St. John's wort oil and applied to the affected area also helps relieve the pain.

Herbal formulas: None.

Healthy habits: My teacher, Paul Bragg, a life-extension specialist, told me that maintaining clean and pure blood and tissues reduces your chances of developing skin cancer. You can protect yourself from the harmful effects of the sun by fasting occasionally throughout the year, eating a wholesome diet, getting enough vitamins and minerals, maintaining a strong immune system, and by wearing protective clothing and a hat. Recent research shows that taking supplements of vitamin E and vitamin C for 2 weeks can offer good protection against sunburn and skin damage. Take the supplement continuously during the time you're exposed to sunlight. Some scientists have suggested that sunscreen isn't the best way to protect yourself from cancer and skin damage due to sun exposure.

Tendinitis

Medical description: Inflammation of a tendon, often occurring following a sports injury or a strain.

Holistic understanding: Possible causes include injury, tight muscles, and chronic, especially repetitive overuse.

Herbal remedies: Take a tea or extract in capsule or tablets of horsetail, to help strengthen and regenerate connective tissue. You can make compresses of plantain leaf, comfrey leaf, or ginger root tea to accelerate healing, and then apply St. John's wort oil to reduce pain and inflammation and reduce nerve trauma. The Chinese herb teasel root (xu duan, pronounced SHOO- dwan) can help speed healing of strained tendons.

Herbal formulas: Simmer 1 tablespoon each of teasel root and horsetail herb in 4 cups water for 20 minutes. Drink 1 cup of the tea, 2 or 3 times daily, before meals. Ready-made products with horsetail extract and other herbs are available in capsules and tablets. Follow the directions on the label.

Healthy habits: Take 1 gram of vitamin C, 400 IU of vitamin E, and 200 to 300 mg of grapeseed extract daily. Eat fresh vegetables and get enough high quality protein, preferably from fish, beans, seeds, and nuts.

Toothache

Medical description: Pain inside or around a tooth, often caused by bacteria eroding the tooth enamel and infecting the tooth pulp, irritating a nerve.

Holistic understanding: Toothaches are a result of bacterial infection due to a weakened immune system and adrenal system, poor dental hygiene, poor mineral absorption, and an imbalanced acid to alkaline balance in your body which can result in a slow reduction of tooth hardness.

Herbal remedies: Use clove oil and echinacea tincture right on a painful tooth to help ease the pain. Take immune tonic herbs like astragalus root, ligustrum berries, and shiitake mushroom to help ward off infections, and adrenal-support herbs like American ginseng root to help protect your teeth.

Herbal formulas: Internally, add 1 teaspoon each of meadowsweet herb and Jamaican dogwood to each 1 cup of water, and drink 1/2 cup, 2 or 3 times daily, for pain. Externally, I find that hot water compresses over the painful tooth are effective for reducing pain.

Healthy habits: For prevention, avoid sugar as much as possible, and eat a balanced diet rich in good quality protein and fresh fruits and vegetables. Dental researchers report that a diet high in refined and junk foods, sugar, and low in vitamins and minerals greatly increases your risk of tooth decay and toothaches. I recommend seeing a holistically-oriented dentist who can give you a comprehensive treatment program, including nutrition and herbs, for better tooth health.

Ulcer

Medical description: An inflammatory lesion which forms in different areas of the gastrointestinal tract. If you have symptoms of severe burning or blood in your stools, consult with your doctor or herbalist.

Holistic understanding: Ulcers are often the result of poor eating habits, stress, and consumption of irritating foods like alcohol. A bacteria known as *Heliobacter pylori* has also been linked with ulcers.

Herbal remedies: You can make teas with soothing herbs, such as chamomile flowers, licorice root, and marshmallow root to help relieve this condition. Herbalists recommend St. John's wort oil, 1 teaspoon, 2 times daily, to help ease the inflammation and speed healing. Echinacea tincture can stimulate your immune system to help eliminate *H. pylori*.

Herbal formulas: Simmer 1 tablespoon of marshmallow root and 1 teaspoon of licorice root in 4 cups water for 30 minutes. Drink 1 cup of the tea, 2 or 3 times daily, before meals. If you prefer, mix 1 teaspoon each of the individual tinctures in 1 cup of water and drink 1/2 cup, 2 times daily.

Healthy habits: Drink up to 1 quart of cabbage juice daily with food.

Vaginal Infections

Medical description: The most common vaginal infections include trichomoniasis, yeast infections, and bacterial vaginosis. They're generally the result of an imbalance in the pH of the vagina, a weakened immune system, or an overgrowth of disease-promoting yeast or bacteria in your vagina and colon. If your vaginal infections are severe or chronic, consult with your doctor and/or herbalist.

Holistic understanding: Common causes of vaginal infections are the use of antibiotics, eating sugar, wearing tight-fitting underwear, bathing in chlorinated pools or hot tubs, and frequent douching.

Herbal remedies: Take antibacterial herbs internally such as the roots of echinacea, and wild indigo. Try herbal douches containing marshmallow root, sage leaf tea and raspberry leaf or a few drops tea tree oil diluted in water or added to the tea.

Herbal formulas: Mix 1 teaspoon each of echinacea root, Oregon grape root, and vitex berries in 4 cups water. Bring herbs and water to a boil, then steep the mixture for 20 minutes. Drink 1 cup of the tea, 2 or 3 times daily, before meals. If you prefer, mix 1 teaspoon each of the individual tinctures in 1 cup of water and drink 1/2 cup, 2 times daily.

Healthy habits: Maintain a strong immune system by getting plenty of exercise and fresh air, eating a healthy diet, regular stretching, deep breathing, and adequate sleep. For recurring infections, exclude sugar from your diet. Also, add yogurt, garlic, ginger, and turmeric to your diet. A good acidophilus supplement, 2 capsules in the morning taken with breakfast, and 1 in the evening with dinner, often helps.

Varicose Veins

Medical description: Varicose veins are distorted veins that occur most commonly in the superficial (near the surface) veins of the legs.

Holistic understanding: Genetics play a role in varicose veins. Women who are overweight or constipated or sit or stand for long periods are more likely to develop them.

Herbal remedies: Herbal vein tonics include horse chestnut extract and butcher's broom herb, stone root, and witch hazel bark or leaf extract. Massage the swollen veins with massage oils containing essential oils of chamomile, frankincense, and cypress to help reduce the inflammation.

Herbal formulas: Simmer 1 teaspoon each of butcher's broom herb, witch hazel bark, and stone root for each 2 cups of water for 30 minutes and let the brew steep for 15 minutes. Drink 1 cup of the tea, 2 or 3 times daily, before meals. If you prefer, mix 1 teaspoon each of the individual tinctures in 1 cup of water and drink 1/2 cup, 2 times daily.

Healthy habits: To maintain a healthy vascular system, eat high-fiber foods such as vegetables, fruits, whole grains, and beans. Make sure cayenne, garlic, onions, and ginger are plentiful in your diet. Regular walking and leg stretches are essential.

Wart

Medical description: Warts are small, sometimes hard growths on the skin associated with a virus infection.

Holistic understanding: Warts often occur when your immune system is weak, for example, after a period of stress.

Herbal remedies: You can apply anti-viral herb preparations such as thuja oil, clove oil, castor oil, or bloodroot tincture or ointment directly on the wart, 2 times daily, to discourage growth. Don't take any of the anti-viral herbs internally.

Herbal formulas: None.

Healthy habits: None.

Weight Loss

Medical description: About one-half of the population of North America is overweight, one-quarter are obese, and a recent survey showed that 75 percent feel they are over their ideal weight. Mild obesity is 20 percent to 40 percent over your ideal weight, moderate obesity is 41 percent to 100 percent over your ideal weight, and severe obesity is over 100 percent over your ideal weight.

Holistic understanding: Being overweight is often linked to genetics, sedentary habits, overeating, weakened digestion, and emotional problems.

Herbal remedies: Digestive strengthening herbs are essential for successful weight management. Take bitter herbs like gentian root, centaury herb, angelica root, artichoke leaf, and wormwood leaf tea, and digestive-warming herbs like ginger rhizome and red ginseng root daily before meals. Long-term use, up to six months or more, brings the best results. Many commercial formulas with various combinations of these herbs are widely available. Take 2 capsules of cayenne fruit powder, 2 times daily, to stimulate your metabolism. You may also want to take capsules of bladderwrack thallus and guggul oleoresin to regulate metabolism and support proper thyroid activity.

Herbal formulas: Simmer 1 teaspoon each of ginger rhizome, cardamom pods, orange peel, cinnamon bark, and gentian root in 4 cups of water for 15 minutes, and let the brew steep for 15 more minutes. Drink 1 cup of the tea, 2 or 3 times daily, before meals. If you prefer, mix 1 teaspoon each of the individual tinctures in 1 cup of water and drink $^1/_2$ cup, 2 times daily, before meals.

Healthy habits: Engage in regular aerobic activity, including walking, running, swimming, or biking. Do gentle stretching exercises before and after to increase your flexibility. Don't eat too late at night, and, even better, have your big meal at noon, and eat lightly in the evening. Keep starches and sugar to a minimum. Lightly increase your intake of high quality protein, and focus on all kinds of fresh raw and steamed vegetables and beans. Also keep dairy, meat, oil, nuts, and eggs to a minimum.

Worms

Medical description: Parasites that inhabit the digestive tract, including roundworms, pinworms, tapeworms, and hookworms.

Holistic understanding: Many people of the world harbor worms in their intestines. People in some cultures believe that worms help break down their food and provide healthful benefits. In industrialized cultures, worms are considered unclean and unhealthy. Your herbalist can give you a complete program to help you eliminate worms. Call Great Smokies Laboratory (800-522-4762) or talk to your herbalist to receive an intestinal worm and parasite test to do at home. In the philosophy of natural healing, when your immune system is strong, worms won't bother you.

Herbal remedies: Take herbs known to kill or discourage the growth of worms, like garlic, quassia bark, sweet annie herb, wormwood tea, and ginger rhizome.

Herbal formulas: Blend 1 teaspoon each of the tinctures of black walnut hull, sweet annie whole plant, and quassia bark for each cup of water and drink $^1/_2$ cup, 2 or 3 times daily. Add a cup of wormwood herb infusion several times daily for stubborn cases.

Healthy habits: Add garlic, onions, pomegranate and pumpkin seeds, and raw carrots to your diet until the worms are eliminated.

Herb Guide

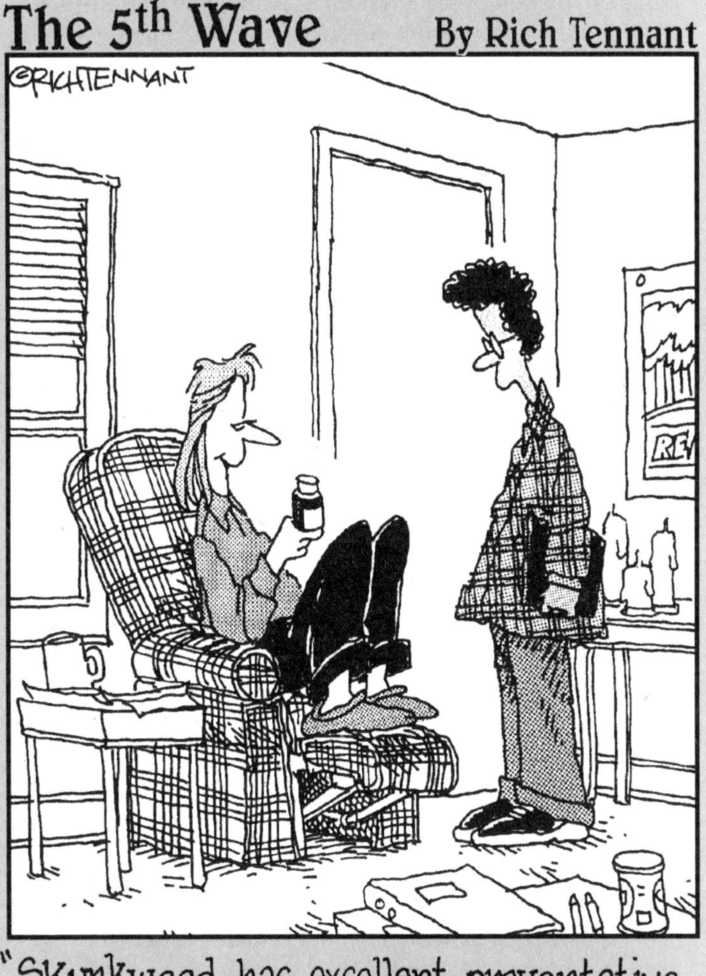

"Skunkweed has excellent preventative properties. It prevents guys from getting too close to me on first dates."

In this guide . . .

For thousands of years, herbs have been safe and effective medicines. Today, modern science is accumulating an impressive body of research on a few healing herbs, such as ginkgo, St. John's wort, feverfew, valerian, ginger, and garlic. The research is still preliminary to many hard-nosed scientists, but even skeptics agree that herbs may just be *the* medicine of the next century — a repeat performance of major proportions.

This *Herb Guide* is an ultra-practical guide that you can take with you on vacations, business trips, in the car, and in the kitchen (or bedroom) for any sudden problems that come up in your life. The guide lists over 100 herbs in alphabetical order and for each one, I include an illustration, a brief description, a listing of medicinal uses, a dosage guide, and any caution.

When you run into a term that stops you dead in your tracks — like *damp heat* — look it up in Appendix A. Also note that spices such as garlic, parsley, sage, and so on are almost always safe in the amounts used in everyday cooking — far less than a therapeutic dose. (Remember that the information in this reference is not intended to substitute for expert medical advice or treatment; it is designed to help you make informed choices. Because each individual is unique, a professional health care provider must diagnose conditions and supervise treatments for each individual health problem. If you're under a doctor's care and receive advice that is contrary to the information provided in this reference, the doctor's advice should be followed, because it is based on your unique characteristics.)

I hope this guide empowers you, helps you find your healing path, fascinates you, and excites you to discover even more about healing herbs.

Alfalfa

Latin name: *Medicago sativa* L.

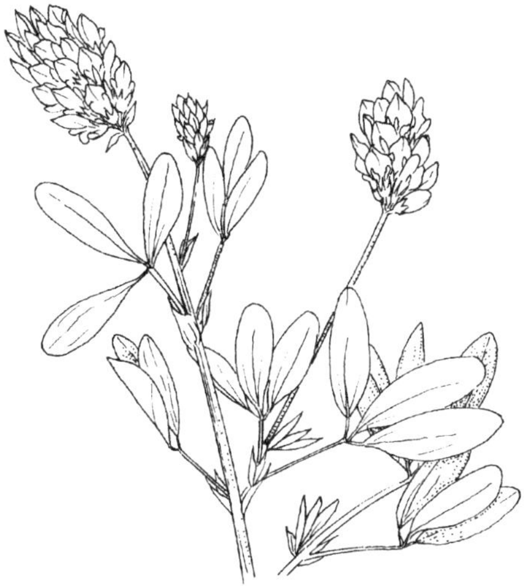

Description: Green herbaceous plant, two to three feet high with short spikes of small purple pea-like flowers. The above-ground parts are used, including the leaves, flowers, and stems. Take the powdered herb in capsules or tablets or make the bulk herb into a light decoction.

Uses: Alfalfa is rich in minerals, and you may consider adding the herb to your supplement regime to help prevent elevated cholesterol. The herb may have cancer-protective properties. Alfalfa contains phytoestrogens and makes a gentle substitute for estrogen after menopause.

Dosage: Take 3 to 5 grams a day as tea or in capsules (5 to 10 double-ought capsules with meals), or make a decoction by simmering 1 teaspoon of the herb in 1 cup of water for 20 minutes. Drink 1 cup, 2 or 3 times daily.

Aloe Vera

Latin name: *Aloe* spp.

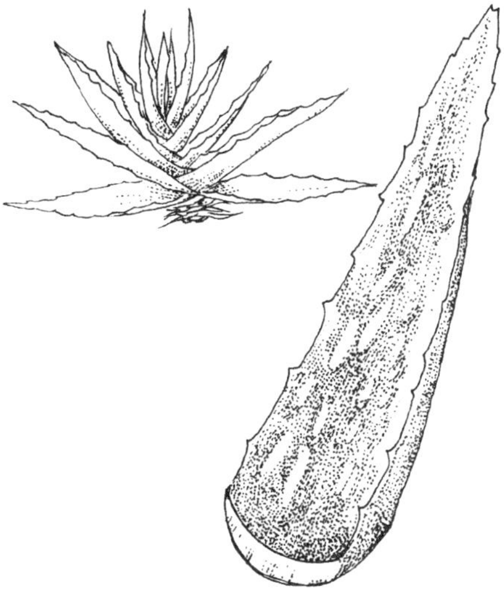

Description: Aloe vera is a spiny, succulent perennial, grown as a houseplant and in gardens. The dried leaf resin and the inner leaf gel are used. You can use the leaf resin in capsule form and the liquid gel as a drink.

Uses: Aloe resin relieves constipation and sluggish or dry bowel movements. The liquid gel is popular as a drink to cleanse the bowels and help clear the skin of acne and rashes. Aloe gel has long been used for burns. It is currently used as a mild anti-viral for people with AIDS and HIV.

Dosage: Take 10 to 300 milligrams per day of the resin, before bed, in capsules or tablets. You can add orange peel or fennel seed to reduce cramping. Follow the label instructions for the liquid gel.

Caution: Aloe resin can cause bowel cramping and diarrhea when you exceed the manufacturer's recommended dose.

Angelica

Latin name: *Angelica archangelica* L.

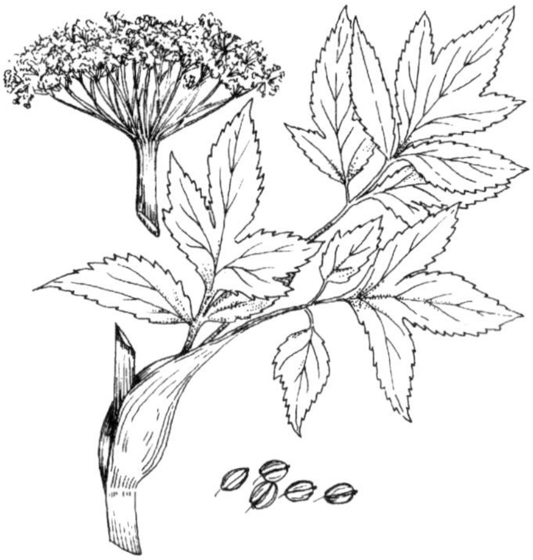

Description: Angelica is a stout, celery-like biennial plant with white umbrella-shaped flowering parts. The pungent seeds and roots are made into elixirs, liqueurs, and bitter tonics. Angelica is available as a bulk herb, in tinctures, and as a powdered herb in capsules and tablets.

Uses: The root and seeds of angelica make an excellent digestive tonic used for poor digestion and gas. This herb can improve your appetite and assimilation of nutrients.

Dosage: You can make a decoction with $^1/_2$ to 1 teaspoon of the herb per 1 cup of water. Drink 1 cup 3 times daily, before meals, as a decoction or $^1/_2$ to 1 teaspoon of the tincture in water, preferably before meals.

Caution: Avoid prolonged sunlight exposure and don't use during pregnancy.

Arnica

Latin name: *Arnica montana* L.

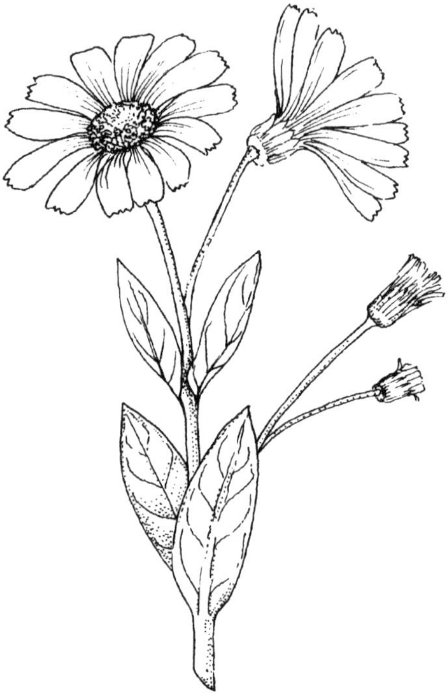

Description: Arnica is an aromatic perennial with opposite leaves and bright yellow flowers that are in the daisy family. The flowers and rhizomes are both active, but the flowers are more renewable than the root, so they're more often used for medicine. Use arnica as a liniment, tincture, or oil.

Uses: Arnica is fantastically effective in liniments and oils for joint and muscle inflammation, sprains, bruises, and varicose veins. You can also use arnica in homeopathic form for shock or trauma to body tissues, or after an accident.

Dosage: Use the diluted tincture or oil externally, 2 or 3 times daily. Take the homeopathic preparation internally as directed on the packaging.

Caution: Don't use on open wounds, because arnica can cause irritation. Don't use arnica preparations internally, except in homeopathic dilution.

Artichoke

Latin name: *Cynara scolymus* L.

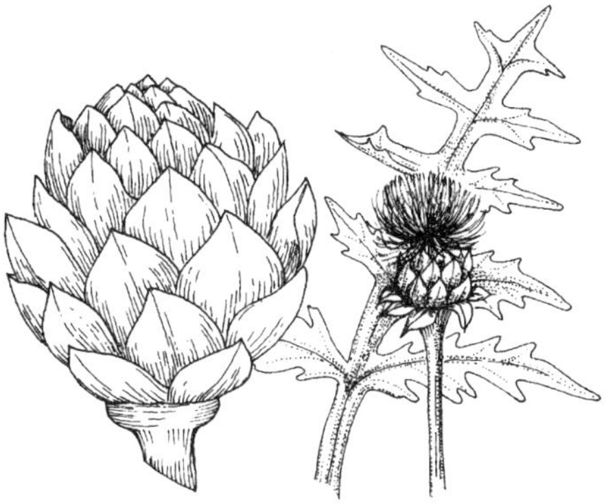

Description: A large, stout, whitish, hairy-leaved perennial that's grown in fields or gardens — it produces the familiar artichoke vegetable. The large sharply-lobed leaves are used. You can buy artichoke extracts in capsules or liquid tinctures and elixirs.

Uses: Use artichoke leaf preparations for poor appetite, weak digestion, and weight loss. Because of its bile-stimulating properties, it's beneficial for gallbladder problems and high cholesterol.

Dosage: Make an infusion by simmering $^1/_2$ cup of the dry or fresh leaves for every 2 cups of water for 5 minutes, then steeping for 15 minutes. Take $^1/_2$ to 1 teaspoon of the tincture, 2 to 3 times daily, preferably before meals. When using the dry extract, take 2 capsules before meals.

Astragalus

Latin name: *Astragalus membranaceus* Bunge.

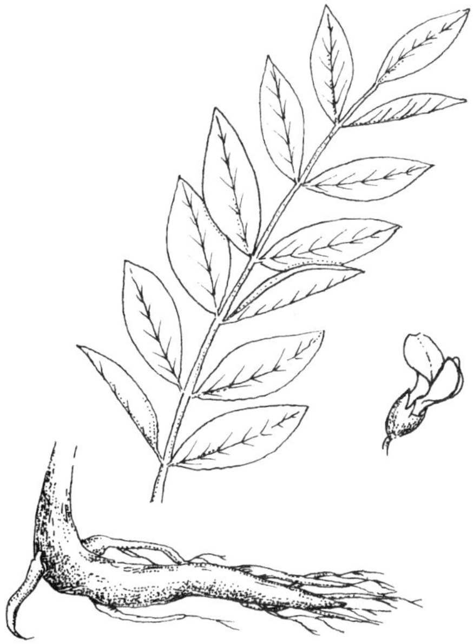

Chinese name: Huang Qi (pronounced HWANG-chee).

Description: Astragalus is a perennial member of the pea family. The small lemon-yellow pea flowers are in elongated spikes. The sliced root is either dried fresh or soaked in honey and dried to form long slices that look like tongue depressors. Astragalus is widely available as a powdered concentrated extract in capsules or tablets, in liquid tinctures, and sweet elixirs in one-dose vials for personal use, but is most often blended with other immune and digestive herbs in formula preparations. If you're taking astragalus for longer than two weeks, avoid the tincture form and instead take teas or dry extracts in capsule or tablet form.

Uses: Astragalus root is an immune tonic and cancer-fighting herb. The root is an ingredient in many products for general immune weakness, digestive weakness with lack of appetite, and as a supportive product — along with chemotherapy and radiation — for the treatment of cancer. Astragalus increases the body's resistance to disease.

Dosage: You can chop up 4 or 5 astragalus sticks with a pair of scissors and decoct the herb for up to an hour in 4 cups of water, drinking 1 strong cup in the morning and 1 cup in the evening. Blend astragalus with other tonic herbs like poria to balance the herb's effects. Follow the directions on the bottle for capsules and tablets.

Caution: Avoid for about a week to ten days during an acute infection such as a flu or urinary tract infection. Otherwise, astragalus is safe.

Bilberry

Latin name: *Vaccinum myrtillus* L.

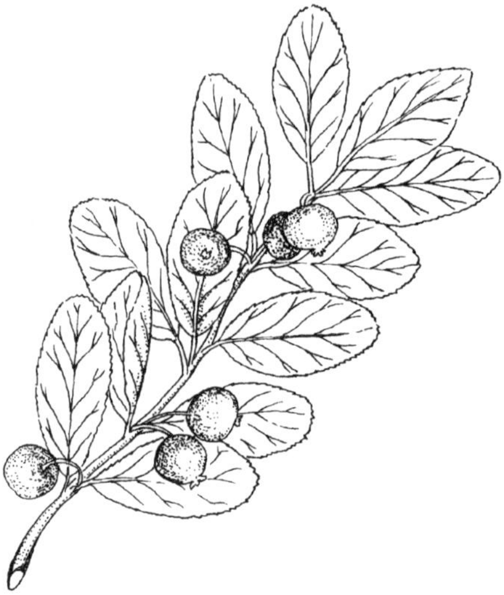

Description: Bilberry is a small, woody shrub native to northern Europe and a close relative of huckleberry and blueberry. The small purple fruits are extracted to make healthful dietary supplements and can be eaten like blueberries. You can buy the standardized extract in capsules and tablets.

Uses: Use bilberry extracts for reducing capillary fragility, improving night vision, counteracting diarrhea, and helping relieve the pain and distension of varicose veins. You may find that regular use of bilberry extract helps keep your eyes clear and youthful. Night flyers of the Royal Air Force noticed they could see better on their night missions when they ate bilberry jam on toast, and a popular remedy was discovered.

Dosage: Take 1 to 2 capsules of the standardized extract, 2 times daily.

Black Cohosh

Latin name: *Cimicifuga racemosa* [L.] Nutt.

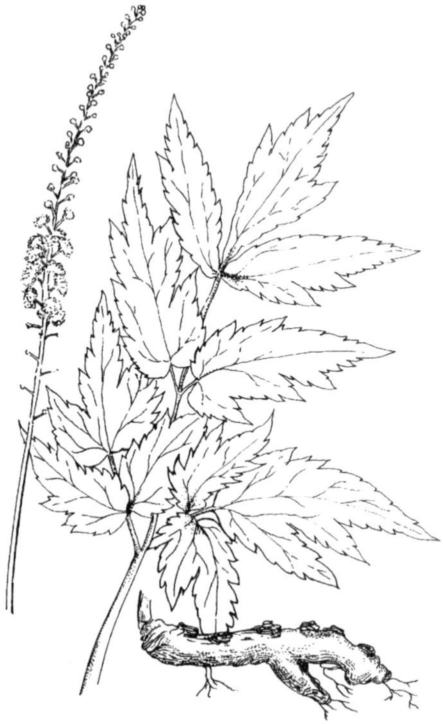

Description: Black cohosh is a stout, bushy perennial plant with tall spires of starry white flowers. The rhizome and roots are the active parts. Herbalists encourage the cultivation of black cohosh because greatly increased demand is stressing natural populations. Black cohosh is available in bulk form to make teas, as a powdered herb in capsules, as a standardized extract, and in tincture form.

Uses: Use black cohosh preparations for hot flashes and depression during menopause. Consider the herb if you have rheumatism or sciatica. Try it as a muscle relaxant.

Dosage: Simmer 1 teaspoon of the cut and sifted herb for every cup of water, and drink 1 cup decoction twice daily. Take 10 to 60 drops of the tincture 2 to 3 times daily, or 1 capsule or tablet, 2 times daily of the standardized extract.

Caution: Avoid use of this herb during pregnancy or nursing without the advice of an herbalist. Don't use for a period longer than six months.

Black Walnut

Latin name: *Juglans nigra* L.

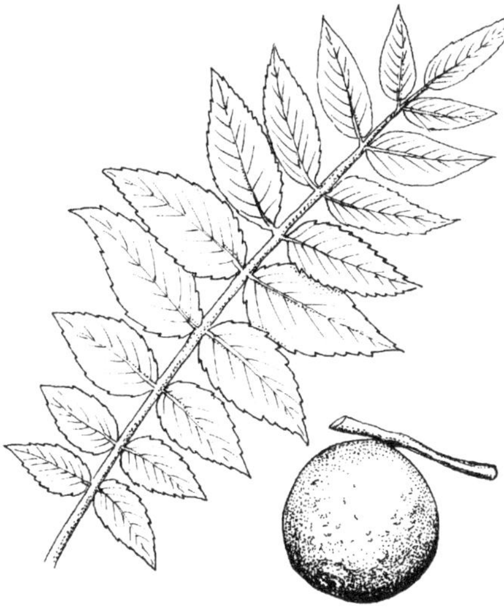

Description: The black walnut tree ranges from medium-sized to very large with dark, deeply furrowed bark. The green walnut fruit hulls contain the antifungal and antiparasitic compound, juglone. The hulls are made into liquid tinctures or are dried and powdered for use in capsules and tablets.

Uses: Black walnut hull liquid tincture is especially helpful to prevent and slow diarrhea, especially due to intestinal parasites like giardia. Herbalists recommend black walnut preparations to help treat candida infections and gastrointestinal irritation.

Dosage: Take 1 to 3 droppersful of the tincture or 2 to 3 capsules, 3 to 5 times daily, depending on the severity of the symptoms.

Caution: Don't use black walnut for more than a month at a time. Consult a qualified herbalist or physician if symptoms persist or are severe.

Bloodroot

Latin name: *Sanguinaria canadensis* L.

Description: A small perennial herb with delicate, vase-like, white flowers that open early in the spring. The rhizomes are harvested to make herbal preparations. The tincture of bloodroot is the most useful form of the herb. A small amount is added to the Viadent mouthwash (produced by Colgate).

Uses: You can use bloodroot to prevent plaque formation or for gum problems. The rhizome extract is an ingredient in medicinal mouthwashes and toothpastes. Bloodroot is a component of many expectorants and cough syrups because of its strong expectorant and antibacterial action. The herb extract can treat skin cancers and fungal infections.

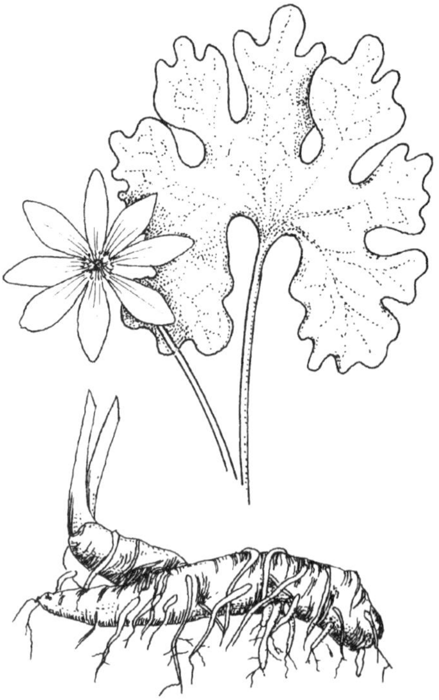

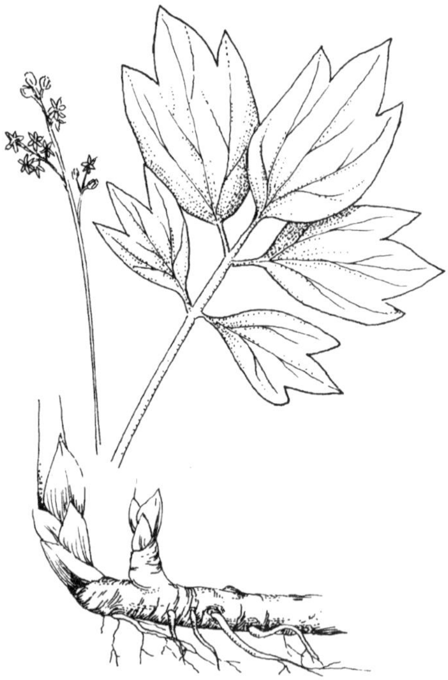

Dosage: Use 1/2 to 1 dropperful in 2 or 3 ounces of water as a mouth rinse or follow the manufacturer's directions for using the mouthwash or toothpaste. Consult a qualified herbalist before attempting to use bloodroot to treat skin cancer. Apply a few drops of the tincture on a wart or rub on 1/2 teaspoon of a commercial cream for athlete's foot.

Caution: Avoid use of this herb during pregnancy. Don't exceed the recommended dose because it can strongly irritate the skin, throat, and intestines. Consult a physician for a diagnosis if you suspect you have a skin cancer lesion.

Blue Cohosh

Latin name: *Caulophyllum thalictroides* L.

Description: Blue cohosh is a stout, perennial with blue-green leaves and bright, china-blue berries. The rhizome and roots are commercially harvested. You can buy powdered rhizome in capsules, bulk dried and cut rhizome, and blue cohosh tincture.

Uses: Blue cohosh is a specific and effective remedy for pain, especially associated with menstruation, ovulation, and childbirth. Blend blue cohosh with black cohosh to help facilitate childbirth.

Dosage: Drink 1 cup of the decoction made by simmering 1/2 teaspoon for every cup of water, 2 to 3 times daily, preferably with a little orange peel or licorice to ease the harsh taste. Take 20 to 30 drops of the tincture, 3 times daily in a little water or tea.

Caution: Avoid use of this herb during pregnancy except in small amounts just prior to giving birth, under the supervision of a qualified health practitioner.

Burdock

Latin name: *Arctium lappa* L.

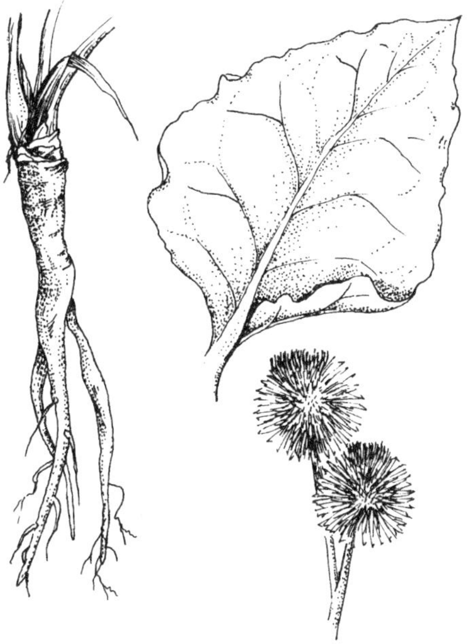

Description: Burdock is a large-leaved, weedy biennial in the daisy family with spiny burr-like fruiting heads. The roots and seeds are used in herbal medicine. The root is available fresh in markets, cut and sifted in herb shops, and in many tincture, capsule, or tablet products. The seed is sold in herb shops that carry Chinese herbs and is found in tinctures, capsules, or tablets.

Uses: Burdock is a blood purifier that you can use for skin problems such as acne, eczema, and psoriasis, especially the seeds. Herbalists universally recommend the root (called gobo in Japan) to help ease liver congestion and difficulty in digesting fats. Use the root or the seeds for rheumatism and arthritis and the root as a protectant against cancer.

Dosage: Make a decoction by simmering 1 teaspoon of the cut root, fresh or dried, for every cup of water for 30 minutes. Drink 1 cup of the decoction, 3 times daily, around mealtimes. Slice 1 or 2 crisp, juicy fresh roots and add to a soup or stew. Take 3 droppersful of the tincture, 2 to 3 times daily.

Butcher's Broom

Latin name: *Ruscus aculeatus* L.

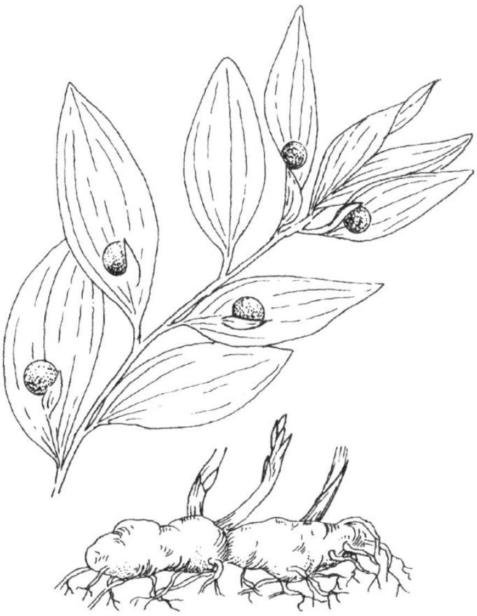

Description: Originally from Eurasia, butcher's broom is a small, stiff, spiny-leaved shrub from the lily family. Large bright red or yellow berries develop on the upper twigs. The herb is available — dried, cut, and sifted — for teas. The tincture, powdered herb in capsules, and standardized extracts are also commonly found.

Uses: Butcher's broom is a popular remedy for varicose veins and hemorrhoids, as a liver regulator for jaundice, and for improving overall circulation and relieving edema.

Dosage: Make a light decoction by simmering one teaspoon of the herb for every cup of water for 15 minutes. Drink 1 cup, or take 2 to 3 capsules with a little water, or take 20 to 40 drops of the tincture, 2 or 3 times daily.

Calendula

Latin name: *Calendula officinalis* L.

Description: A member of the daisy family, calendula is a stout herb with elongated, tongue-shaped leaves. The beautiful, bright-orange flowers are abundant when they're harvested regularly. The entire flowering heads are dried and used in herbal medicine. Calendula is available as a bulk herb to make creams, salves, teas, and tinctures; and in commercially-made creams, lotions, and salves.

Uses: Internally, calendula flower tea or tincture is effective for speeding the healing of ulcers in the digestive tract; to ease gallbladder inflammation and enlarged, sore lymph glands; for measles; and for painful menstruation. Use a calendula cream or salve for healing cuts, sunburns, skin cancers, diaper rash, sores, ulcers, varicose veins, chapped dry skin and lips, and insect bites. Calendula can prevent infections after an operation.

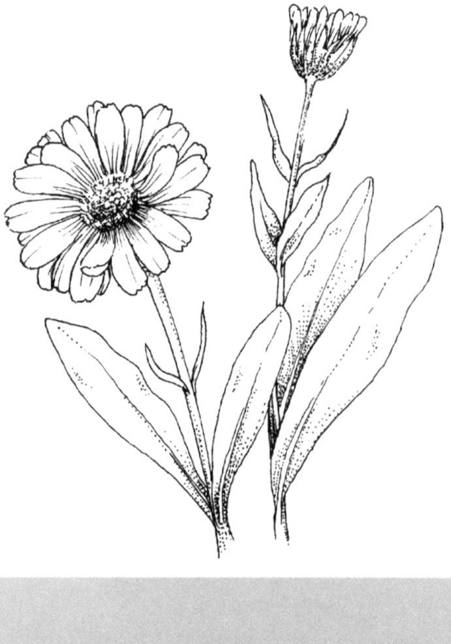

Dosage: Use externally as needed. Drink 1 cup of the infusion made with a heaping teaspoon of the petals of chopped-up flower heads. Take 1 to 3 droppersful of the tincture in a little water, several times daily.

California Poppy

Latin name: *Eschscholzia californica* Cham.

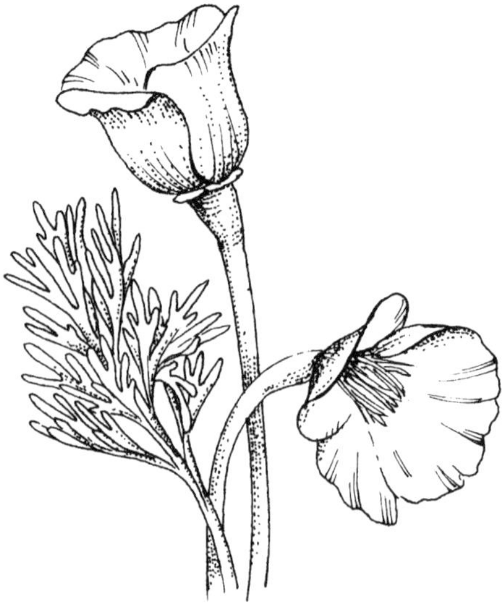

Description: The golden California poppy is a wild annual or perennial with finely dissected leaves that are tinged with red. The plant produces bright, cup-shaped, golden flowers that bloom profusely for a month or two at a time, and later produces long, spear-shaped pods. The bright orange translucent root is the strongest medicinal part, but the leaves and flowers are also used. You can find California poppy tincture as an ingredient in relaxing and sleep-promoting blends.

Uses: Modern herbalists recommend extracts for easing anxiety, nervousness, sleeplessness, stomach cramps, bronchial constriction, and toothaches. I've had success giving it to children with hyperactivity disorders, instead of Ritalin — consult a qualified herbalist before using it for this purpose.

Dosage: Take 2 to 4 droppersful, or a teaspoon of the tincture in a little water or herb tea as needed, up to 3 or 4 times daily.

Caution: Avoid use of this herb during pregnancy.

Caraway

Latin name: *Carum carvi* L.

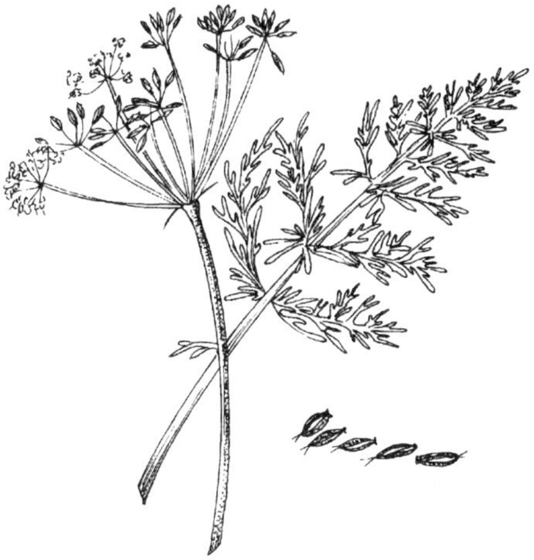

Description: Caraway is a slender, annual member of the parsley family with finely dissected, filament-like leaves, white umbrella-shaped flower parts, and pungent ribbed fruits. The bulk seed is widely available as a spice and is used to make teas.

Uses: Use caraway for easing colic, painful digestion, bloating and a feeling of uncomfortable fullness after eating, flatulence, diarrhea, and to increase lactation. Caraway tea is safe for children and adults.

Dosage: You can make the infusion by steeping a heaping teaspoon of the seed for 15 to 20 minutes in freshly boiled water and drink 1 cup, 2 or 3 times daily.

Cascara Sagrada

Latin name: *Rhamnus purshiana* DC.

Description: Cascara is a large shrub to small tree with yellowish-green oval leaves and red stems. The bark is collected from the two- or three-year old branches and aged for about nine months. Buy cascara in tincture form, as a powdered herb or extract in capsules and tablets, and as a sweet elixir.

Uses: Cascara sagrada means *sacred bark*. If you've ever been really constipated, you know how it got its name! Cascara is an official drug plant in many countries for relieving constipation and moistening the bowels for dry, hard bowel movements, and especially non-movements. Cascara is also helpful as an addition to herbal formulas for gallstones and hemorrhoids.

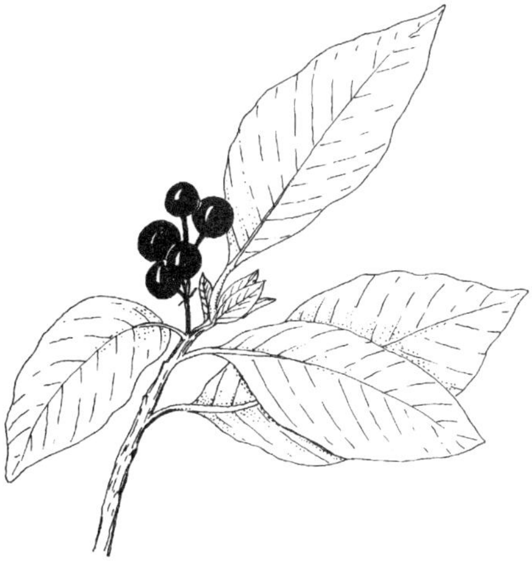

Dosage: Take 2 to 4 capsules of the powdered herb or 1 to 3 droppersful of the liquid tincture in a little water before bedtime. For other kinds of extracts, follow the manufacturer's directions. You should experience a good bowel movement the next morning. If your cascara preparation doesn't work, try increasing the dose by 50 percent for a few days. If constipation persists, see your herbalist.

Caution: Avoid use of this herb if you're pregnant, when you have persistent pain or obstruction of the intestines, or if you have a history of kidney stones. Children under twelve years old should use the herb no longer than one week. Sensitive people who start with more than the recommended dose may experience diarrhea and bowel cramps. Reduce your dose by fifty percent and continue if you have persistent trouble with constipation, or consult your herbalist. To use cascara for other uses mentioned above, consult with a qualified health care practitioner.

Castor Oil

Latin name: *Riccinus communis* L.

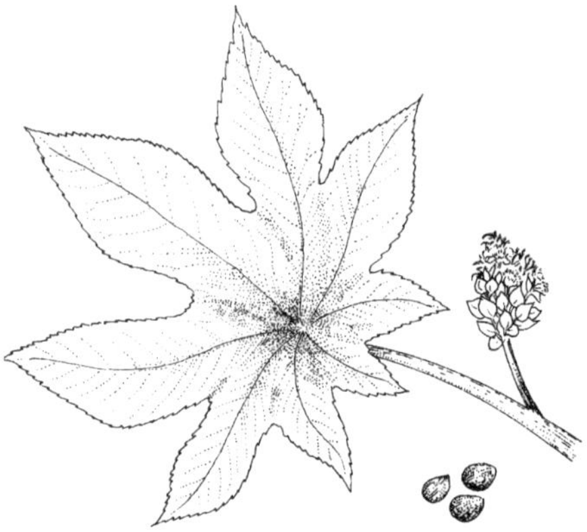

Description: Castor is a small tree with red bark and sharply palmately compound leaves. The colorfully-marked castor beans are enclosed in spiny pods. Castor is a common weed in many warm parts of the United States, Europe, Africa, and other continents. You can buy quality castor oil from your local herb shop.

Uses: Castor oil is a favorite old-time remedy for constipation. Today, the external use of castor oil is more common than the internal use. The famous psychic healer, Edgar Cayce helped make the castor oil pack popular for healing cancerous and benign tumors of all kinds. Herbalists often recommend the poultice for treating uterine fibroids and breast cysts.

Dosage: Take 1 to 2 tablespoons of the oil before bedtime, depending on age and weight. Turn to Chapter 4 to find out how to make a castor oil pack.

Caution: Don't take castor oil internally longer than one week. Don't use this herb if you're pregnant. Avoid use of this herb if you have intestinal obstruction or abdominal pain.

Catnip

Latin name: *Nepeta cataria* L.

Description: Catnip is an aromatic herbaceous plant that cats love. My cats have been hooked ever since they discovered it. The plant readily spreads and also reseeds itself. It's a common weed in damper parts of the United States and Europe. Catnip is easy to grow and is available in bulk from your local herb shop — look for a green color and an aromatic smell. Tinctures are sometimes available, but you may find them rather weak. Catnip is delicate, so don't expect too much from the dried herb in capsules.

Uses: Makes a mild, aromatic tea for colds, flu, fever, and fussiness in children. The herb has mild calming, sweat-releasing, and digestion-promoting effects.

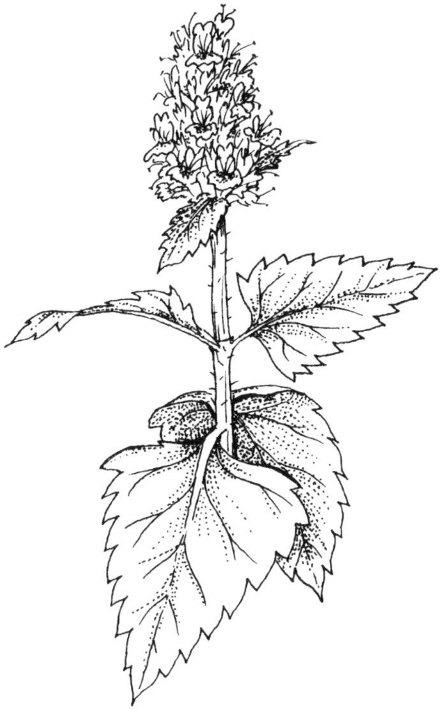

Dosage: Drink 1 cup of the strong infusion made with 1 tablespoon of the dried or fresh herb, 2 to 3 times daily.

Caution: Avoid use of this herb during pregnancy.

Cayenne

Latin name: *Capsicum annum* var. annum.

Description: The red pepper, or cayenne, is a small perennial shrub in its native South America, or other warm parts of the world. In northern gardens, it dies back each year. This pepper plant has white flowers, and then green, and eventually red or yellow pods. Take cayenne powder in capsules and tablets, tincture form, and sprinkle it on your food (if you can take the heat).

Uses: Use cayenne powder or tincture if you have a cold, poor circulation, or weak digestion. In hotter climates, the use of cayenne actually helps cool the body by promoting sweating. Cayenne is an ingredient of commercial over-the-counter and prescription salves or liniments that you can buy for shingles, arthritis, carpal tunnel syndrome, and sore muscles. One of its active ingredients, capsaicin, is effective for blocking the transmission of the pain impulse in the body.

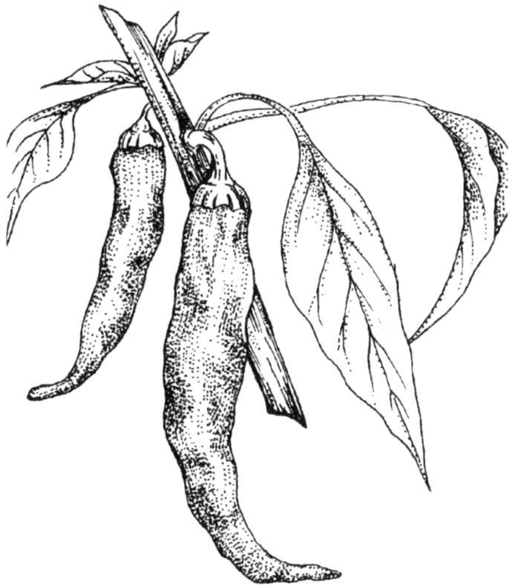

Dosage: Take 1 to 4 capsules powder, 2 times daily. Follow the manufacturer's directions for other products.

Caution: Avoid getting cayenne near your eyes, because it can burn, though it won't cause damage. Some herbalists recommend putting cayenne in your eyes for cataracts and other problems, but don't try this at home without first consulting your herbalist. The burning sensation you sometimes feel after ingesting cayenne won't hurt you either. In fact, studies show that cayenne can help heal an ulcer rather than aggravate one.

Chamomile, German

Latin name: *Matricaria recutita* L.

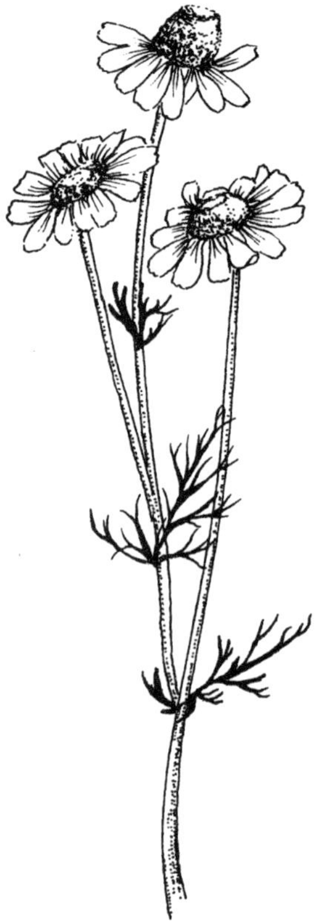

Description: German chamomile is a feathery-leaved garden plant with abundant, small, daisy-like flowers that are reminiscent of pineapple. The flowers are harvested and sold worldwide for making tea. The bulk flowers are widely available, but make sure that the flowers are white and yellow-colored, not brown or dingy. Smell the flowers, too — you should detect a fresh fruity smell, rather than a musty odor.

Uses: Drink chamomile tea liberally to help ease intestinal cramps or irritation, indigestion, and nervousness. Use chamomile tea (called manzanilla in Spain, Mexico, Central America, and South America), for colic, fever, and teething in children. Externally, you can apply a chamomile cream for soothing skin inflammation, burns, and bites.

Dosage: Drink 1 cup of the infusion, made with 1 tablespoon of the herb, 3 to 5 times daily. You can make a strong instant tea by adding 1/2 to 1 teaspoon of the tincture to a cup of warm water.

Caution: Allergic reactions to the pollen in the flowers are rare.

Chaparral

Latin name: *Larrea tridentata* [DC] Cov.

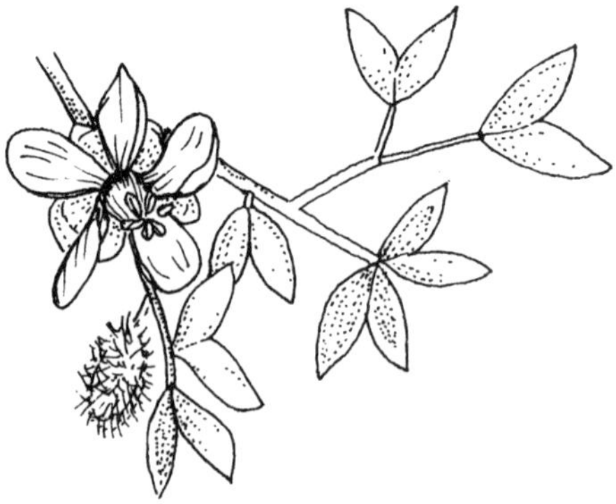

Description: Chaparral is a common desert shrub that grows up to twelve or fifteen feet high with small resinous leaves; bright-yellow flowers; and small, white, hairy fruits. The fresh, flowering twigs are harvested for medicine. You can find chaparral in capsules, tablets, and as a bulk herb.

Uses: Chaparral promotes sweating; improves elimination of toxins from the liver and skin; and eases the symptoms of colds, flu, and bronchitis. Although herbalists recommend chaparral for the prevention and treatment of cancer, clinical studies are lacking. A concentrated extract is sometimes used externally for skin cancer. Chaparral may have potent antioxidant properties.

Dosage: Make a light decoction with 1 teaspoon of the chopped herb for every cup of water, and drink 1/2 to 1 cup of the infusion, twice daily. Take 2 capsules or droppersful of the tincture, 2 times daily.

Caution: Don't use chaparral if you have a pre-existing kidney or liver condition like hepatitis. Don't use for more than two weeks except under the advice of your herbalist. I consider the herb safe when you follow these guidelines.

Cinnamon

Latin name: *Cinnamomum zeylanicum* Blume.

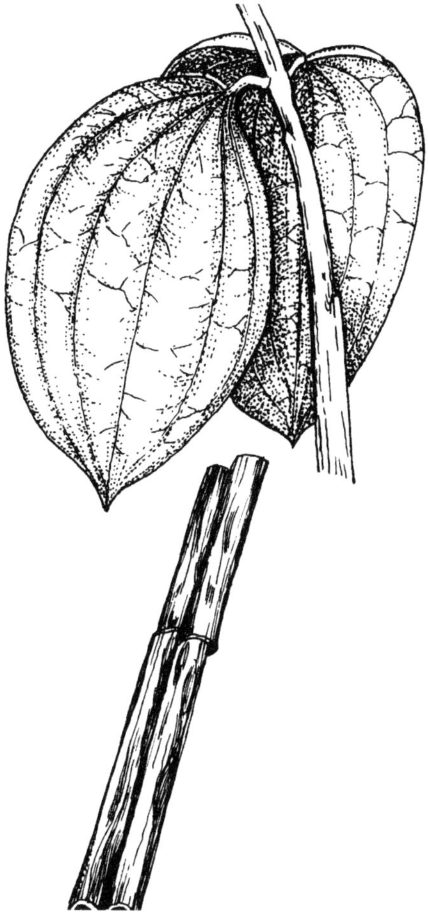

Description: Cinnamon bark comes from a small tropical tree of the laurel family. The twigs and bark are harvested for tea and for extracting the essential oil. Cinnamon is available as a bulk tea, in tea bags, as an ingredient of tinctures and herbal formulas that are in capsule and tablet form, and as an essential oil.

Uses: Cinnamon bark tea is a popular remedy for relieving the symptoms of colds, mucus congestion, and digestive problems. The warming tea helps induce sweating, clearing a feeling of coldness in your body. Cinnamon has an astringent effect and you may find it effective for easing diarrhea. When diluted, cinnamon essential oil is an ingredient in mouthwashes, toothpastes, breath mints, and candy.

Dosage: Make a light decoction by simmering 1 teaspoon of the bark for every cup of water for 10 minutes, then steep for 15 minutes. Drink 1 cup, 1 to 3 times daily. The milder cinnamon twig tea is available from herb shops that feature Chinese herbs.

Caution: Cinnamon is a warming herb, so avoid the tea if you run hot all the time.

Cleavers

Latin name: *Galium aparine* L.

Description: Cleavers (also called bedstraw or goosegrass) is a weak, climbing plant with whorls of narrow leaves arranged around the main stem covered with small hooked hairs that makes the plant *cleave* or stick onto clothing and animals (a way of dispersing the seeds). The whole fresh plant is collected before flowering. Because the herb loses its properties soon after harvest, capsules and tablets containing the dried herb are mostly ineffective. I recommend using only tinctures of the fresh plant or freshly-dried herb for teas. Add a handful or two of the fresh plant to your juicer when you make vegetable juices.

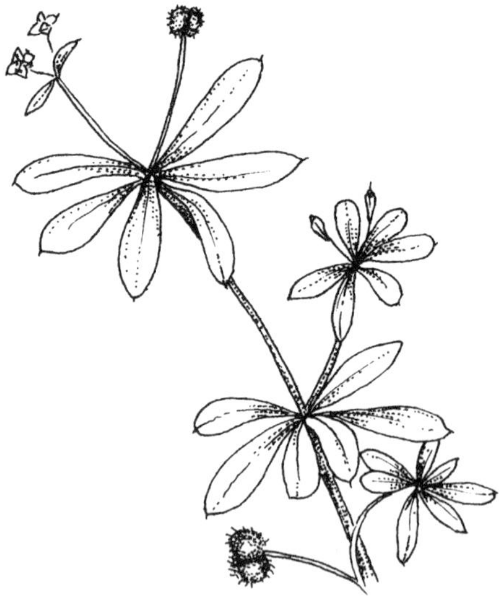

Uses: Cleavers is useful for cleansing the lymphatic system and shrinking swollen lymph glands. Consider using the herb if you have tonsillitis, psoriasis, or other skin conditions. It can be an effective herbal diuretic to clear bladder infections, cleanse the urinary tract, and help prevent small kidney stones (also called *gravel)* from forming.

Dosage: Drink 1 cup of the infusion or take up to 1 teaspoonful of the tincture in a little water, 2 to 3 times daily.

Codonopsis

Latin name: *Codonopsis pilosula* [Franch.] Nannf.

Description: A mint-green, vine-like perennial in the bellflower family. The long, white, and sweet root is harvested, soaked, and dried to make the famous Chinese tonic herb, dang shen. Codonopsis is available in bulk form from herb shops and also in capsule, tablet, and liquid form.

Uses: Codonopsis is used to strengthen digestion, the respiratory tract, and the immune system. Try using codonopsis for fatigue, poor appetite, chronic lung infections, shortness of breath, asthma, and general weakness. The herb has similar effects to ginseng, but is milder, so is often substituted for ginseng in Chinese herb formulas.

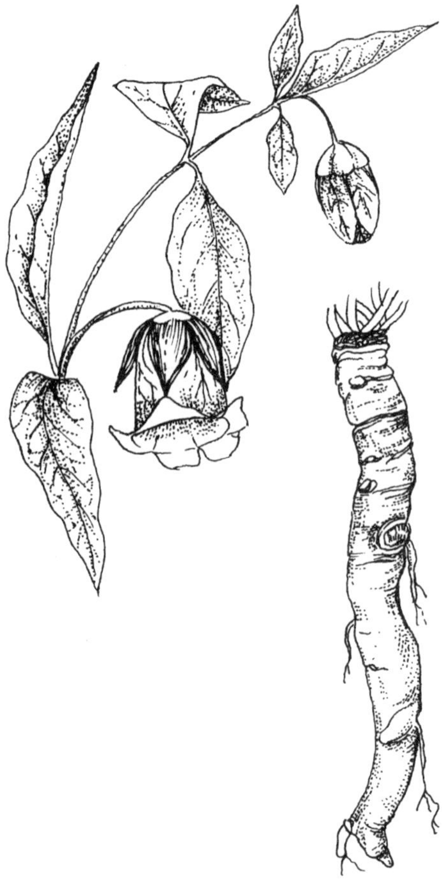

Dosage: Make a decoction with about 9 to 25 grams of the roots to 3 or 4 cups of water, and simmer down to 2 or 3 cups. Drink 1 strong cup, 2 times daily. Follow the manufacturer's recommendations for other products.

Comfrey

Latin name: *Symphytum officinale* L.

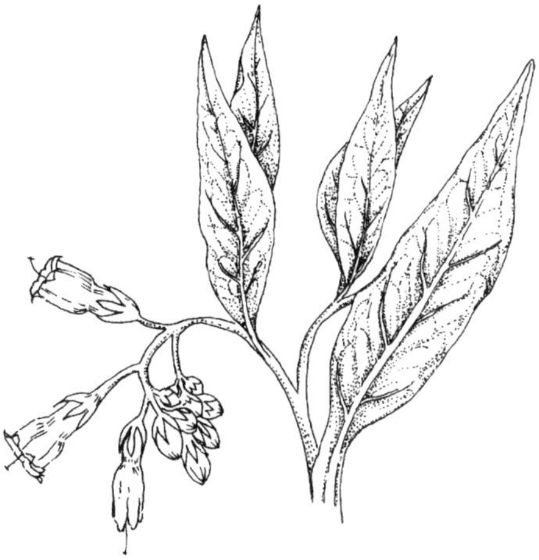

Description: A vigorous, perennial garden plant of the borage family. A profusion of large acutely-pointed, coarsely-hairy leaves spring up from stout, spreading roots. Give comfrey plenty of room in the garden, and keep the roots trimmed back if you don't want it to spread. You can purchase the dried leaves and roots in natural food stores and can grow the fresh plants easily in your garden.

Uses: Comfrey is a favorite with herbalists to help heal burns, bites, stings, and cuts, as well as strains, sprains, and broken bones.

Dosage: Make a light decoction with the leaves, and drink 1 cup, 2 or 3 times daily for up to ten days. Blend the leaves or roots with a little water to make a slimy paste, and apply to external injuries for as long as needed on unbroken skin and up to a week on broken skin under the advice of an herbalist.

Caution: Avoid using comfrey if you're pregnant or nursing. Don't use comfrey leaf preparations internally longer than one week, twice a year, under the advice of a qualified herbalist. Comfrey roots are high in toxic alkaloids, and I don't advise using them internally or on broken skin.

Cramp Bark

Latin name: *Viburnum opulus* L.

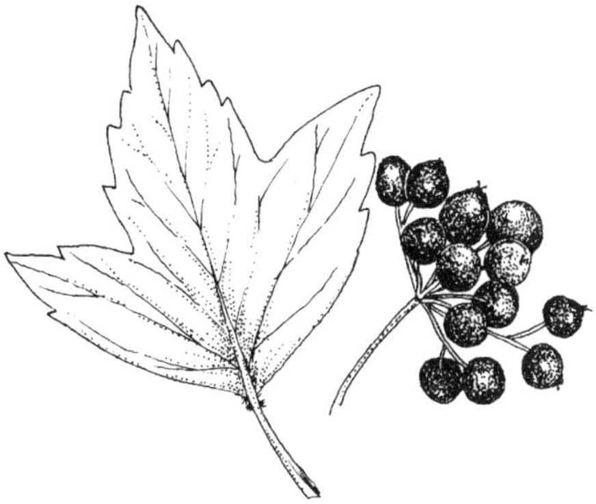

Description: A native shrub of the eastern United States, cramp bark has showy white snowball-like flower clusters. The bark is harvested for medicine. You can purchase cramp bark in capsule or tablet form, in liquid tinctures, and in bulk as a tea.

Uses: Cramp bark is a renowned herbal remedy for easing menstrual cramps and intestinal cramps.

Dosage: Drink 1 cup of the decoction made with 1 teaspoon of the chopped herb per cup of water, or 2 droppersful to 1 teaspoon of the tincture in a little water, 2 or 3 times daily.

Cranberry

Latin name: *Vaccinium macrocarpon* Aiton.

Description: Cranberry is a low, trailing plant in the heather family that grows in wet and boggy places. Cranberry standardized extracts are available in capsule and tablet form. You can buy the unsweetened juice in natural food stores.

Uses: Regular use of cranberry juice helps cleanse your urinary tract, is recommended for preventing bladder infections, and can help prevent kidney stones. Cranberry helps to deodorize the urine and is useful for incontinence.

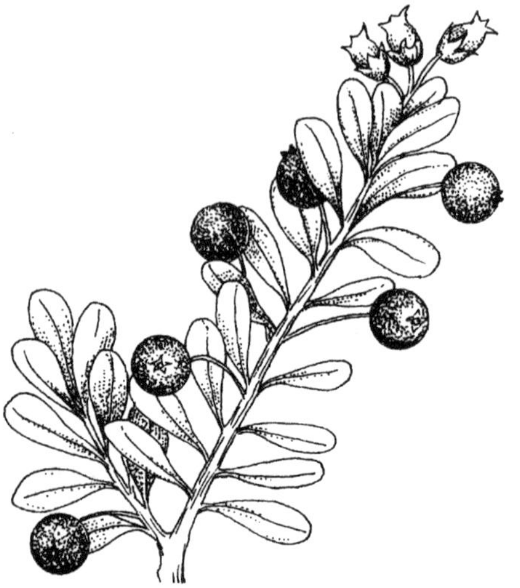

Dosage: Drink 1 cup of unsweetened (if you *really* like sour) or lightly-sweetened cranberry juice, 1 or 2 times daily. Increase to 3 to 5 cups to help eliminate a urinary tract infection. Or take 2 to 4 capsules of an extract in capsule or tablet form. Use cranberry for several weeks to get the best results.

Dandelion

Latin name: *Taraxacum officinale* Wiggers.

Description: The ever-present dandelion is easy to confuse with other plants, like sow thistle or false dandelion, that have solid yellow daisy-like flowers commonly found in lawns and gardens. Dandelion is the only one of the three that has single flowering heads on hollow, unbranched stalks and hairless, large-toothed leaves. All three plants exude milky juice when cut. Dandelion root and leaf are available in capsule or tablet form, in liquid tinctures, and in bulk for making tea.

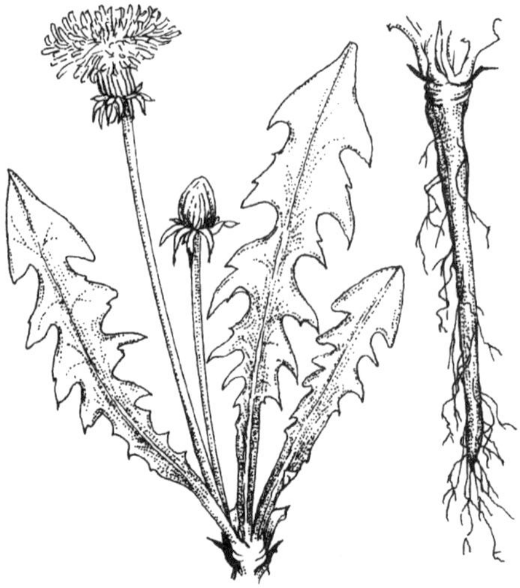

Uses: Dandelion is a famous liver cooler and cleanser and a favorite with herbalists since ancient times. Consider using dandelion for liver-related problems, such as hepatitis, cirrhosis, and liver toxicity, as well as poor appetite and constipation. The leaves are a powerful diuretic and are used for water retention and to increase lactation.

Dosage: Make a decoction by simmering 1 tablespoon of the leaf or root for every cup of water. Drink 1 cup, 2 or 3 times daily, or 2 to 4 droppersful of the tincture, 1 to 3 times daily.

Caution: Don't use dandelion if you have bile duct blockage, gallbladder inflammation, or intestinal blockage, except under the advice of an experienced herbalist.

Dong Quai

Latin name: *Angelica sinensis* [Oliv.] Diels.

Description: A small, fern-leafed, aromatic plant from the parsley family, native to China. The roots are dried or soaked in wine and then dried. Dong quai is an ingredient in many liquid and encapsulated tonic formulas. You can buy the fragrant celery-scented root crowns and thin *palm slices* in herb shops and Chinese grocery stores to add to soups and stews — a traditional way to use the herb.

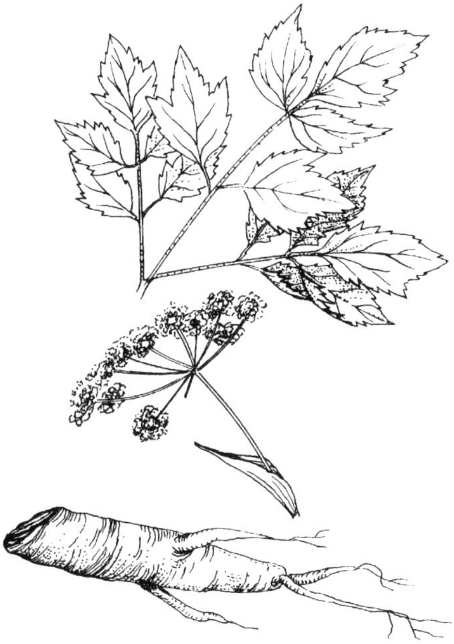

Uses: Dong quai is commonly taken by women for strengthening the blood and female organs. Herbalists recommended the herb for anemia, PMS, and menopause. Consider using dong quai if you're experiencing general weakness and debility and circulatory disorders, such as angina. The herb is useful for coronary problems and for mild anemia in both men and women.

Dosage: Make a decoction by simmering 1 crown or 3 or 4 of the palm slices in 2 or 3 cups of water for 45 minutes. Drink 1 cup 2 or 3 times daily. Take 1 to 3 droppersful of the tincture, 2 times daily.

Caution: Avoid use of this herb during pregnancy.

Echinacea

Latin name: *Echinacea* spp.

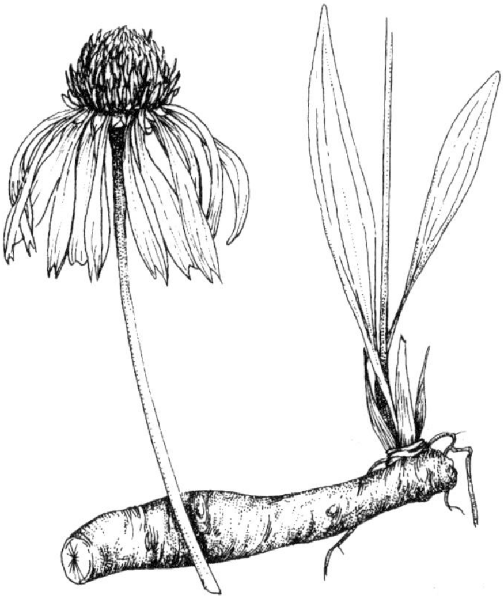

Description: Also called purple coneflower, echinacea belongs to a group of native North American perennial plants in the daisy family with large purple flowers and cone-shaped spiny seed heads that grow in the wild. Nine species are known, but only three are important in commercial trade — *E. purpurea, E. pallida,* and *E. angustifolia. Echinacea purpurea* is a renewable resource because it's easy to cultivate organically. While *E. angustifolia* is considered more potent by some herbalists, it isn't widely cultivated, and native stands are disappearing rapidly. I've found that *E. purpurea* is just as potent as other species. The leaves, flowers, and roots are harvested for making a variety of preparations. Echinacea is an ingredient in tinctures, skin creams, throat sprays, mouthwashes, and soaps.

Uses: Research shows that echinacea possesses strong immune-stimulating activity to help prevent and treat infections of all kinds. The herb is especially useful for colds, flu, urinary tract infections, and skin infections like impetigo and boils. Echinacea is also used as a mouthwash for gum problems.

Dosage: Take 2 droppersful to 1 teaspoon of the tincture, 3 or 4 times daily taken in cycles of two weeks on and one week off. Make a tea by simmering 1 teaspoon of the chopped root or leaf in 1 cup of water for 10 minutes, and then steeping for 15 minutes. Drink 1 cup, several times daily. Follow the label instructions for other products.

Caution: No known side effects, but use echinacea cautiously under the advice of an herbal practitioner if you have an autoimmune condition like lupus or an immune-compromised condition like AIDS.

Elder

Latin name: *Sambucus* spp.

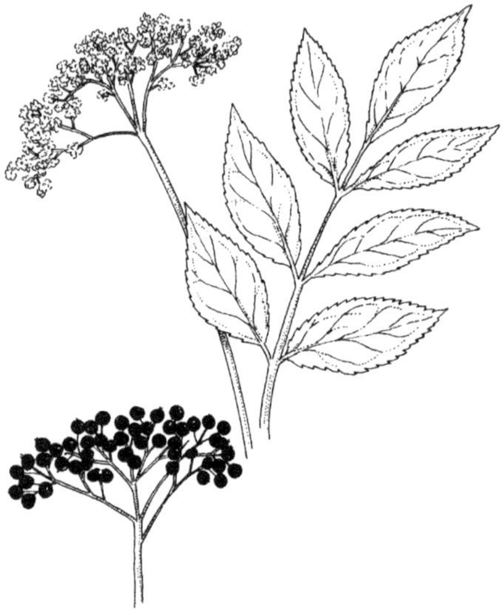

Description: Blue elder is a shrub to small tree with masses of creamy-yellow, umbrella-shaped, flowering parts and bright-blue, edible berries. You can find elder flowers in herb shops as a bulk herb. High-quality flower tinctures are also available. Other kinds of preparations, such as standardized extracts, may or may not be as active, because some of the constituents break down within a week after harvest.

Uses: Elder's anti-viral properties make it effective for relieving colds, flu, and fevers. The herb is an excellent detoxifier and helps clear infections like acne, boils, skin rashes, and other forms of dermatitis. Modern research also shows that elder flowers can help strengthen resistance against infections by supporting immune function. Herbalists sometimes also recommend elder for hay fever and sinusitis. The extracts, made from the ripe blue fruits of the elderberry, can be an excellent remedy for chronic rheumatism, neuralgia, and sciatica.

Dosage: For colds and fever, take 2 to 3 cups of the infusion, 2 to 3 times daily to induce sweating. Soaking in a hot bath or wrapping up in a sheet and a sleeping bag or blankets helps bring on a good flow of sweat, eliminating toxins and speeding the healing process. Follow the manufacturer's instructions for berry syrups and extracts in capsule or tablet form.

Eleuthero (Siberian Ginseng)

Latin name: *Eleutherococcus senticosus* [Rupr. ex Maxim.] Maxim.

Description: While not a true ginseng, eleuthero is often called Siberian ginseng because it's a tall spiny shrub from the ginseng family. Eleuthero is available as a bulk herb to make tea, in tincture form, and as a standardized or concentrated extract in capsules and tablets.

Uses: Consider taking eleuthero if you're feeling tired, run-down, are going through major changes in your life, are under stress, or if you're serious about sports. Eleuthero is an herbal remedy from a group of natural remedies called

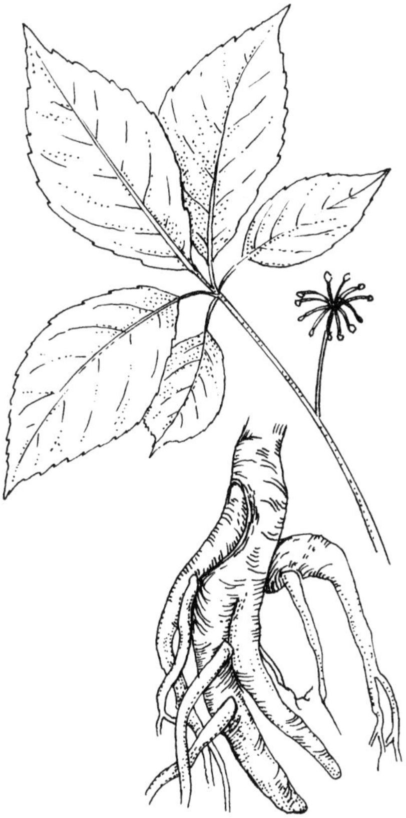

adaptogens — they help you adapt to stress and changes in your life. Studies show that you may have more energy, get sick less often, have better workouts, or let stress roll off your back more easily with eleuthero. I travel a lot to teach herb classes, and eleuthero helps me avoid jet lag.

Dosage: Make a decoction with 1 teaspoon of the herb for every cup of water by simmering for 30 minutes. Drink 1 cup of the tea, or add 1/2 teaspoon of the tincture to a little water, and drink, 2 times daily. Follow the label directions for other kinds of products.

Evening Primrose

Latin name: *Oenothera biennis* L.

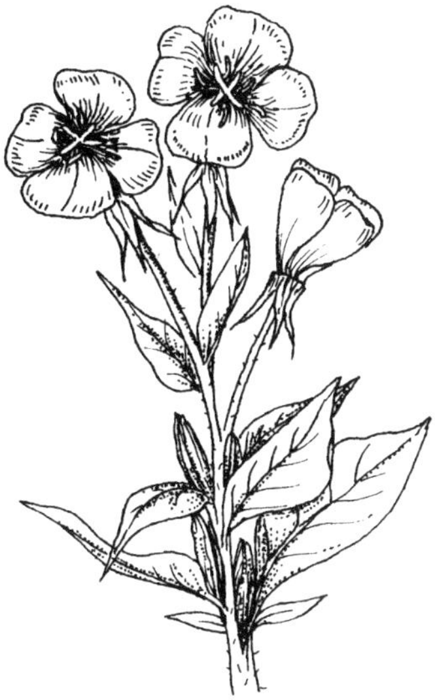

Description: A tall biennial weed found in gardens, roadsides, and fields. Evening primrose has large, bright-yellow flowers turning into short spike-like capsules that produce an abundant crop of small brown seeds. The oil, extracted from the seeds, is rich in gamma linolenic acid (GLA). You can find evening primrose oil in capsules.

Uses: Consider taking evening primrose to help you ease the symptoms of arthritis and skin problems (like eczema and psoriasis). I've seen uneven results for PMS and breast tenderness, but I'm more optimistic about its effectiveness when evening primrose is added to other herbal remedies like vitex, black cohosh, or skullcap.

Dosage: Take 250 to 500 mg of the oil daily, in capsules.

Eyebright

Latin name: *Euphrasia* spp.

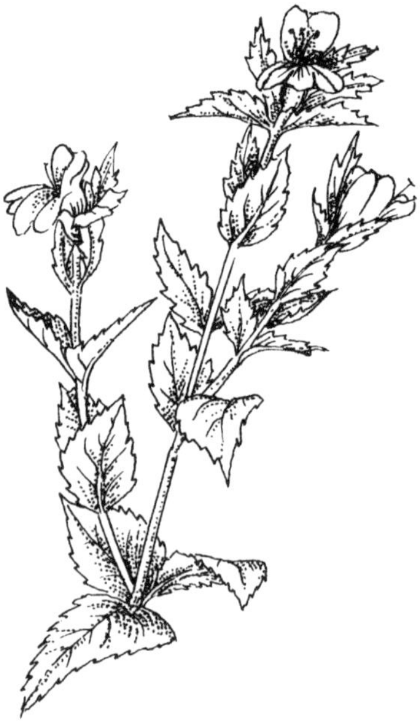

Description: Eyebright is a small perennial found in grasslands and pastures. The above-ground parts are harvested when the plant is in full flower. Eyebright herb is available in capsule form, in liquid tinctures, and in bulk as a tea for internal use and to make compresses.

Uses: Although the active constituents or mechanism of action of eyebright isn't known, the herb has a long history of use for eye infections like pink eye and styes, as well as for eye irritation, sinus infections, and hay fever. Consider using eyebright for its anti-inflammatory and mild decongestant properties.

Dosage: Take 2 to 4 droppersful of the tincture, 2 to 3 cups of the infusion, or 3 to 5 capsules of the herb, 2 to 3 times daily.

Fennel

Latin name: *Foeniculum vulgare* Mill.

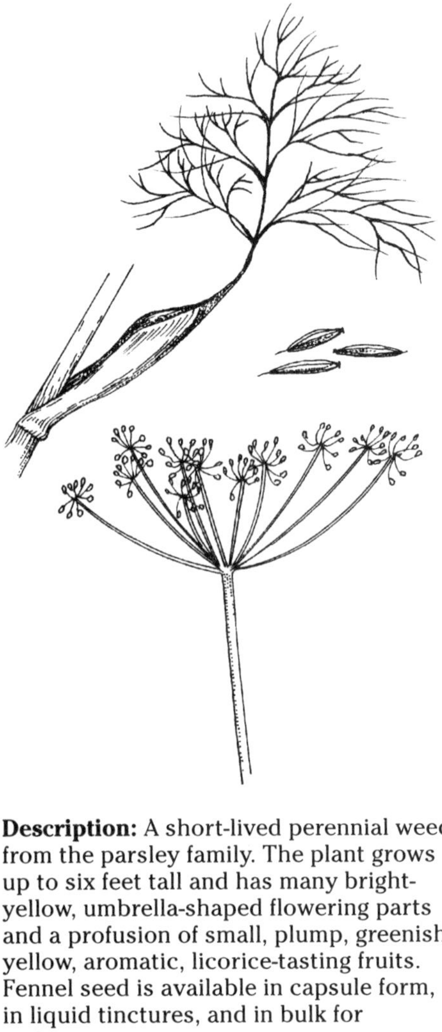

Description: A short-lived perennial weed from the parsley family. The plant grows up to six feet tall and has many bright-yellow, umbrella-shaped flowering parts and a profusion of small, plump, greenish-yellow, aromatic, licorice-tasting fruits. Fennel seed is available in capsule form, in liquid tinctures, and in bulk for making tea.

Uses: Fennel is an ancient and popular modern herbal remedy for dyspepsia, flatulence, nausea, and stomachache and for easing the pains and spasms of colic and diarrhea of babies and young children. Herbalists recommend fennel to mothers for increasing lactation after a child is born. An infusion of the seeds is used externally as a compress for conjunctivitis.

Dosage: Drink 1 cup of the light decoction or infusion, made by steeping 1 teaspoon of the herb for every cup of water, or take 3 or 4 capsules or 2 to 4 droppersful of the tincture, 2 to 3 times daily.

Fenugreek

Latin name: *Trigonella foenum-graecum* L.

Description: Fenugreek is a simple-stemmed, hairy, white-flowered plant in the pea family that grows one- to two-feet tall. Fenugreek seed is available in capsule form, and you can also find it in liquid tinctures and in bulk for making tea. I recommend the tea or poultice as the most effective way to use the herb.

Uses: Crush the seeds and simmer them to make a thick, slimy tea, then spread the mass onto a piece of cloth, and place over boils and sores to help draw out waste products and speed healing. This preparation is called a *cataplasm*. A tea of fenugreek is an excellent remedy to help relieve atherosclerosis, bronchitis, diabetes, and to increase lactation.

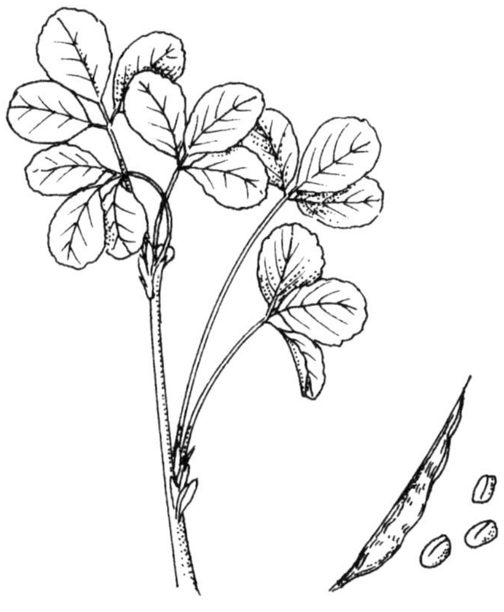

Dosage: Simmer 1 to 2 tablespoons of the ground or crushed seeds in 4 cups of water for 15 minutes and let the decoction steep for another 15 minutes. Drink 1/2 to 1 cup, 2 or 3 times daily.

Caution: Avoid use of this herb during pregnancy.

Feverfew

Latin name: *Tanacetum parthenium* [L.] Schulz-Bip.

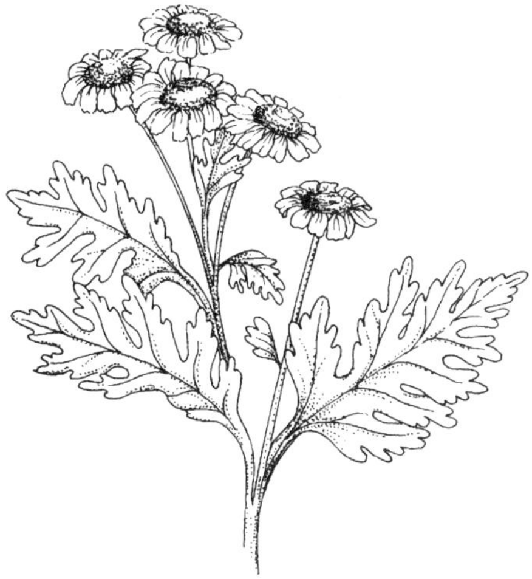

Description: A common aromatic garden plant, feverfew has delicate leaves and a profusion of small daisy-like flowers. Feverfew is available in extract form, or dried and powdered in capsules, in liquid tinctures, and in bulk for making tea. You can purchase the herb as a standardized extract, and you may get a more consistent effect, because certain feverfew varieties contain very little, if any, of the active compounds.

Uses: As the name implies, feverfew is an excellent remedy for flu and other respiratory infections that are accompanied by a fever. As a bitter, aromatic herb, the Italians favor the plant as an herb to use in cooking for stimulating the appetite. Because of its strong anti-inflammatory properties, feverfew is a popular remedy for migraine headaches and arthritis.

Dosage: Take 1 to 3 droppersful of the tincture, 1 to 2 times daily, or 2 capsules of the powder or standardized extract daily.

Caution: Avoid the use of feverfew if you're pregnant.

Flaxseed

Latin name: *Linum usitatissimum* L.

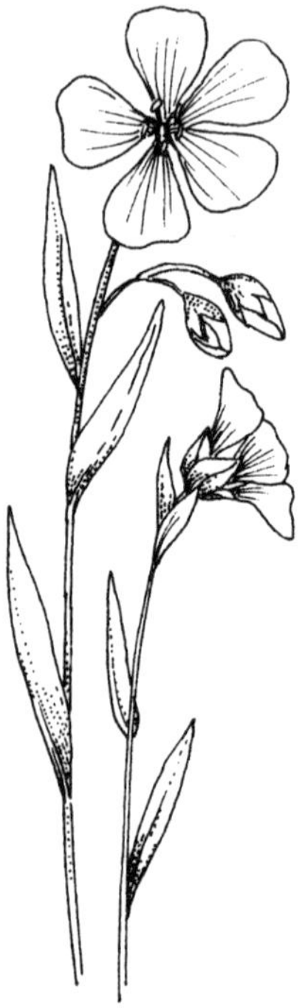

Description: Flax is a slender, branching, annual plant with blue or white flowers. The small, round, fruiting capsules contain the sharp-pointed glossy-brown seeds that are used for food and medicine. Crude flaxseed oil is called *linseed oil* and is a component of paints and the original linoleum tiles. The stalk fiber is durable and was formerly used to make linen. Always buy whole, organic flaxseeds and grind them fresh for daily use. The organic high lignan oil is available in bulk or in capsules.

Uses: Flaxseed is useful for easing constipation, inflammation, and irritation of the stomach and intestines and the respiratory tract. Applied externally, it can draw out toxins, reduce inflammation, and speed healing. Flaxseed meal and some commercial oil products are high in lignans, which act as weak estrogens in the body. The regular use of these preparations may help you to balance your estrogen activity, reducing the risk of some cancers and heart disease and benefiting women who are going through menopause.

Dosage: Simmer 1 tablespoon of flaxseeds or flaxseed meal in 2 cups of water, and drink 1 cup, 2 times daily, as needed. Sprinkle flaxseed meal on cereals and other foods. Grind 1 or 2 tablespoons of flaxseeds in a seed grinder or blender to a powder and soak in $^1/_4$ to $^1/_2$ cup of hot water until a slimy mass forms. Spread the gel into a small piece of cloth and apply to boils and sores.

Caution: Don't use flaxseed if you have bowel obstruction. Always drink plenty of water, about 2 eight-ounce glasses, when taking this herb.

Garlic

Latin name: *Allium sativum* L.

Description: Garlic is an onion-like aromatic plant with hollow, round leaves and umbrella-shaped, flowering parts with starry purple flowers. The bulbs are harvested in the summer and stored for use in cooking and to make medicinal products. You can buy garlic bulbs from your local grocery store or natural food store. Garlic is also available as a powder or granules in bulk and in many commercial *odor-controlled* capsules, either as oil or powder.

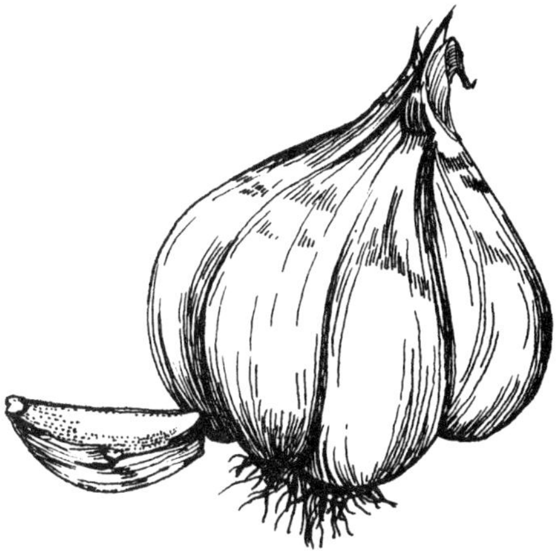

Uses: Garlic is warming to your digestion and respiratory tract and is an important antibiotic and anti-viral remedy for colds, flu, bronchitis, pneumonia, and other infections. Consider garlic preparations for protecting the blood and cardiovascular system. With regular use, the herb can help to slightly lower your high blood pressure, reduce high cholesterol, and help prevent atherosclerosis. Garlic is famous for killing and clearing intestinal parasites.

Dosage: Take 2 to 4 perles of a garlic product daily or follow the manufacturer's directions. The therapeutic dose of whole garlic is 2 to 3 cloves daily with meals, either cooked or raw.

Caution: Avoid the use of garlic if you're nursing. Raw garlic can sometimes irritate your stomach if you eat too much.

Gentian

Latin name: *Gentiana lutea* L.

Description: A tall and stout perennial plant with whorls of yellow flowers. Gentian root is available as a powdered herb in capsule or tablet form, in liquid tinctures, and as a bulk herb for making tea. You can find the root extract as an ingredient of many commercial digestion-promoting products.

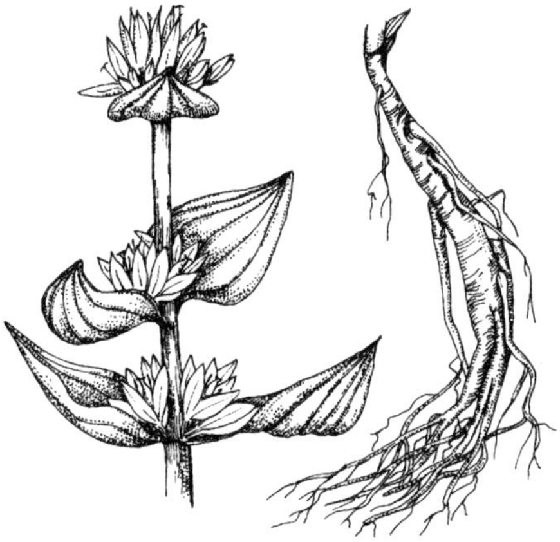

Uses: The roots contain pure bitter compounds so intense that you can still taste the bitter at a dilution of 1 drop of the tincture in 20,000 parts water. Because the root doesn't contain tannins or other digestive irritants, it's recommended for daily use and can be taken for years. The herb is prescribed for weak digestion, poor appetite, anemia, and if you're recovering from an illness.

Dosage: Make a decoction by simmering $^1/_2$ teaspoon of the herb for every cup of water for 10 minutes, then steeping for 15 minutes. Drink $^1/_2$ cup of the decoction or take 10 to 30 drops of the tincture, 2 to 3 times daily, in a little water before meals.

Caution: Avoid the use of this herb if you have an ulcer or gastric irritation or inflammation.

Ginger

Latin name: *Zingiber officinale* Roscoe.

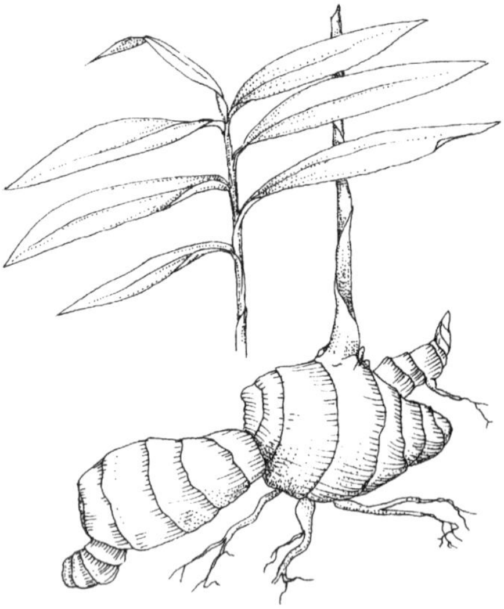

Description: The ginger plant, with yellow or tan fragrant flowers, grows to three or more feet high from masses of knobby underground rhizomes. You can find the fresh rhizome nestled in with garlic in natural food stores and supermarkets, and herb shops carry every kind of preparation and formula, including tinctures, syrups, capsules, and tablets. You may enjoy pickled or candied ginger, which is available in herb shops and grocery stores.

Uses: Ginger is arguably the most important digestive herb in world commerce. Consider using ginger if you feel nauseous or to settle your stomach if you have morning sickness, motion sickness, or other intestinal problems. I've found ginger to be an important aid for easing nausea and discomfort common in patients who are going through chemotherapy. Ginger's warming and blood-moving effects are helpful if you have poor circulation. The herb's sweat-promoting properties can help ease and shorten unpleasant symptoms you experience during colds and flu, such as coughs and mucus congestion. I often recommend ginger tea to help prevent colds in the first place. My patients report that a hot compress of ginger tea is remarkably beneficial for arthritis, sore joints after a joint replacement procedure, and for strains, sprains, sore backs, and other injuries. Cool ginger tea is effective for easing the pain of minor burns and rashes.

Dosage: You can make a strong ginger tea by simmering several slices of the fresh rhizome or one teaspoon of the cut and sifted dried herb for every cup of water. Drink 1 cup of decoction, 2 or 3 as needed, preferably around mealtimes. You can also take 2 capsules of the powder or 2 to 4 droppersful of the tincture, 2 to 3 times daily.

Caution: Avoid taking more than 2 or 3 cups a day during pregnancy. The fresh rhizome is safer to use during pregnancy than the dried root.

Ginkgo

Latin name: *Ginkgo biloba* L.

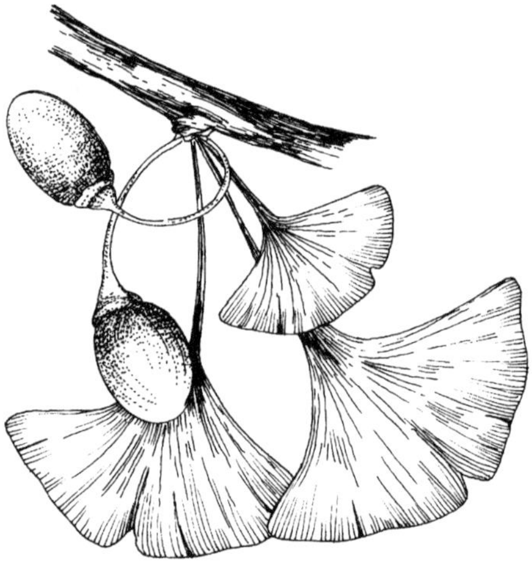

Description: A large tree originally from the mountains of China, ginkgo has fanciful fan-shaped leaves, often with two lobes. Ginkgo is widely available as a standardized extract in capsule or tablet form and as a liquid tincture. In my experience, you probably won't enjoy the taste of the tea, and it isn't really effective for moderate to severe symptoms. You're better off using the tincture for mild conditions or prevention, or the standardized extract for moderate to severe conditions, especially for long-term use.

Uses: Research and clinical experience show that ginkgo extract is effective for improving blood circulation to the brain which makes it useful for improving your memory, for mental alertness, and for mental energy. Ginkgo is often recommended for helping to slow the progression of Alzheimer's disease. Extracts of ginkgo help restore circulation to your legs if you have blocked arteries and experience pain when you walk. The extract can also improve circulation to your eyes and ears. This improved blood flow, coupled with ginkgo's powerful antioxidant action, makes it useful as a remedy for reducing ringing in the ears (tinnitis), for protecting your eyesight, and even for preventing and treating macular degeneration. I find ginkgo an important herb for autoimmune conditions like some forms of hepatitis and asthma.

Dosage: Take 2 to 3 droppersful of the tincture for up to a month or two for daily prevention or mild to moderate symptoms. For longer-term use or moderate to severe symptoms, I recommend 1 capsule or tablet containing 60 mg of the standardized extract, 2 to 3 times daily.

Caution: The highly purified extract containing 24 percent flavone glycosides can cause mild gastrointestinal irritation if you're sensitive.

Ginseng

Latin name: *Panax ginseng* C. A. Mey.

Description: Ginseng is a small perennial herb with symmetrical branches at the top of the stem, each palmately compound with coarsely-toothed, sharply-pointed leaflets. The single flowering stalk comes out of the top of the plant and produces bright red berries. You can find ginseng in capsule or tablet form as a powder, in capsules as a standardized extract, in liquid tinctures, and as whole root or powder in bulk for making tea.

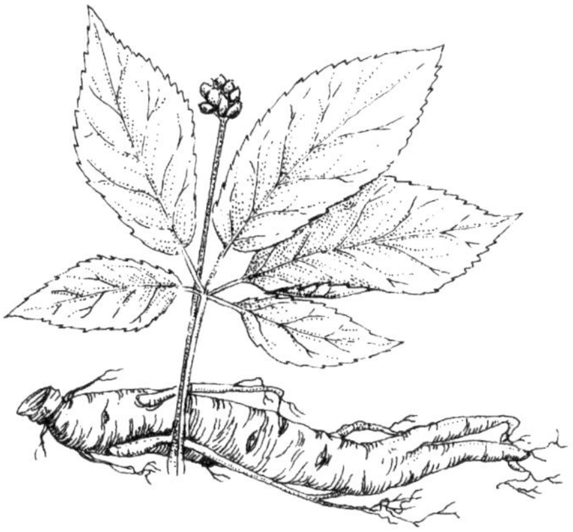

Uses: Consider taking ginseng if you have digestive problems like gas or malabsorption or if you commonly experience a feeling of fullness, even after eating only small meals. Use ginseng for chronic fatigue, convalescence, lethargy, depression, and chronic infections related to immune weakness, especially if you're over forty-five. Ginseng is particularly revered for its digestive-strengthening powers. Because your digestion is the source of daily vitality, by improving its efficiency you also strengthen your immune system and hormone balance.

Dosage: Make a decoction by simmering 1 level teaspoon of the ground-up root for every cup of water, and drink 1 cup, 2 to 3 times daily. Take 1 to 3 droppersful of the tincture, or 1 to 2 capsules of the standardized extract, 2 to 3 times daily.

Caution: Avoid use of this herb if you have hypertension. Use American ginseng or eleuthero (Siberian ginseng) if you're under forty years old, unless prescribed by a practitioner of Traditional Chinese Medicine.

Ginseng, American

Latin name: *Panax quinquefolius* Meyer.

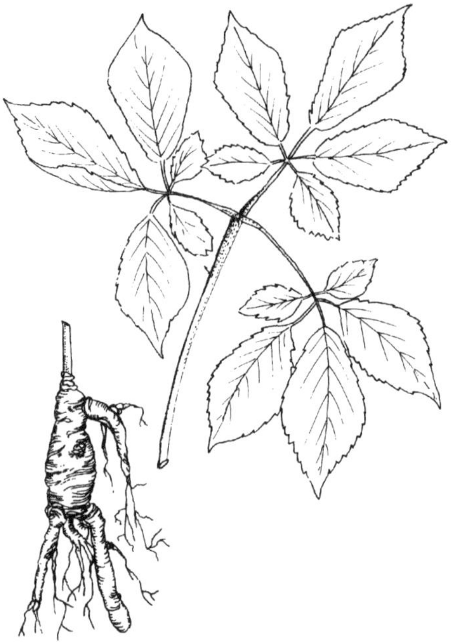

Description: American ginseng is an upright, three-pronged plant of hardwood forests of the eastern United States and southern Canada with up to five leaflets on each prong. The plant produces red berries in the fall. Many wild populations are depleted because of its popularity for the last 400 years. Your best bet is to buy whole roots and products containing organically cultivated, woods-grown, or commercially-grown roots.

Uses: American ginseng supports hormone balance, cools the body, and protects the adrenals against stress. Use it for adrenal fatigue, chronic fatigue, chronic rashes, arthritis, digestive weakness with inflammation, irritable bowel syndrome, certain kinds of insomnia, and nervousness.

Dosage: Take 2 to 4 grams daily as a decoction, $^{1}/_{2}$ to 1 teaspoon of the tincture in a little water, or 2 capsules or tablets containing a powdered extract that you take morning and evening with meals.

Caution: Don't use if you feel anxious — it's slightly stimulating.

Goldenrod

Latin name: *Solidago* spp.

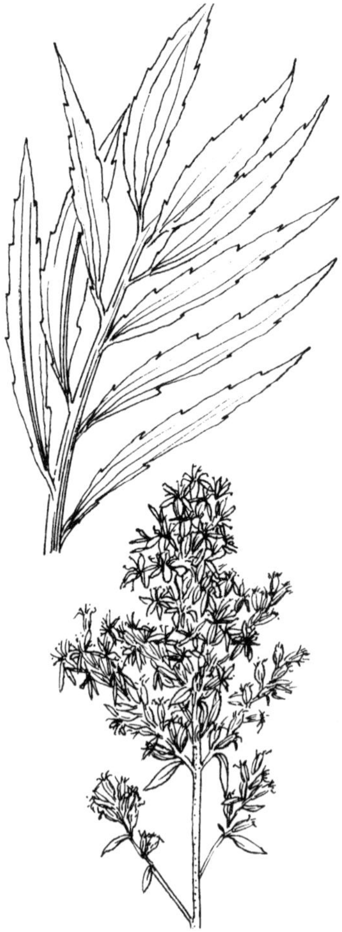

Description: The goldenrods are tall perennial plants growing in large colonies in fields and open places with long arching sprays of small yellow flowering heads. The flowering parts of the aromatic plant are harvested for medicine. You can find goldenrod in liquid tinctures, in capsules, and in bulk for making tea.

Uses: Goldenrod herb is an effective remedy for stimulating kidney function and increasing the flow of urine output. I recommend this herb for strengthening the prostate gland and urinary organs and reducing inflammation, especially blended with saw palmetto extract. German herbalists recommend goldenrod for varicose veins due to its rich store of flavonoids. Blend goldenrod herb with echinacea and ginger for colds.

Dosage: Make a light decoction with 1 teaspoon of the herb for every cup of water, and drink 1/2 cup several times daily. Take 2 to 4 droppersful of the tincture, 2 or 3 times daily.

Caution: Avoid goldenrod if you have chronic kidney problems. See your herbalist and a physician if you suspect that you have a kidney infection.

Goldenseal

Latin name: *Hydrastis canadensis* L.

Description: Goldenseal is a small perennial plant that grows to about one foot high, with several five to nine-lobed leaves, a cluster of small white flowers, and crimson-red berries. The rhizomes are harvested for making medicinal preparations. Goldenseal is available in capsule form, in liquid tinctures, and as whole root or powder in bulk for making tea.

Uses: Internally, take goldenseal preparations to reduce inflammation, for bacterial infections of the upper respiratory tract and urinary tract, and for bacterial or amebic infections of the digestive tract, like giardia and dysentery. The herb isn't as effective for viral conditions like colds and flu, gastritis, and sinus infections. Externally, use goldenseal tea as a wash for conjunctivitis and gum problems and as a douche for vaginal infections from candida or trichomonas.

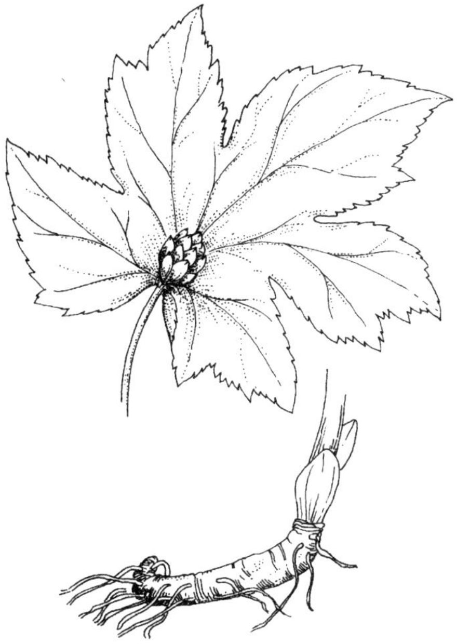

Dosage: You can take 1 to 2 droppersful of the tincture, or 1 to 2 capsules 2 times daily. Make a light decoction with 1/2 teaspoon of the herb for each cup of water, and drink 1 cup, up to 3 times daily, as needed.

Caution: Don't use goldenseal if you're pregnant. Contrary to popular belief, goldenseal isn't effective for clearing drugs out of the body to help you pass a drug detection test. The plant is overharvested and was recently added to a national list of endangered plants. Herbalists often recommend alternative herbs with the same active compound, the yellow alkaloid berberine, like barberry and the Chinese herb coptis.

Gotu Kola

Latin name: *Centella asiatica* [L.] Urban.

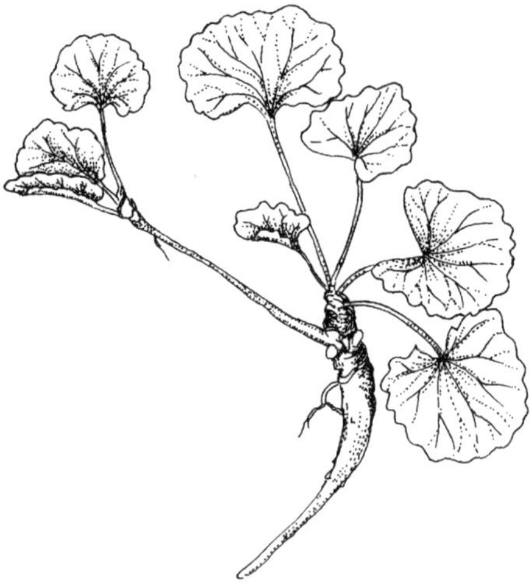

Description: A creeping and spreading herbaceous perennial from the parsley family, gotu kola has round leaves and trailing stems. The entire herb is collected for making tonic drinks and other preparations. You can buy gotu kola in capsule form, in liquid tinctures, and in bulk as leaf or powder for making tea.

Uses: Use gotu kola internally for improving your memory and supporting your mental functions and nervous system. Use creams and external preparations for healing eczema, wounds, and other skin conditions.

Dosage: Take 2 to 4 droppersful of the tincture made from the fresh plant or 2 to 3 cups of the infusion made from the dried herb, 2 to 3 times daily.

Grapeseed

Latin name: *Vitis vinifera* L.

Description: Grapeseed comes from the grape vine. The seed extract contains potent antioxidant compounds called oligomeric proanthocyanidins (OPCs), which some researchers claim may slow down the aging process. Grapeseed extract is available as a standardized extract in capsule or tablet form. When you eat grapes, choose varieties containing seeds and chew and swallow them along with the sweet pulp to receive the best health benefits.

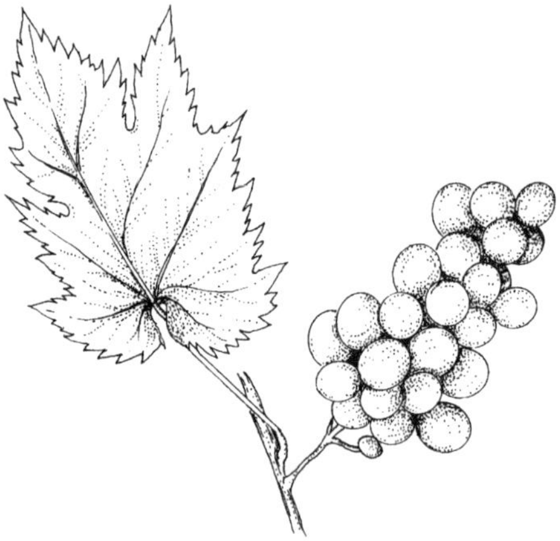

Uses: Grapeseed extract can help protect the skin and internal organs against the ravages of stress and environmental toxins. Regular use of grape skin and seed extracts may help protect you from developing cancer.

Dosage: Follow the manufacturer's instructions on the packaging. I often recommend that you take 1 or 2 capsules of the extract, 1 or 2 times daily, depending on your need.

Green Tea

Latin name: *Camellia sinensis* [L.] Kuntze.

Description: Green tea comes from a large bush or small tree. Green tea is available as a standardized extract in capsule or tablet form, and in bulk and teabags for making tea. Decaffeinated tea is available in capsules and tea.

Uses: Green tea may protect you against heart disease, ulcers, and cancer. You can use tea as a mouthwash to prevent plaque formation. Green tea contains antibacterial and antioxidant properties. It's used in many countries to help relieve diarrhea, reduce pain, and invigorate the mind and the nervous system.

Dosage: Make a cup of tea with one teaspoon of loose herb for every cup of water, and drink 2 to 3 cups infusion daily. Follow the manufacturer's instructions for other products, but generally I recommend 1 or 2 capsules a day of the standardized extract. Try substituting green tea for coffee.

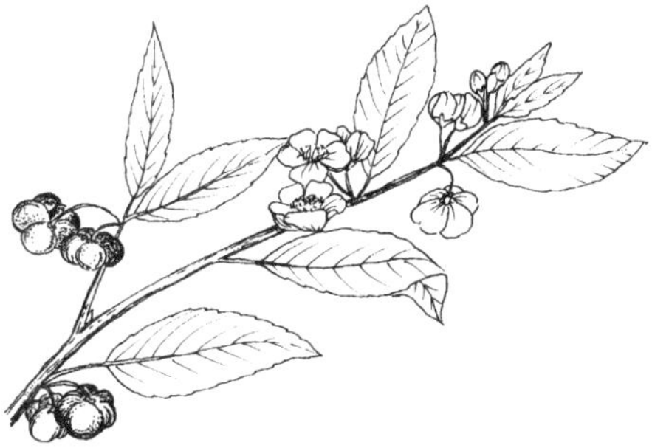

Caution: Green tea contains four or five percent caffeine. Avoid using the herb if you have heart palpitations or experience insomnia or anxiety. Remember that the tea and standardized extract are available without the caffeine.

Hawthorn

Latin name: *Crataegus laevigata* [Poir] DC.

Description: Hawthorn is a small to medium-sized tree with umbrella-shaped clusters of white or pink flowers and dark, glossy-green, toothed leaves. Hawthorn flowers, leaves, and fruits are available as a powder in capsule or tablet form, or you can buy standardized extract in tablets, in liquid tinctures, and in bulk for making tea.

Uses: Take hawthorn preparations for heart irregularity and palpitations, atherosclerosis, angina, hypertension, and nervousness, and to support and strengthen your heart. Herbalists enthusiastically recommend extracts of hawthorn for steadying the heartbeat and increasing blood flow to the heart muscle. When used over months and years, you may find the herb has a pronounced strengthening effect on the heart and blood vessels.

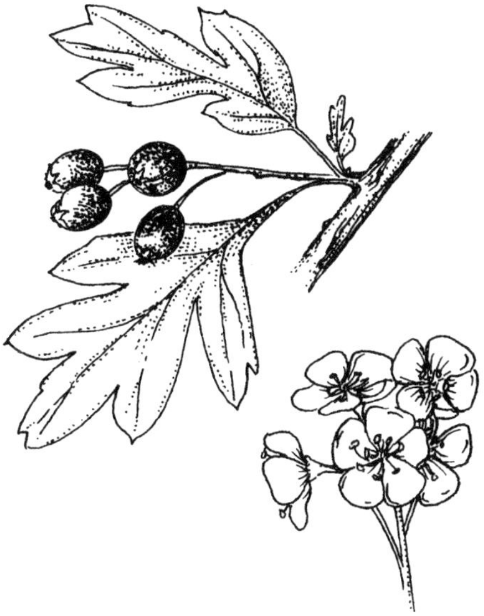

Dosage: Take 2 to 3 droppersful of the flower and leaf tincture, 1 cup of the decoction, or 3 to 4 capsules of the powder, 2 to 3 times daily.

Caution: Hawthorn can potentize the effects of digitalis preparations (such as digoxin). See your doctor if you're taking digoxin or related compounds.

Hops

Latin name: *Humulus lupulus* L.

Description: The hops vine is fast-growing, rough, and sandpaper-like in texture, and forms small female and male *cones* (called strobiles) on stalks from the area just above the upper leaves. The female cones, which produce a golden yellow resinous powder called lupulin, are collected for medicine and for the brewing of beer. Hops is available in capsule form as an extract or powder, in liquid tinctures, and in bulk for making tea.

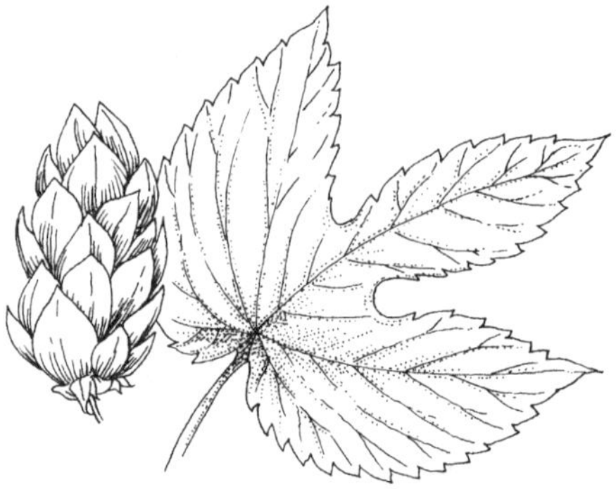

Uses: Hops cones are an ancient remedy for relieving nervousness, insomnia, restlessness, excitability, and excessive sexual excitement. I've observed excellent results with this herb for easing heart palpitations. You can also use hops for nervous digestion and insufficient breast milk. Hops may have weak estrogenic properties, but this isn't proven.

Dosage: You can take 1 to 3 droppersful of the tincture, 2 to 3 times daily, or 1 cup of the infusion made with 1 tablespoon of hops, as needed.

Caution: Avoid hops if you're depressed.

Horehound

Latin name: *Marrubium vulgare* L.

Description: Horehound is a hairy, greenish-white garden perennial from the mint family. The whole herb is harvested for medicinal use — it's certainly far too bitter to make a pleasant beverage. Horehound is available in liquid tinctures and in bulk for making tea. The extract is added to candies and syrups.

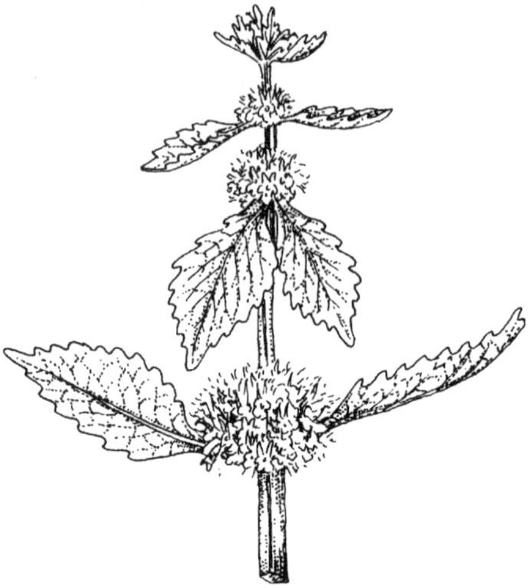

Uses: Horehound herb is famous for relieving coughs. It has antispasmodic and expectorant properties, and you may find it effective for easing the congestion, wheezing, coughs of colds and asthma, sore throats, and fevers.

Dosage: Make an infusion by steeping 1 teaspoon of the dried herb in 1 cup of boiled water and drinking $^1/_2$ to 1 cup, or 2 to 4 droppersful of the tincture in a little water, 2 or 3 times daily. You can suck on a horehound candy, several times daily, to relieve coughs.

Caution: Avoid horehound when you're pregnant.

Horse Chestnut

Latin name: *Aesculus hippocastunum* L.

Description: Horse chestnut is a large tree with palmately compound leaves with five coarsely-toothed leaflets and long spikes of fragrant pinkish-white flowers. The two-inch nuts are harvested and extracted to produce liquid extracts, standardized capsules, and in creams for external use.

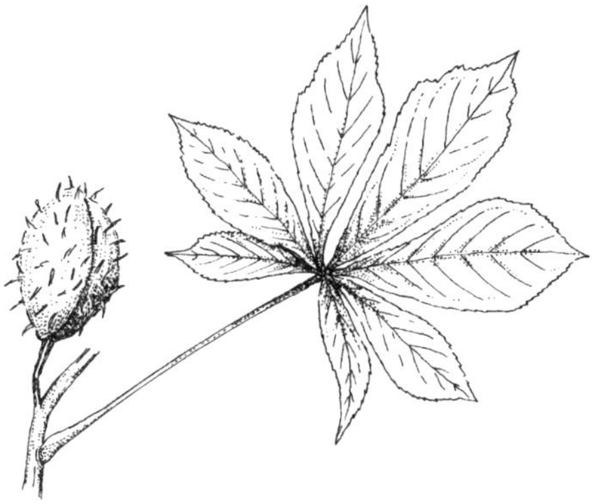

Uses: Internally, horse chestnut tinctures or standardized extracts in capsules are popular in Europe for treating varicose veins, hemorrhoids, and sports injuries. Externally, horse chestnut creams are effective for easing the pain and swelling of sports injuries, sprains, strains, bruises, and varicose veins.

Dosage: Take 5 to 20 drops of the tincture, 3 times daily. Follow the manufacturer's directions for other products.

Caution: Don't exceed the recommended dose. The raw nuts of the horse chestnut tree are irritating to the gastrointestinal tract and are considered toxic if not processed. Commercial preparations are safe when the label instructions are followed.

Horsetail

Latin name: *Equisetum arvense* L.

Description: Horsetail is a non-flowering plant that looks like a green horse's tail. The straight, ribbed stems are often covered with whorled, radiating branches, but some species aren't. Branchless shoots, which are not as likely to be harvested for herbal remedies, are often capped with an arrowhead-shaped cone at the top that produces a prolific amount of spores. You can find horsetail as a bulk herb for making teas, as a tincture, or in capsules or tablets. I recommend adding nettle herb to horsetail for extra minerals. Products standardized to organic silicic acid are often effective.

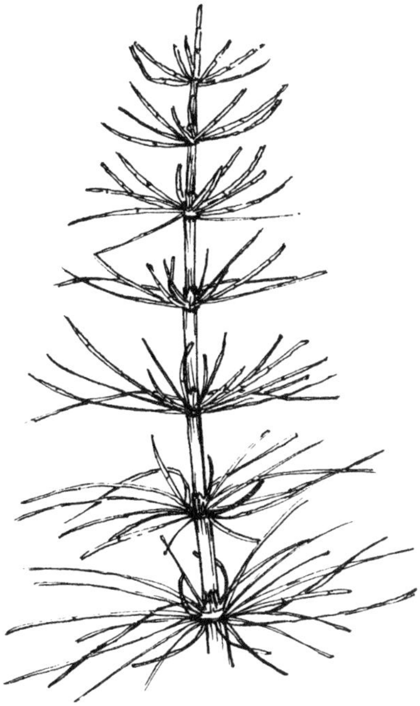

Uses: Consider taking horsetail herb internally for cystitis, prostatitis, and to strengthen and regenerate connective tissue. The herb is high in organic silica and is useful for strengthening bones, hair, and nails. I recommend using horsetail extracts in capsule form if your nails or hair are brittle and break easily. In Europe, extracts of horsetail are used for easing inflammation and to speed healing of rheumatism and arthritis. The tincture or tea is a useful diuretic and helps cleanse the urinary tract and remove excess mucus.

Dosage: Drink 1 cup decoction several times a day made by simmering 1 or 2 tablespoons of the cut and sifted herb for each cup of water for up to 3 hours to extract the organic silica. Take 2 or 3 droppersful of the tincture, 2 or 3 times daily. Follow the manufacturer's directions for taking the standardized extract.

Caution: Consult with an herbalist before taking horsetail if you have chronic heart or kidney problems.

Juniper

Latin name: *Juniperus communis* L.

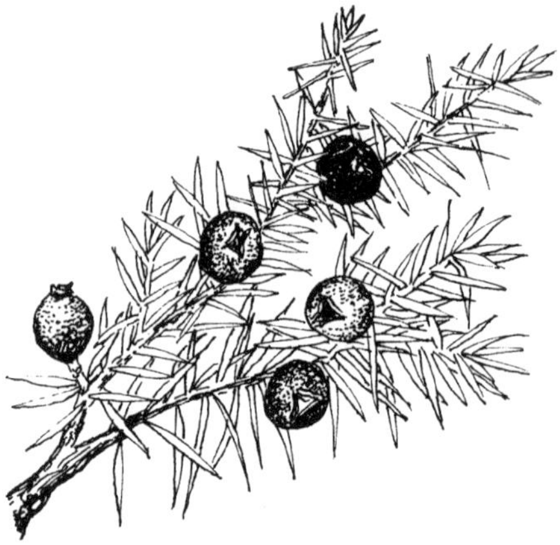

Description: Junipers are small to medium-sized evergreen trees of dry places with whorls of sharp needles on the branches, shredding bark, and purple-green berry-like cones. Juniper is available in capsule form, in liquid tinctures, and in bulk for making tea.

Uses: Use the berries to help ease the symptoms of urinary tract infections because of their antibiotic and cleansing effects. Herbalists recommend the berries for cystitis, gout, and weak digestion with gas. You may find that rubbing the tincture on sore rheumatic joints helps to ease pain and inflammation.

Dosage: Make a tea by infusing 1 teaspoon of the berries with 6 cups of freshly boiled water for 20 minutes. Drink $1/2$ cup of the tea, several times daily. Take 20 to 30 drops, or 1 to 2 capsules of the ground berry powder with a little water, several times daily.

Caution: Avoid the use of juniper berries when you're pregnant or if you have preexisting kidney disease.

Kava

Latin name: *Piper methysticum* G. Forster.

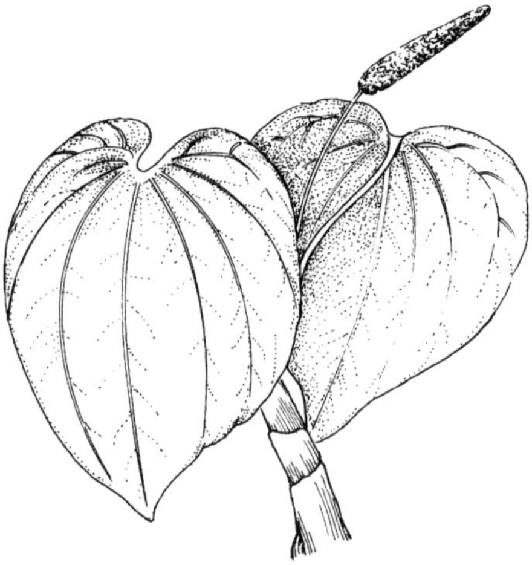

Description: A relative of black pepper, kava is a large-leaved perennial shrub with angled jointed stems. The spicy rhizomes, roots, and the leaves are all harvested. Kava powder and standardized extracts are available in capsule or tablet form, along with liquid tinctures, and the bulk powder or cut and sifted herb is available for making teas.

Uses: Drink a cup of kava when you feel tense, overtired, nervous, or have trouble sleeping. Herbalists recommend kava drinks and tinctures for fatigue, insomnia, tight muscles, and mild depression, as well as for bladder infections and prostate inflammation with decreased urination.

Dosage: Take 2 to 4 droppersful of the tincture, or swallow 1 or 2 tablets or capsules of the standardized extract, 2 or 3 times daily, with a little water. Make a decoction by simmering 1 teaspoon of the herb for every cup of water, and drink 1 cup several times daily as needed. My experience with the herb shows me that the tincture is best for relaxing tight, tense muscles. Either the powdered extract or tea is better for a euphoric and mentally-relaxing effect.

Caution: Avoid use of this herb during pregnancy and nursing. Don't exceed the recommended dose. If you drink kava — be careful if you drive. A kava user was recently cited for driving while under the influence of kava — and fined!

Lavender

Latin name: *Lavandula angustifolia* Mill.

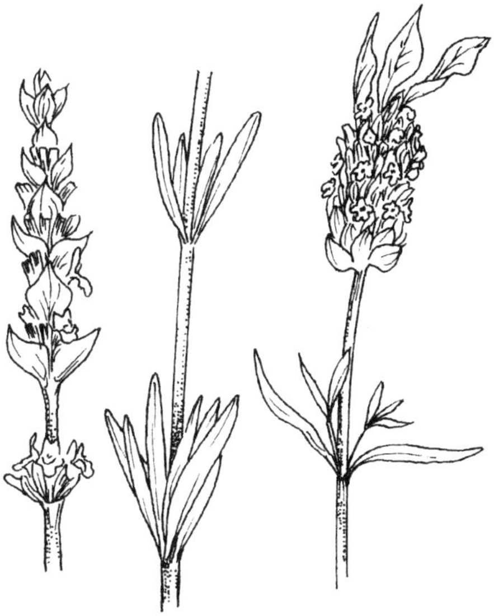

Description: Lavender is a small shrub of the mint family with tall, purple-spiked flowering parts. Lavender is available in liquid tinctures, in bulk for making tea, and as an essential oil, which is an ingredient in soaps, bath products, and hair products.

Uses: Lavender is best-known for helping to lift the spirits, relax the body, and settle the stomach. Herbalists recommend lavender for nausea, depression, and colic. Use lavender oil topically for burns and add a few drops to baths for relaxation.

Dosage: You can make the infusion with 1 teaspoon of the flowers for every cup of tea and drink 1 cup, 2 to 3 times daily.

Lemon Balm

Latin name: *Melissa officinalis* L.

Description: Lemon balm has lush, green, lemony foliage and fresh white flowers that attract bees. Lemon balm is available in liquid tinctures and in bulk for making tea.

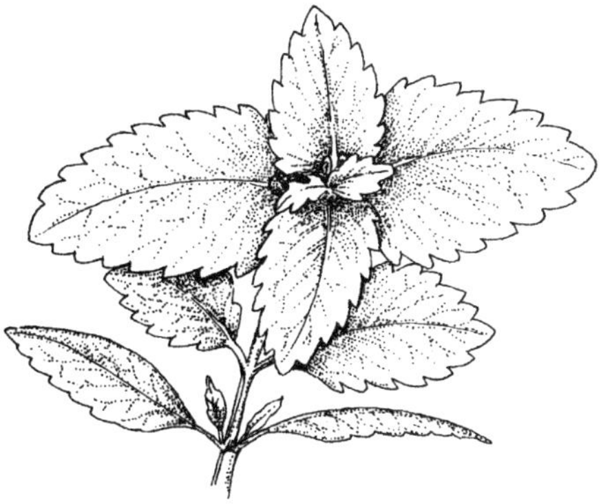

Uses: Use lemon balm if you want a refreshing and relaxing tea that is good for settling the stomach. Herbalists recommend preparations of this herb for calming the nervous system, for nervous heart, tension and insomnia, and for relaxing spasms of the stomach and intestines. Lemon balm is one of my favorite remedies for *nervous stomach,* often accompanied by burning, heartburn, and a feeling of pressure or knots in the stomach. Combine it with other soothing remedies, like marshmallow root and licorice root, for ulcers. Lemon balm creams are widely used in Europe and increasingly in North American and other countries for treating genital and oral herpes sores. I have seen good results when my patients apply a strong decoction of the herb as a compress to areas of the body that are affected by herpes.

Dosage: Make an infusion with 1 tablespoon of the dry leaves and tops for every cup of water, and drink 2 or 3 cups during the day, as needed. Boil the herb for 30 to 60 minutes, let it steep for 15 minutes, and soak a washcloth in the warm tea for external application.

Licorice

Latin name: *Glycyrrhiza glabra* L.

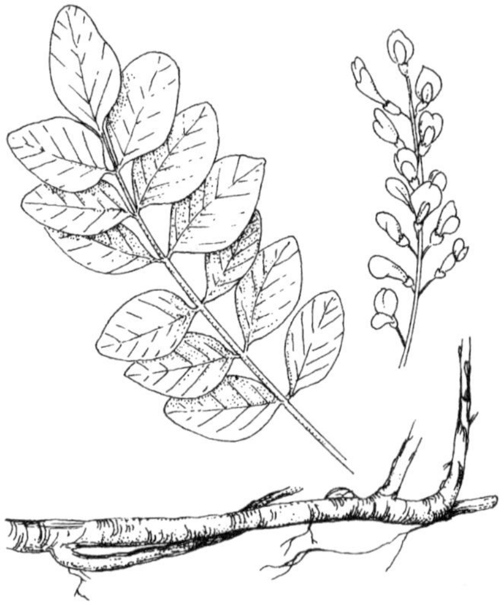

Description: Licorice is a small shrubby perennial plant in the pea family. The roots are harvested after three years of growth for making medicines and food flavoring preparations. Licorice root is available in capsule form, in liquid tinctures, and in bulk for making tea. A special, standardized extract with less potential for causing high blood pressure is available in capsules and tablets under the name DGL.

Uses: Licorice has potent soothing, anti-inflammatory, and anti-viral effects. You can take licorice tea or other preparations for digestive weakness, especially when accompanied by fatigue and shortness of breath. You can also use this herb for ulcers, irritable bowel and bowel inflammation, bronchitis, coughs, and adrenal weakness due to stress or overwork.

Dosage: Make a decoction by simmering 1 teaspoon of the herb for every cup of water for 30 minutes. Drink 1 cup of the decoction or take 1 or 2 droppersful of the tincture, 2 to 3 times daily. Follow the manufacturer's directions for DGL products or standardized extracts.

Caution: Avoid the use of licorice if you're pregnant or have diabetes or hypertension. When taken for prolonged periods, licorice may potentially cause potassium depletion and sodium retention. Licorice is available in a deglycyrrhizinised form, which doesn't cause these side effects.

Ligustrum

Latin name: *Ligustrum lucidum* Ait.

Description: Ligustrum (or wax privet tree) is a shrub or small tree with dark, thick, glossy green leaves and clusters of small creamy flowers. The purple berries are harvested and dried for tea and making prepared medicines. Ligustrum is available in liquid and powdered extracts and in bulk for making tea.

Uses: Take ligustrum for chronic adrenal weakness due to stress and overwork — low back pain, ringing in the ears, and premature greying. Science has supported the traditional use of ligustrum berries for strengthening the immune system during the treatment of cancer.

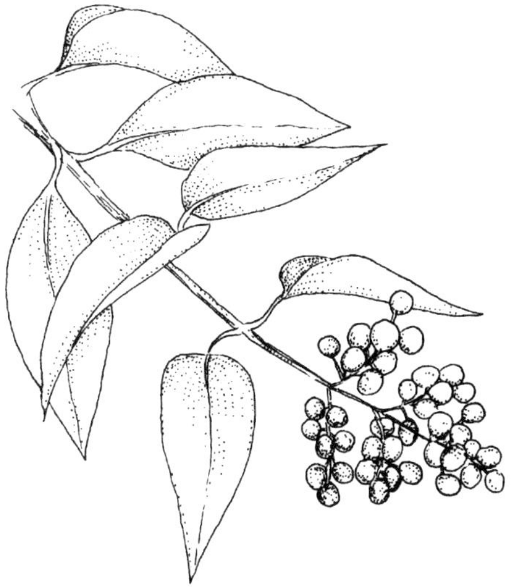

Dosage: Make a decoction by simmering 1 teaspoon of the dried berries 40 to 60 minutes for every cup of water. Drink 1 cup, or take 1/2 to 1 teaspoon of the tincture in a little water, 2 or 3 times daily.

Linden

Latin name: *Tilia* x *europaea* L.

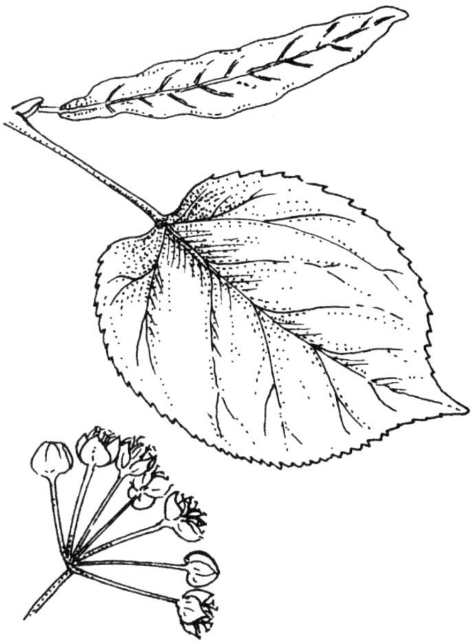

Description: Linden, also called basswood or lime tree, has masses of fragrant, nectar-producing cream-colored flowers arising from special tongue-shaped bracts (small leaf-like appendages). The flowers are collected for making teas and other remedies. Linden flowers are available as liquid tinctures and in bulk form for making tea.

Uses: Linden can bolster your immune system and induce sweating and elimination to relieve symptoms of colds and flu. The flowers also have mild sedative properties and are often added to products for calming your nervous system and reducing blood pressure.

Dosage: Make an infusion by steeping 1 tablespoon of the herb for every cup of boiled water for 20 to 30 minutes, and drink 1 cup, 2 or 3 times a day. Commercial extracts of linden are available but aren't as effective as the tea.

Ma Huang

Latin name: *Ephedra* spp.

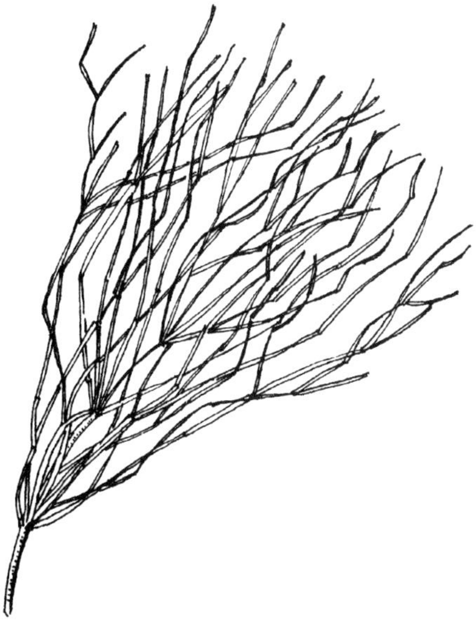

Description: Ma huang is a leafless shrub with grey-green stems. The twigs and branches are harvested for medicine, and some species contain the stimulant alkaloids ephedrine and pseudoephedrine. Ma huang is available as a liquid tincture, powdered extracts in capsules and tablets, and in bulk for making tea.

Uses: Use ma huang for relieving temporary symptoms of asthma, colds with no fever or sweating, hay fever with nasal congestion, and coughs. A strong decongestant, this herb is also useful for earaches. Many commercial formulas are available with ma huang for increasing energy and weight loss, but I discourage this nontraditional use.

Dosage: Make a decoction using 1 tablespoon of the herb for each cup of water, and drink 1/2 to 1 cup, 2 to 3 times daily. Follow the label instructions of other products.

Caution: Avoid ma huang when you're pregnant. Note that ma huang is a nervous system stimulant and may cause anxiety, nervousness, or sleeplessness. Several people have died from using excessive quantities of this herb to stimulate energy. Regular use of ma huang products robs the digestion of the energy it needs to properly digest and assimilate important nutrients and can adversely affect your energy and immune function, nervous system, and cardiovascular system.

Marshmallow

Latin name: *Althaea officinalis* L.

Description: Marshmallow is a shrubby perennial plant, with grey-green, hairy, arrowhead-shaped leaves and pink flowers. All parts of the plant contain a thick mucilage, but the roots contain the highest concentration and are harvested for medicine. (This herb no longer has any connection to the modern marshmallow made with sugar, gelatin, and white flour.) Marshmallow root is available in capsule form, in liquid tinctures, and in bulk for making tea.

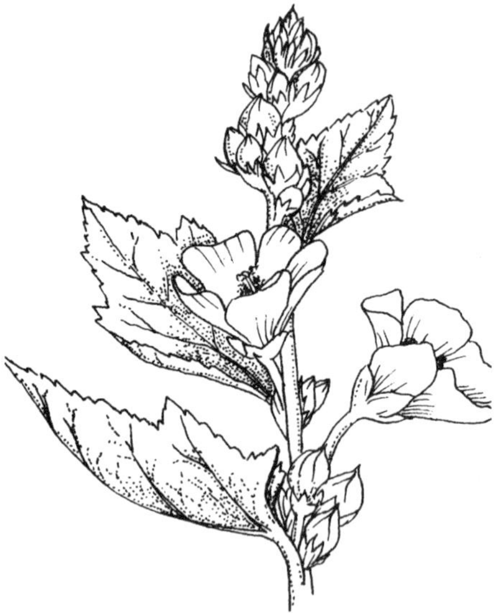

Uses: Marshmallow root is effective for reducing irritation and inflammation of bronchitis and other respiratory tract infections with sore throat. Herbalists also recommend the herb to help soothe an inflamed urinary tract with cystitis or your stomach and colon for gastritis, ulcers, and colitis.

Dosage: Blending 1 teaspoon of the root for each cup of cool water for 5 minutes, steeping for 30 minutes, and straining and drinking 1 cup, several times daily, is an effective way to take the remedy. You can add plantain leaf or calendula flowers to increase the healing powers of the tea. Follow the label instructions for other kinds of products.

Caution: Strong marshmallow tea may interfere with the absorption of some pharmaceutical medications, so take them separately.

Meadowsweet

Latin name: *Filipendula ulmaria* [L.] Maxim.

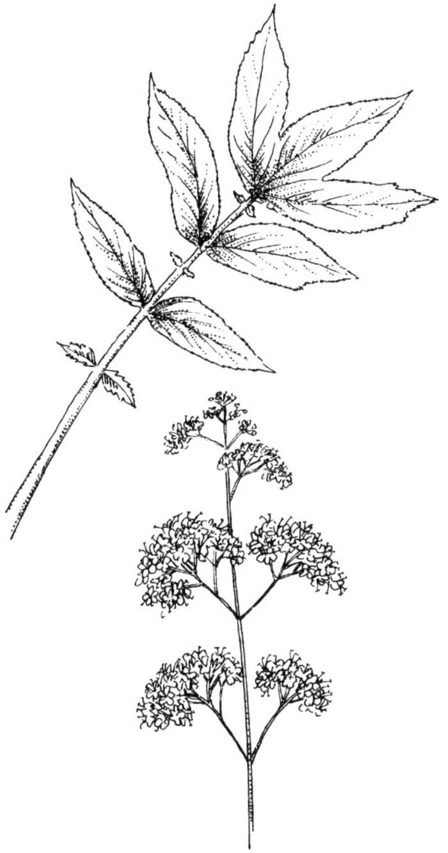

Description: Also called queen of the meadow, meadowsweet is a stout perennial in the rose family, growing up to three to six feet high in large clumps. The plant produces dense sprays of small white flowers. The entire herb is harvested for medicine. Meadowsweet is available in liquid tinctures and in bulk for making tea.

Uses: Meadowsweet contains salicin, a natural form of aspirin, and is recommended by herbalists for headaches, heartburn, fevers, rheumatism and arthritis, gastritis, or ulcers. Meadowsweet preparations soothe the digestive tract, relieving nausea and hyperacidity.

Dosage: Make an infusion by steeping 1 or 2 teaspoons of the herb for 20 minutes for each cup of water. Drink $^1/_2$ to 1 cup, 2 to 3 times daily. Take 2 to 4 droppersful of the tincture, 2 to 3 times daily.

Milk Thistle

Latin name: *Silybum marianum* [L.] Gaertner.

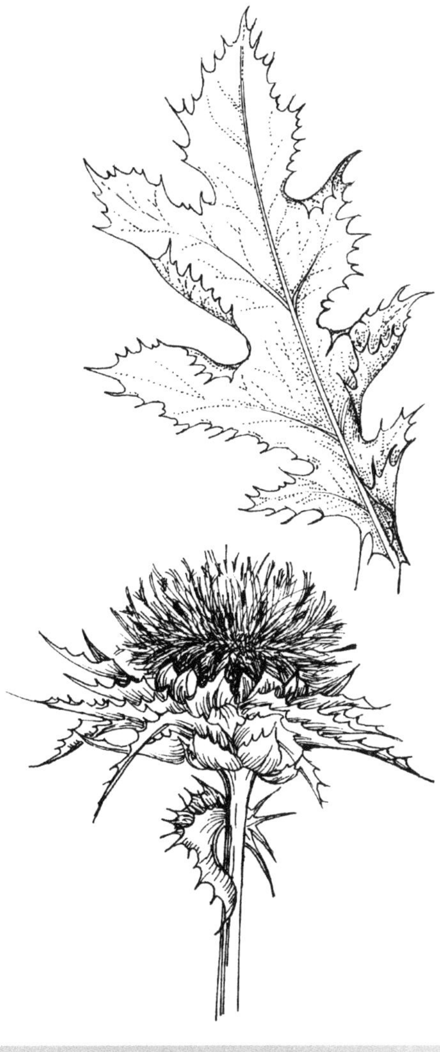

Description: Milk thistle is a tall stout spiny thistle with bright purple flowering heads. The leaves are covered with wavy milky bands, hence its name. The shells of the plump purple seeds are made into medicines. Milk thistle seed is available in capsule or tablet form as a standardized extract, in liquid tinctures, and in bulk for grinding up and sprinkling on food.

Uses: Take milk thistle for protecting your liver from toxins and drugs and for building liver health. Herbalists recommend standardized seed extracts and tinctures for cirrhosis, hepatitis, and jaundice. Known as "the liver herb," milk thistle protects the liver from substances such as alcohol, aspirin, acetominophen, and pharmaceutical drugs.

Dosage: Take 2 to 4 droppersful of the tincture, or 1 to 2 capsules or tablets of the standardized extract, 2 to 3 times daily. If you have a chronic liver condition like hepatitis or cirrhosis, avoid using the tincture of milk thistle — I recommend taking the standardized extract in tablets or capsules only.

Motherwort

Latin name: *Leonurus cardiaca* L.

Description: Motherwort is a medium-sized garden perennial with sharp-toothed leaves and whorls of small pink two-lipped flowers. The whole upper flowering part of the plant in flower is harvested for making herbal preparations. Motherwort is available in liquid tinctures and in bulk for making tea.

Uses: Use motherwort for the cardiovascular system, as a heart tonic for easing palpitations, helping hypertension, strengthening the heart, and helping relieve pain of mild angina. The herb is equally beneficial for the female reproductive system and is effective for painful, delayed, or suppressed menstruation and premenstrual tension (PMS).

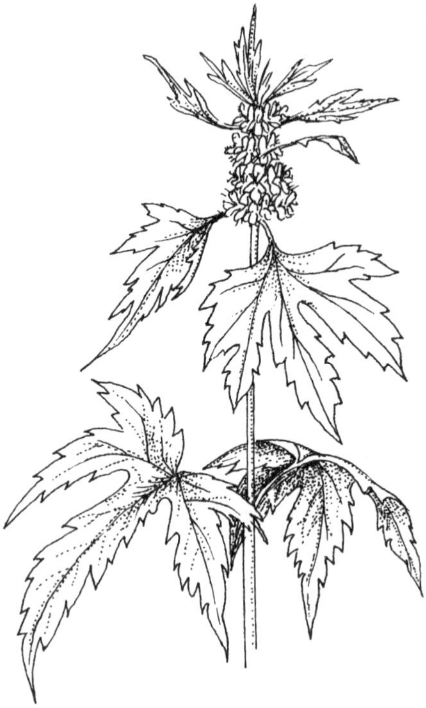

Dosage: Make an infusion by steeping 1 teaspoon to 1 tablespoon of the herb for every cup of freshly boiled water. Drink 1 cup, or take 2 to 4 droppersful of the tincture, 2 to 3 times daily.

Caution: Avoid use during pregnancy.

Mullein

Latin name: *Verbascum thapsus* L.

Description: Mullein is a triennial herb — the leaves are harvested at the end of the first year or beginning of the second year of growth, and the flowers are collected as they open. Mullein is available in capsule form, in liquid tinctures, as an oil, and in bulk for making tea.

Uses: Herbalists recommend mullein leaves as one of the safest and most useful herbal lung tonics. The leaves have an expectorant and soothing action on the mucous membranes of the respiratory tract. Mullein is also a useful lymphatic cleanser, and you may find it effective for helping to relieve skin problems like psoriasis. Take mullein for easing the symptoms of asthma, chronic bronchitis, dry coughs, and laryngitis. Use the flower oil in your ears for inflammation, earaches, and infections of the eustachian tubes, inner ear, and ear canal. See your doctor or herbalist if you have an ear infection.

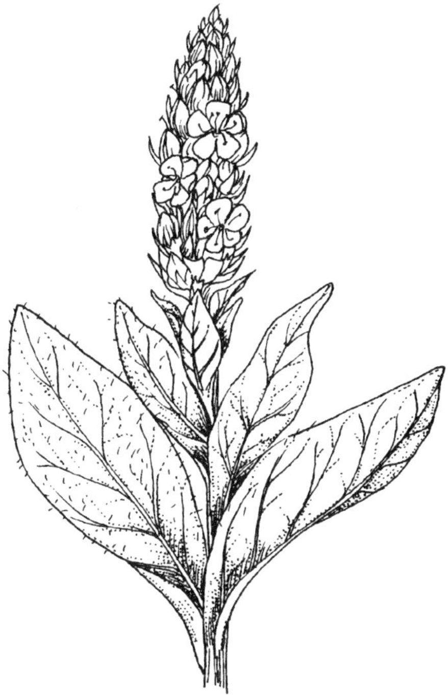

Dosage: Make a light decoction by simmering 1 tablespoon of the herb for every cup of water for 15 minutes. Drink 1 cup, up to several times daily, as needed. Use 2 to 4 drops of the oil in the ear, morning and evening.

Nettle

Latin name: *Urtica dioica* L.

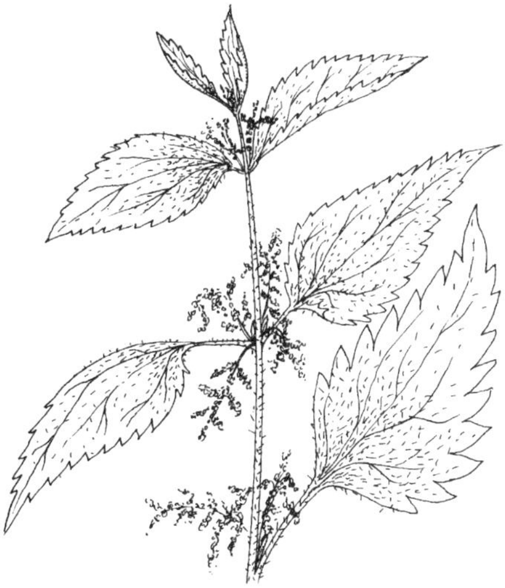

Description: Found on most continents, nettles are upright perennial herbs covered with stinging hairs and spreading from creeping underground stems. The plants have round-toothed leaves and sprays of nondescript flowers. Nettle leaf and rhizomes are both available in powder or extract form in capsules and tablets and in bulk for making tea.

Uses: Nettle has diuretic, cleansing, antihistamine, and anti-inflammatory properties. Consider using nettle herb for hay fever, arthritis and rheumatism, anemia and weak blood, cystitis and water-retention, and gout. The rhizomes are increasingly used to reduce prostate inflammation and improve symptoms like painful urination that occur with benign prostatic hyperplasia (BPH).

Dosage: Make a decoction with 1 tablespoon of herb or rhizome for every cup of water by simmering for 20 or 30 minutes. Drink 1 to 2 cups, 2 or 3 times daily. Follow the label instructions for other products.

Orange Peel

Latin name: *Citrus aurantium* L.

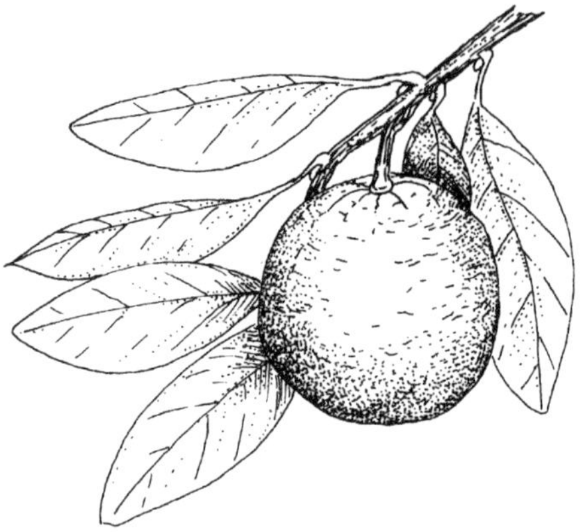

Description: The orange tree has dark glossy green leaves and fragrant white flowers. The peel of organic fruit is dried and used for medicine. Orange peel is available in bulk for making teas and in tinctures and some ready-made Chinese herbal formulas in pill form. An essential oil comes from the peel and is used to flavor foods and as an ingredient in herbal medicines.

Uses: Orange peel is a flavorful herb for enhancing digestion and relieving symptoms like nausea, vomiting, burping, and a feeling of fullness after eating even small amounts. You may find orange peel effective for assisting the body to get rid of excess mucus and relieving coughs and a feeling of fullness in the chest.

Dosage: You can make a light decoction in a covered pan by gently simmering 1/2 cup of the fresh or 1/4 cup of the dried peels in 5 cups of water. Drink 1 cup, 2 or 3 times a day, after meals.

Oregon Grape Root

Latin name: *Mahonia aquifolium* [Pursh] Nutt.

Description: Oregon grape root is a perennial native plant with stiff prickly leaves, clusters of lemon yellow flowers, and sour bright blue berries. The roots contain the yellow alkaloid berberine and are harvested for making teas and prepared medicines. Oregon grape is available in capsule form, in liquid tinctures, and in bulk for making tea.

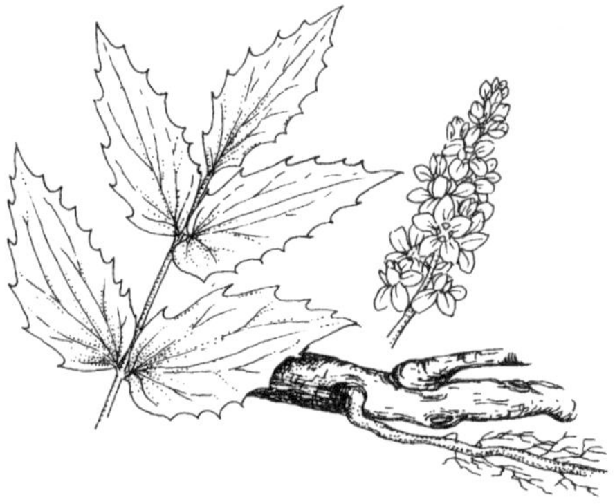

Uses: Use Oregon grape root for cooling the liver, stimulating bile flow, reducing inflammation in the intestines, and benefiting symptoms of dermatitis. My experience shows that Oregon grape root extracts are effective for clearing skin disorders (such as acne, cysts, or psoriasis), gastritis and ulcers, vaginal yeast infections, and bowel infections.

Dosage: Make a decoction by simmering 1 teaspoon of the cut and sifted herb for every cup of water. Drink 1/2 to 1 cup, or 1 to 2 droppersful of the tincture, 2 or 3 times daily.

Caution: Avoid use of this herb during pregnancy.

Parsley

Latin name: *Petroselinum crispum* [Mill.) Nym. Ex A.W. Hill.

Description: Parsley is a familiar addition to many restaurant dishes, where it's mostly pushed aside and neglected. The parsley plant has dark green curly and dissected leaves, insignificant greenish flowers, and plump aromatic fruits that

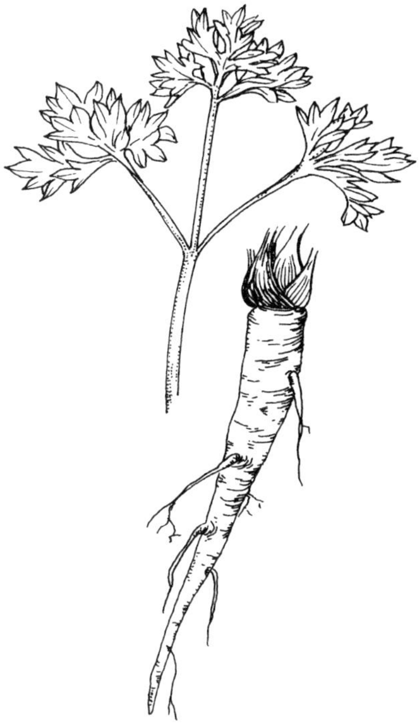

look like caraway seeds. The fruits and roots are used in herbal medicine. Parsley root and fruits are available in capsule form, in liquid tinctures, and in bulk for making tea.

Uses: Parsley seed tea is a potent diuretic. The roots are less potent, but are also used. European herbalists and doctors recommend parsley fruit and root tea for relieving water retention and edema.

Dosage: Make a tea by steeping 1/2 teaspoon of the fruits or 1 teaspoon of the cut and sifted root for every cup of water for 15 minutes. Drink 1/2 cup of the preparation, 2 to 3 times daily.

Caution: Avoid using parsley root or fruits in medicinal doses during pregnancy. Don't use parsley fruit tea for more than two weeks at a time without consulting an experienced herbalist.

Passion Flower

Latin name: *Passiflora incarnata* L.

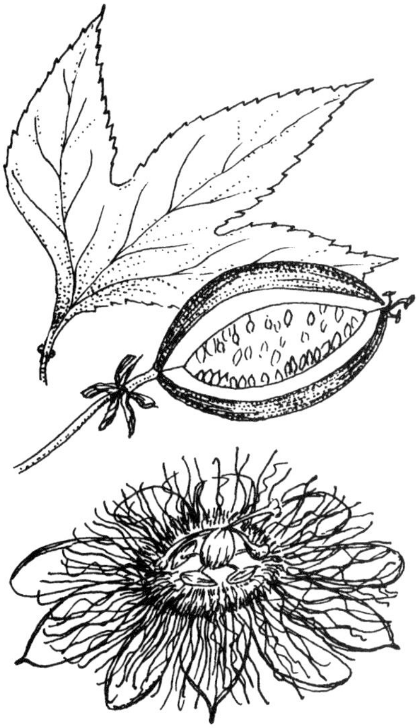

Description: The North American native passion flower, *Passiflora incarnata,* is also called *maypop.* It's a wild vine with beautiful fringed purple flowers and palmately five-lobed leaves. The leaves and flowers are harvested to make herbal remedies. Passion flower is available in capsule form, in liquid tinctures, and in bulk for making tea.

Uses: Herbalists recommend passion flower for easing anxiety and insomnia, especially caused by hypertension, premenstrual syndrome, and neuralgia. You may find that passion flower is most effective when used in a supporting role with other calming herbs like California poppy and valerian.

Dosage: Take 2 to 4 droppersful of the tincture in a little water, several times daily as needed.

Pau d'Arco

Latin name: *Tabebuia heptaphylla* (Vell.) Toledo.

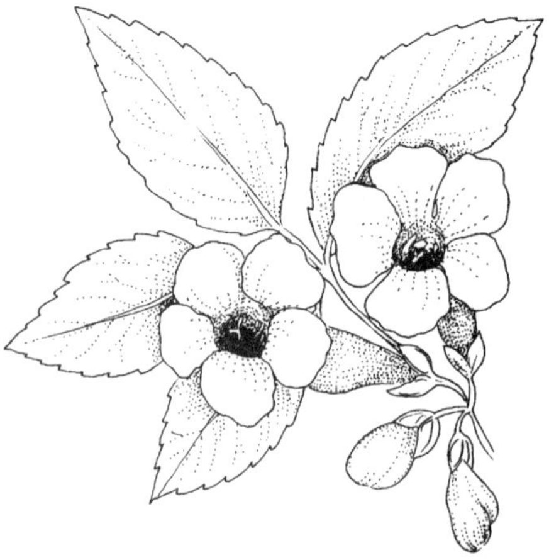

Description: Pau d'arco is one of a number of large trees in the bignonia family from South America with large, two-lipped pink or yellow flowers. The vanilla-scented cinnamon red inner bark is collected for medicine. Pau d'arco is available in capsule form, in liquid tinctures, and in bulk for tea.

Uses: Herbalists recommend pau d'arco for its proven antifungal and cancer-fighting properties and possible immune strengthening qualities. Consider using the bark for helping to prevent and eliminate candida yeast infections.

Dosage: Make a decoction by simmering 1 teaspoon of the dried bark for every cup of water for 20 minutes. Drink 1 cup of the tea or 1 to 3 droppersful tincture in a little water, 3 or 4 times daily.

Peppermint

Latin name: *Mentha* x *piperita* L.

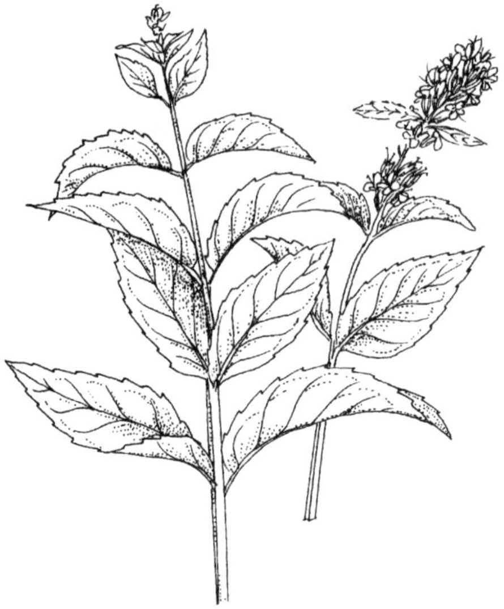

Description: Peppermint is a familiar fragrant garden herb also widely cultivated for its oil, with dark green opposite leaves and purple stems. The whole plant is harvested. Peppermint is available in enteric-coated capsule form, in liquid tinctures, as an essential oil, and in bulk for making tea.

Uses: Peppermint is a favorite remedy for relaxing the intestinal tract and relieving gas pains. The herb is effective for easing nausea, vomiting, heartburn, morning sickness, irritable bowel syndrome, and colitis. Try peppermint tea for helping to relieve symptoms of the common cold, fevers, and headaches.

Dosage: Make an infusion by steeping a small handful of the fresh herb or 1 tablespoon for every cup of water, and drink 1 cup, 2 to 3 times daily.

Pipsissewa

Latin name: *Chimaphila umbellata* Nutt.

Description: A short plant with dark green, leathery, sharply-toothed leaves and greenish purple cup-shaped flowers.

The entire above-ground herb is harvested for medicine and as a flavoring for some commercial beverages. You can buy pipsissewa herb in capsule form, in liquid tinctures, and in bulk for making tea.

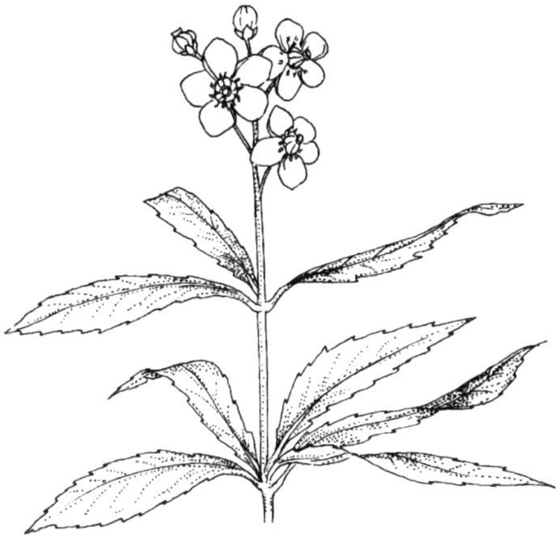

Uses: Herbalists recommend the herb for bladder and kidney weakness, cystitis, arthritis, and rheumatism.

Dosage: Simmer 1 teaspoon for every cup of water for 20 minutes. Drink 1 cup or take 2 to 4 droppersful of the tincture, 2 times daily.

Plantain

Latin name: *Plantago lanceolata* L.

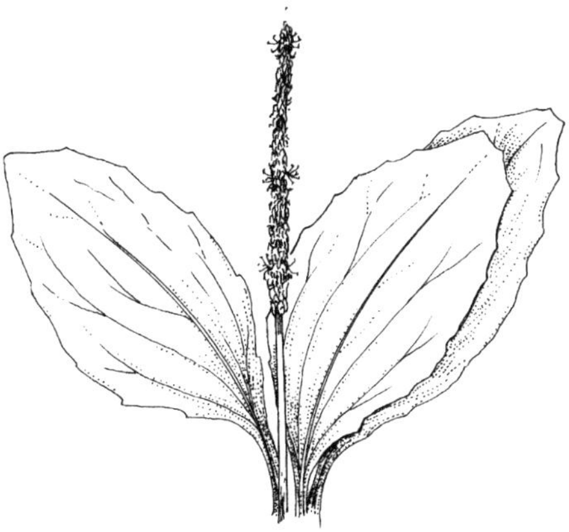

Description: A common weed of gardens, fields, and meadows. One species has long, ribbed lance-shaped leaves and the other has larger eliptic leaves. Both species have long flowering spikes with a brown dense tuft of flowers and seed-bearing capsules. The leaves and seeds are harvested to make herbal medicines. Plantain is available in capsule form, in liquid tinctures, and in bulk for making tea. I don't find the tincture effective, because the active compounds aren't soluble in alcohol.

Uses: Internally, plantain leaves are an important remedy to soothe inflamed and infected tissues of the respiratory, urinary, and digestive tracts. Take the tea liberally for relieving coughs, ulcers, irritable bowel, colitis, cystitis, and painful urination. Externally, the fresh leaves are amazing for quickly reducing the pain of bites, stings, cuts, scrapes, and burns. I recommend using a slimy wad of the herb inside the mouth for easing the inflammation and pain of infected gums, gum disease, and abscesses.

Dosage: You can easily make a poultice for external use by blending the fresh leaves with a little water to form a slimy paste. Apply to the affected spot, cover with a bandage or adhesive tape, and leave in place for an hour or two. Replace the poultice several times a day, keeping it wet, and apply before bedtime. Make a decoction by simmering $^1/_2$ cup of the fresh or dried leaves in 2 or 3 cups of water for 30 or 40 minutes. Drink 1 or 2 cups of the tea, several times daily. Juice the fresh leaves and add the juice to carrot, celery, apple, or other juices.

Caution: You can substitute plantain for comfrey during pregnancy or for long-term use because it contains similar active constituents and effects.

Psyllium

Latin name: *Plantago* spp.

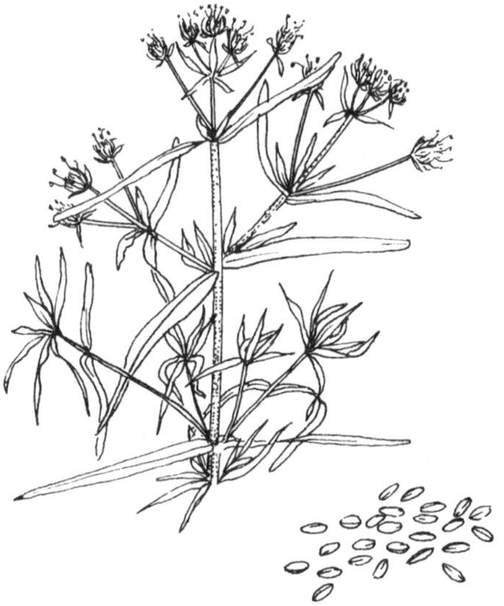

Description: Psyllium seed comes from a large plantain herb. The seed husks and whole seeds are widely available in bulk, and you can find them in many commercial bowel-cleansing and laxative formulas. Wild plantain seeds collected from a grassy meadow have similar effects.

Uses: Psyllium seed is used as a gentle bulk laxative. Herbalists and doctors recommend the husk and seeds to help relieve constipation, diarrhea, hemorrhoids, irritable bowel syndrome, Crohn's disease, and high cholesterol.

Dosage: Soak 1/2 to 2 teaspoons in 1 cup of warm water and drink 1 or 2 times daily, especially first thing in the morning and before bedtime. Follow the label instructions of any commercial products.

Caution: You must take psyllium seed with at least eight ounces of water. When taking other drugs, wait an hour before taking psyllium.

Raspberry

Latin name: *Rubus idaeus* L.

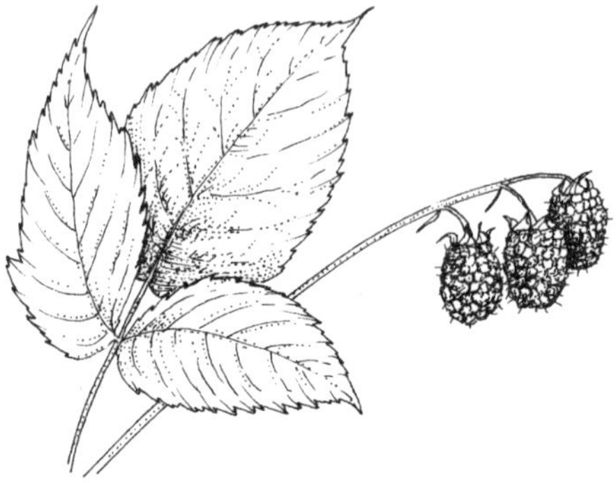

Description: The plant is thorny and prickly with white or rose-colored flowers. The leaves of the familiar garden raspberry are harvested and used to make herbal teas. The berries aren't bad either! The bulk herb is available to make light decoctions.

Uses: Raspberry leaf tea is the safest and least controversial tea to use during pregnancy. Herbalists and midwives recommend raspberry leaf for tonifying the uterus and facilitating labor. You may find the herb effective for easing painful menstruation and slowing diarrhea when used regularly.

Dosage: Make a light decoction by simmering a small handful of the dried or fresh herb in 2 cups of water for a few minutes and steeping the herb for 15 minutes or so. Drink 1 cup, 2 or three 3 daily.

Red Clover

Latin name: *Trifolium pratense* L.

Description: Red clover is a stout clover, with large pinkish red heads containing numerous small pea-like flowers and a small leafy brack just below each of the heads. Red clover flowers are available as a bulk herb for making teas, in tincture form, and as a component of many kinds of extracts in capsule and tablet form.

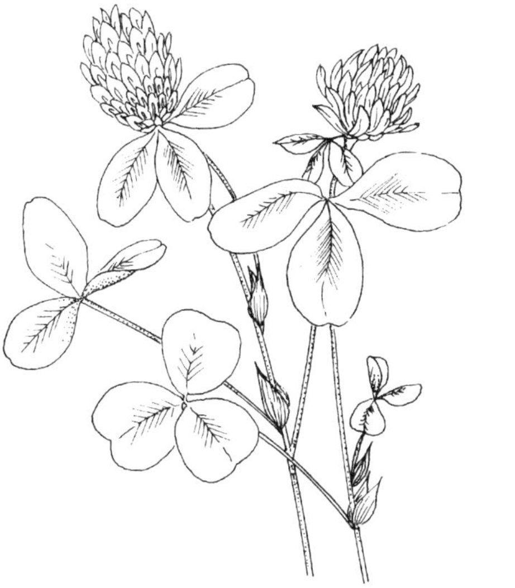

Uses: The flowering heads are recommended to eliminate toxins by the liver and bowels, and to stimulate immune function to assist the body to remove toxic waste products. You may find red clover helpful for relieving skin problems such as eczema, psoriasis, acne, and other kinds of dermatitis. The flowers are also effective as a mild expectorant and cleanser for the respiratory tract for helping to heal lung problems, such as dry coughs, laryngitis, bronchitis, and whooping cough. Rich in phytoestrogenic compounds like genistein, red clover is an important component of well-respected formulas for assisting the body in its fight with cancer and for helping to prevent the disease.

Dosage: Make a tea by simmering 1 tablespoon of the herb for each cup of water for 15 to 20 minutes. Drink 1 cup or take 1/2 to 1 teaspoon of the tincture in a little water, 2 or 3 times daily. Follow the label instructions of commercial capsules or tablets.

Caution: Avoid the use of this herb during pregnancy.

Reishi

Latin name: *Ganoderma lucidum* [Leyss. Ex Fr.) P. Karst.

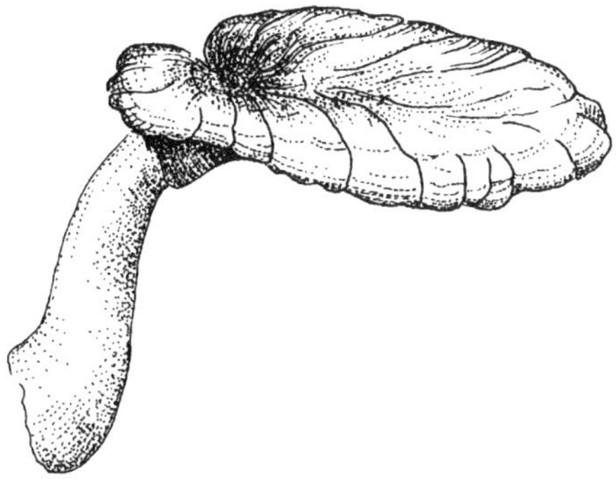

Description: Reishi is a beautiful red- or black-varnished, hard mushroom that grows with a long stalk on dead trees — mostly hardwoods and hemlock. Reishi grows wild on most continents of the world and is extensively cultivated for medicine. It's available in bulk to make teas, in tincture form, and as an extract in capsules and tablets.

Uses: Reishi is an ancient and revered herb, effective for calming the nervous system, strengthening the blood and cardiovascular system, and supporting the immune system, especially for people who have cancer and are undergoing western treatments like chemotherapy and radiation therapy. Take reishi also for helping to relieve the symptoms of anxiety, allergies, general weakness, heart problems, insomnia, and chronic fatigue syndrome. I prescribe reishi extensively in my clinic, with excellent results.

Dosage: Make a decoction by first grinding the whole mushroom in a blender or cuisinart, then simmering 1 cup of the herb for every 4 cups of water for an hour. Drink 1 cup of the tea, or take 3 tablets or capsules, 2 to 3 times daily. Follow the label instructions for other products.

Rosemary

Latin name: *Rosmarinus officinalis* L.

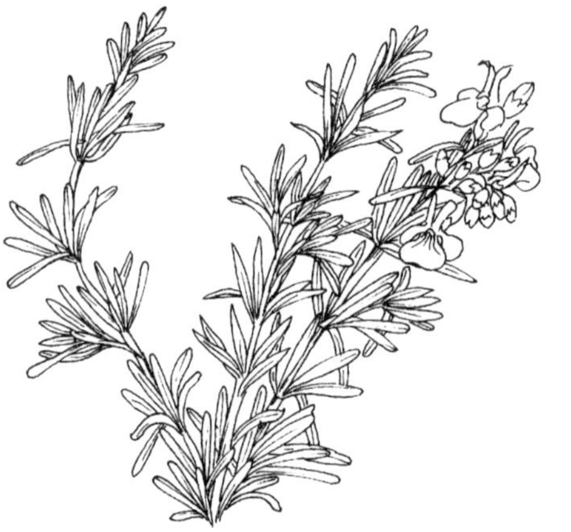

Description: Rosemary herb is a resinous, aromatic woody shrub with narrow, aromatic leaves and masses of pale blue or violet flowers. Rosemary is available as a bulk herb, in tinctures, and as a powdered herb in capsules and tablets.

Uses: Consider using rosemary if you have nervous system or cardiovascular weakness, your period is sluggish or stopped, or if you want a good-tasting herb with powerful antioxidant effects to slow the aging process and reduce the risk of heart disease and cancer. Herbalists recommend rosemary for headaches, chronic fatigue, poor appetite, low blood pressure, and weak circulation. Rosemary is a great tonic for the elderly to invigorate their nervous system, digestion, and help preserve good health.

Dosage: Make an infusion of rosemary by steeping one teaspoon of the herb for each cup of water for 20 minutes. Drink 1 cup of the tea, or take 10 to 30 drops of the tincture, 2 or 3 times daily. Add a pot of tea to your bath to make a rosemary bath, which is invigorating and restorative. Rosemary tea hair rinses are excellent for keeping your hair shiny and healthy.

Caution: Avoid using rosemary if you're pregnant.

Sage

Latin name: *Salvia officinalis* L.

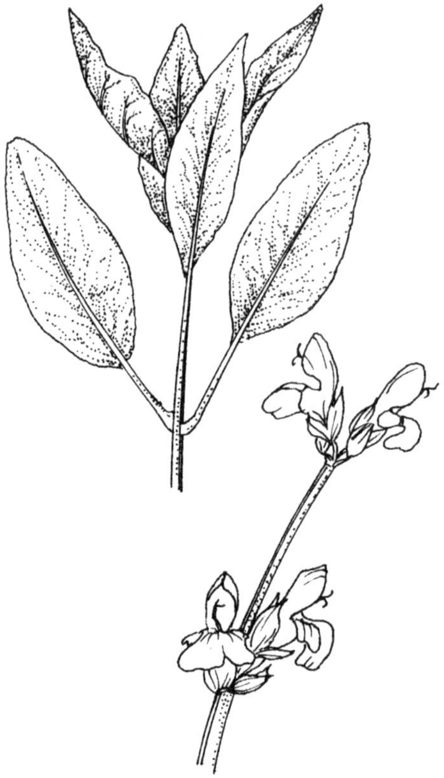

Description: Sage is a silvery-green perennial that is a favorite garden plant. The leaves, stems, and flowers are harvested for medicine.

Uses: Consider using sage if you have a cold, especially with a sore throat or excessive perspiration. Herbalists recommend the herb for its antibacterial and drying qualities. Sage is an ingredient of herbal preparations used externally in antiperspirant formulas to reduce body odor and as a gargle and spray to ease the pain and inflammation of a sore throat. Nursing mothers use sage to help dry up the last flow of milk.

Dosage: Make an infusion by steeping 1 teaspoon of the herb for every cup of boiled water for 15 minutes. Drink 1 cup of the tea, or take 20 to 30 drops of the tincture in a little water, several times daily, as needed. Follow the label instructions for externally-applied products.

Caution: Avoid use of this herb during pregnancy. Avoid long-term use and don't exceed the recommended dose.

St. John's Wort

Latin name: *Hypericum perforatum* L.

Description: St. John's wort is an upright, perennial, weedy herb with bright-yellow flowers and small, elliptical leaves with translucent dots that you can see through. Now that St. John's wort is a superstar herb, it's available in many forms — the tincture, standardized extracts in tablets or capsules, and as a bulk herb.

Uses: Consider taking St. John's wort internally if you're depressed or have insomnia. Herbalists also recommend the herb for relieving chronic nerve pains like peripheral neuropathy, and for trauma and injuries involving nerve damage. Herbalists specifically recommend St. John's wort for children who wet the bed. Externally, the herb is invaluable for reducing inflammation and the pain of scrapes, bruises, strains, burns, and other trauma.

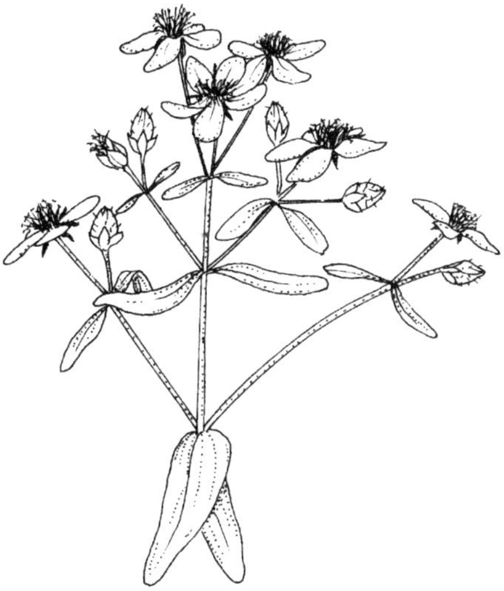

Dosage: Based on my clinical experience, and that of other herbalists, the effective dose of St. John's wort is about 4 droppersful of the tincture in the morning and 3 in the evening in a little water, or 2 capsules of a standardized extract in the morning and 1 in the evening. You can go up to 1 teaspoon of the tincture, or 2 capsules or tablets, morning and evening, as needed. A recent review of several commercial standardized extract products in capsules and tablets showed that the products actually delivered from 30 percent to 80 percent of the advertised levels of active constituents. For this reason, if you have tried capsules with no results, try taking a teaspoon of the dark rich red tincture in the morning and 1/2 to 3/4 teaspoon in the evening, for a month. You can make an infusion of St. John's wort if you want to, but it isn't as effective as the other preparations. Apply the oil, or any other external preparation, liberally as needed, preferably at least twice a day.

Caution: Avoid regular use of this herb when taking pharmaceutical MAO-inhibitors or if fair-skinned.

Saw Palmetto

Latin name: *Serenoa repens* [Bart.] Small.

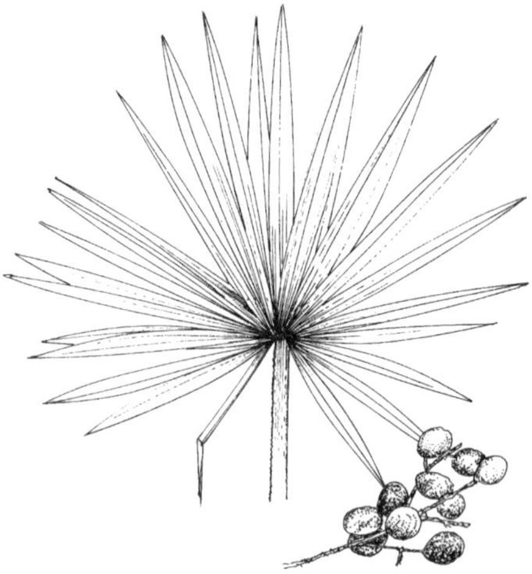

Description: Saw palmetto is a scrubby, trailing palm with fan-shaped leaves and purple berries, which are harvested to make an extract of great demand. Saw palmetto is available as a powdered herb in capsules and as a special extract called a *hexane-free* or *supercritical* extract. Look for this kind of extract in gel caps. I don't recommend extracts made with the industrial solvent hexane. The bulk dried fruits are also available. You can grind these up to a powder and either add it to your food or pack it into double-ought capsules. The fruit naturally has a rather rancid smell. Don't worry, the fruit isn't bad — it just smells that way.

Uses: Use saw palmetto for easing symptoms of prostate inflammation and enlargement (benign prostatic hypertrophy, or BPH), like burning or incomplete urination and reduced flow. I find saw palmetto effective for strengthening and improving the nutrition of the urinary and genital organs. I get good clinical results using saw palmetto with women who have repeated bladder infections. It seems to help prevent the infections. I know women who have experienced relief with neurogenic and irritable bladder conditions using this herb.

Dosage: Take 2 capsules powdered extract twice daily or 2 droppersful tincture, 2 times daily. Consider taking a double dose of saw palmetto if you're on the verge of a bladder infection, especially if they're common, or if you have persistent prostate enlargement and restricted urine flow. See your doctor if symptoms persist.

Schisandra

Latin name: *Schisandra chinensis* [Turcz.] Baill.

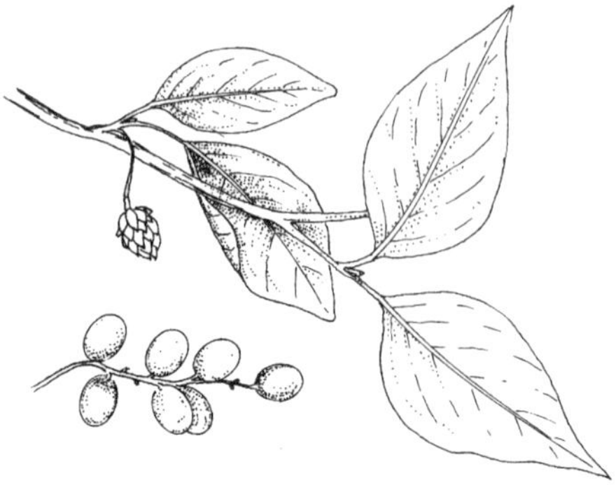

Description: Schisandra is a woody vine from the forests of northern China, cultivated for the sour bright red berries. Schisandra is available as a bulk herb for making teas, in tinctures, powdered herbs in capsules, and extracts in capsules or tablets.

Uses: Consider using schisandra if you have chronic coughs from lung weakness, incontinence from a weak bladder, or excessive sweating during menopause or during chronic infections like AIDS. Herbalists recommend schisandra for protecting the liver with conditions like hepatitis.

Dosage: Make a decoction by simmering 1 teaspoon of the dried fruits for every cup of water for 30 minutes. Drink 1 cup of the tea or 1/2 teaspoon of the tincture in a little water, several times daily.

Shiitake

Latin name: *Lentinus edodes* (Berk.) Singer.

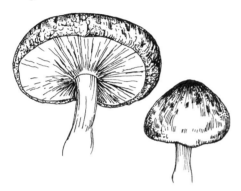

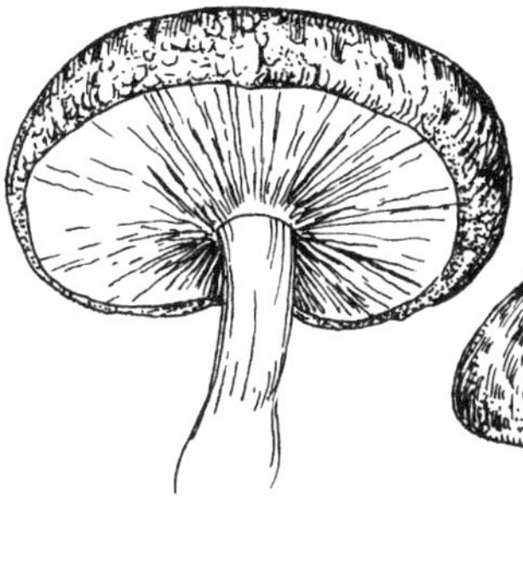

Description: Shiitake is a gilled mushroom with a tan- to cinnamon-colored cap and solid stalk. Eating shiitake, which is widely available as a food in grocery stores and natural food markets, is a great way to get the benefit with the flavor. You may find that powdered extracts in capsules and tablets are the most convenient way to get the therapeutic benefits.

Uses: Consider taking an extract of this mushroom for helping ease symptoms associated with high cholesterol, lowered immune function, hepatitis, environmental allergies, candida, AIDS, and cancer. Scientific studies show that shiitake is a potent immune booster, cancer-fighter, and anti-viral herb. Shiitake is an approved drug in Japan, where it's routinely prescribed to help support the immune system in cancer patients who are undergoing chemotherapy and radiation treatment, and as a treatment for patients with hepatitis, especially hepatitis C.

Dosage: Take 3 or 4 tablets or capsules of a concentrated extract, 2 times daily, with meals. Take half that amount for prevention and general health-promoting benefits.

Skullcap

Latin name: Scutellaria lateriflora L.

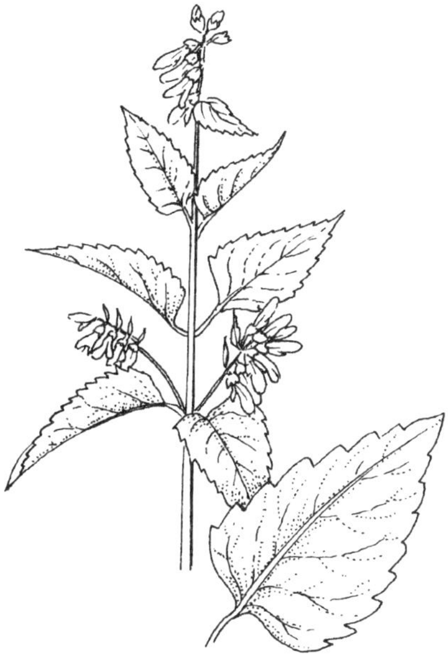

Description: Skullcap is an herb that's native to eastern North American, grows in wet places, and has opposite leaves and small, two-lipped, blue flowers. Skullcap is a member of the mint family, but has no smell. Native American Indians and herbalists have used the flowers and upper leaves for over a century as an herb to calm the nervous system and ease spasms.

Uses: Skullcap is a relaxing herb that you can use for insomnia, headache, nervous exhaustion, muscle spasms, and the nervous tension and irritability associated with premenstrual syndrome. This herb is also used to ease the discomfort of withdrawal from drugs or alcohol and is considered helpful to alleviate excessive sexual desire. Skullcap is a safe herb that may be used long-term to regulate the nervous system. I recommend skullcap most for relieving muscle cramps, tics, menstrual cramps, and as an aid to help eliminate tobacco and drug addictions.

Dosage: Take 3 to 5 droppersful of the liquid tincture in a little water or tea, several times daily. To make a tea, simmer 1/4 ounce of the herb for every 2 ounces of water for 5 minutes, and let the brew steep for 20 minutes. Strain and drink 1 cup, several times a day.

Slippery Elm

Latin name: *Ulmus fulva* Michx.

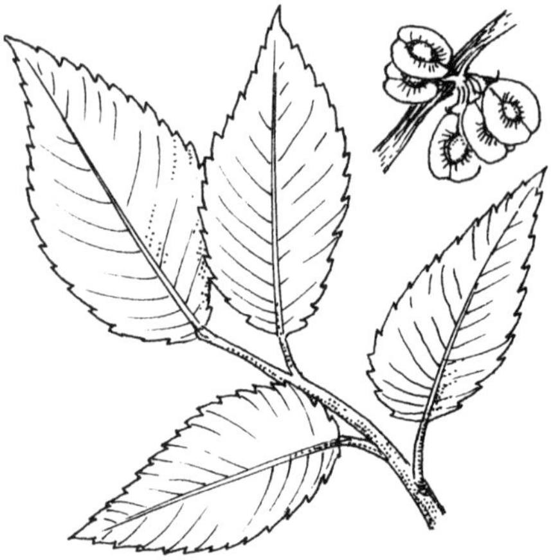

Description: Slippery elm is a large tree that grows to sixty feet high. The inner bark is harvested for making medicinal teas and other preparations. Slippery elm is available as a bulk tea, prepared teas, and in soothing cough lozenges.

Uses: Try a slippery elm lozenge or warm tea when you have a sore throat or any irritation or inflammation of the digestive tract. Herbalists recommend slippery elm for soothing ulcers, gastritis, colitis, coughs, and easing diarrhea. Native American Indians made a nutritious gruel from a powder of the inner bark, a remedy still recommended for convalescence.

Dosage: Make a decoction of the bark by simmering one tablespoon for every cup of water for 15 minutes. Drink 1 cup, 2 or 3 times daily.

Caution: Strong slippery elm tea may interfere with the absorption of some pharmaceutical medications, so take them separately.

Thyme

Latin name: *Thymus vulgaris* L.

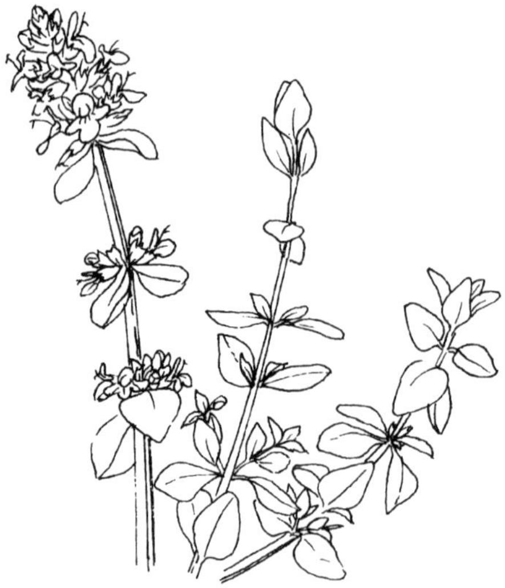

Description: Thyme is a low-growing, aromatic plant from the mint family that forms dense mats. Thyme is available in bulk tea form, in tincture form, and in a wide variety of lozenges, syrups, and other cold and flu preparations.

Uses: Consider a cup of strong, antiseptic, thyme tea to help you eliminate symptoms like coughs, mucus congestion, or sore throat from a cold or flu. You can also take this herb for bronchitis or pneumonia. Use thyme sprays, syrups, or lozenges externally for soothing a sore throat and inhibiting the infection.

Dosage: Make an infusion with 1 teaspoon of the dried herb or 1 tablespoon of the chopped fresh herb for every cup of water for 15 or 20 minutes. Follow the label directions for other products.

Turmeric

Latin name: *Curcuma longa* L.

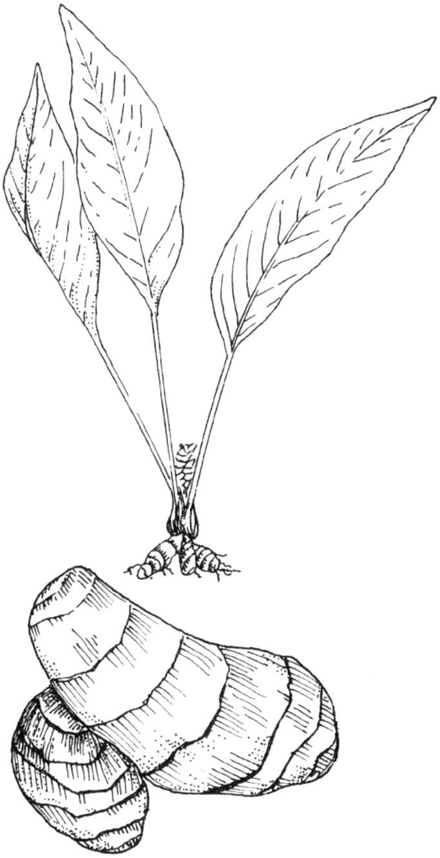

Description: A relative of ginger, turmeric is a large-leafed, aromatic plant. Turmeric is available as a spice, either in powder form or in the produce section as whole fresh rhizomes. You can also buy many ready-made products like tinctures and standardized extracts in capsules and tablets.

Uses: Consider turmeric if you have an inflammatory condition like arthritis, pain after an injury, gallbladder inflammation, liver inflammation associated with hepatitis, or for menstrual pain. Turmeric is known to help protect you against cancer.

Dosage: Make a light decoction with 1 teaspoon of the herb powder or cut and sifted herb, or 1 tablespoon of fresh slices of the rhizome, for every cup of water by simmering for 15 or 20 minutes. Drink 1 cup, or take 1 to 4 droppersful of the tincture in a little water, several times daily. Follow the label instructions on other products.

Caution: Avoid use of this herb during pregnancy. Don't use turmeric if you have an obstructed bile duct, gallstones, stomach ulcers, or hyperacidity, without the advice of an experienced herbalist.

Usnea Thallus

Latin name: *Usnea barbata* [L.] Wigg.

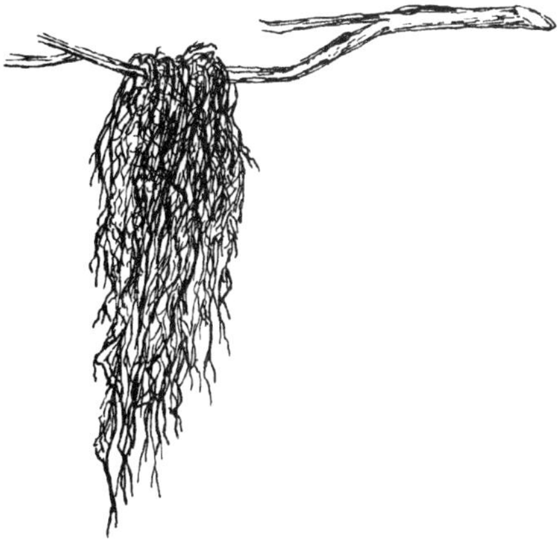

Description: Usnea is a grey-green hair-like organism formed by the union of a green algae and a fungus, called a lichen. Usnea hangs in trees but isn't actually tapped into its sap. Many lichens, usnea included, produce strong antibiotic compounds. Usnea is available in tincture form only. The antibiotic compounds aren't water-soluble, so you may find usnea tea is mostly ineffective for treating infections.

Uses: Consider using usnea when you have conditions like strep throat, a staph infection (like impetigo), urinary tract infections, and pneumonia. I have many years of experience with usnea and find it to be a useful addition to formulas for any bacterial infection of the urinary tract and respiratory tract.

Dosage. Take 2 to 4 droppersful of the tincture, 2 to 3 times daily.

Uva Ursi

Latin name: *Arctostaphylos uva-ursi* [L.] Spreng.

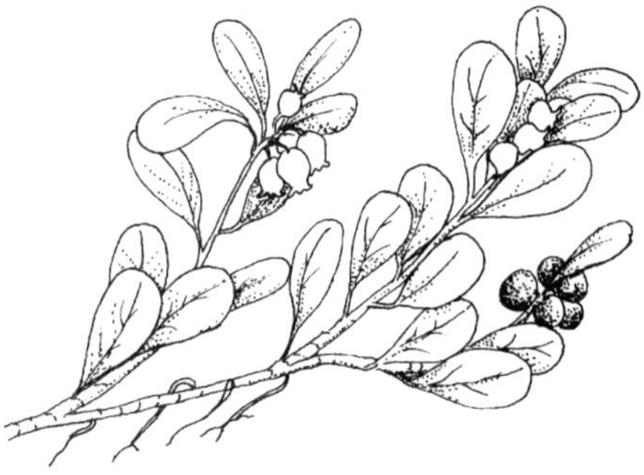

Description: Uva ursi is a low-growing or creeping evergreen woody shrub with red branches, pink urn-shaped flowers in clusters, and bright red berries. The name uva ursi means "bear grapes," presumably because bears like to eat them. The tender young leafy shoots are collected for making teas and other herbal preparations. Uva ursi leaves are available in bulk or as a liquid tincture.

Uses: Consider taking uva ursi if you have a bladder infection or mild kidney infection.

Dosage: Make a tea by simmering 1 tablespoon of the leaves in 2 cups of water for 30 to 40 minutes, until the water is reduced to one cup. Drink 1/2 cup of the tea, 2 times daily. Add 1 teaspoon of the tincture to a cup of water and drink 1/2 of the cup morning and evening. For persistent infections you may find a double dose effective, but consult an experienced herbalist first. Because uva ursi works better when the urine is acidic, take the tea or tincture concurrently with cranberry juice or tablets.

Caution: Avoid use of this herb during pregnancy. Don't use in cases of chronic kidney disorders or digestive irritation, without the advice of an experienced herbalist.

Valerian

Latin name: *Valeriana officinalis* L.

Description: Valerian is a perennial herb that forms clumps with strongly-scented underground rhizomes and tall flowering stalks capped by small white or pink flowers. The rhizomes are collected to make teas and other herbal remedies. Valerian is available in bulk to make teas, in tincture form, and as a powdered herb in capsules. Purchase valerian tincture made from the fresh rhizomes — this should be indicated on the label. Standardized extracts of valerian are available in capsules or tablets, but I don't recommend them, because the active ingredients of valerian are mostly unstable and are often broken down when the rhizomes are so highly processed.

Uses: Take valerian if you feel nervous, anxious, upset, or have trouble sleeping. Also try the herb for menstrual cramps (with cramp bark), heart palpitations (with hawthorn or hops), or for pain (with Roman chamomile or Jamaican dogwood). Valerian is the first remedy herbalists think of for calming the nervous system and to promote healthy sleep. The smell alone is enough to put some people out, but the rhizome also has compounds that science shows work directly on the higher centers of the brain.

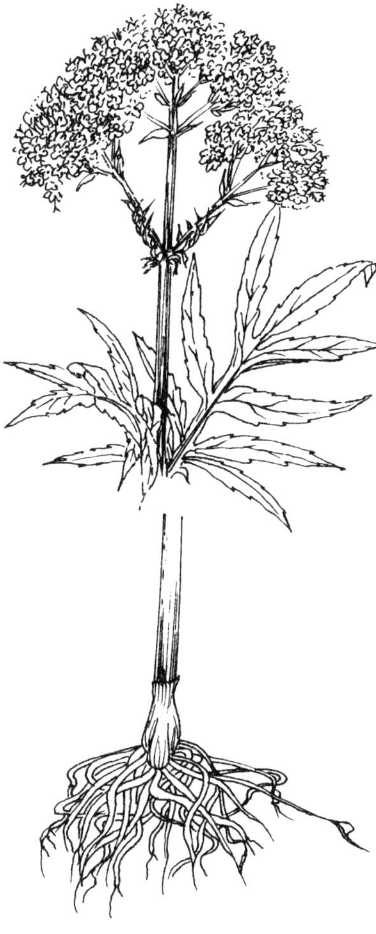

Dosage: You have to take valerian in a strong dose to be effective. Start with 1/2 teaspoon of the tincture, several times daily in a little water, and increase to 1 teaspoon if this isn't working. The tea is also effective. Make an infusion with 1 tablespoon of the cut and sifted herb for every cup of water. Steep the valerian for 30 minutes in a closed pot, and drink 1 cup, several times daily.

Caution: Valerian has few side effects, but some people find the rhizome can cause stimulation rather than a feeling of calm. You can reduce the chance of this happening if you avoid valerian (try California poppy or passion flower instead) when you have chronic fatigue or depression, without first consulting an herbalist.

Vitex

Latin name: *Vitex agnus-castus* L.

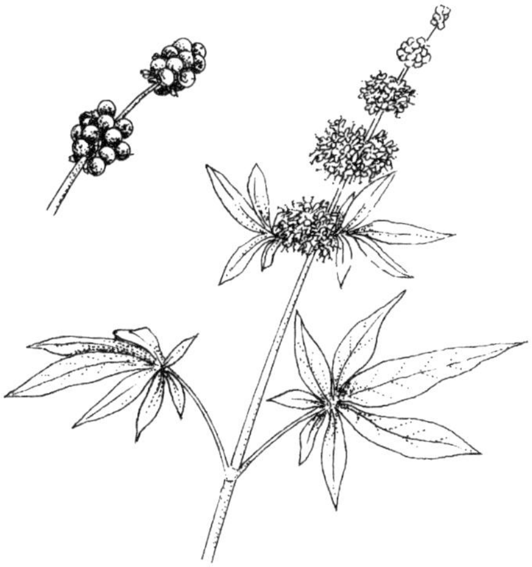

Description: Vitex is an ancient shrub that is often cultivated as an ornamental and medicinal plant for the garden and for its abundant purple or lavender flowers. The small brown fruits are harvested for making medicines. You can find vitex in liquid tincture form, which is the preparation I prefer. Capsules and tablets are also effective, but teas are seldom used.

Uses: Consider taking vitex if you have any of the unpleasant symptoms associated with premenstrual syndrome (PMS) and menopause. Vitex is effective for helping a woman ease off of birth control pills. Herbalists have recommended vitex as an effective *galactagogue* (an herb that increases the flow of mother's milk) for nearly two thousand years. You may consider taking vitex if you're nursing and wanting to increase milk flow. Teenage acne is another medical use of vitex in Germany, and I've seen good results for this condition with some of my patients. It doesn't work as well for teens with a strong family history of acne, who are continuously broken out.

Dosage: Take 1 to 2 droppersful of the tincture daily, first thing in the morning, or 2 to 4 capsules containing the powdered herb, 2 times daily. You can try a double dose if the regular dose doesn't work after 2 or 3 months. Follow the label instructions for standardized extracts.

Caution: Avoid using vitex during pregnancy or if you are taking birth control pills, except under the advice of an experienced herbalist.

White Willow

Latin name: *Salix* spp.

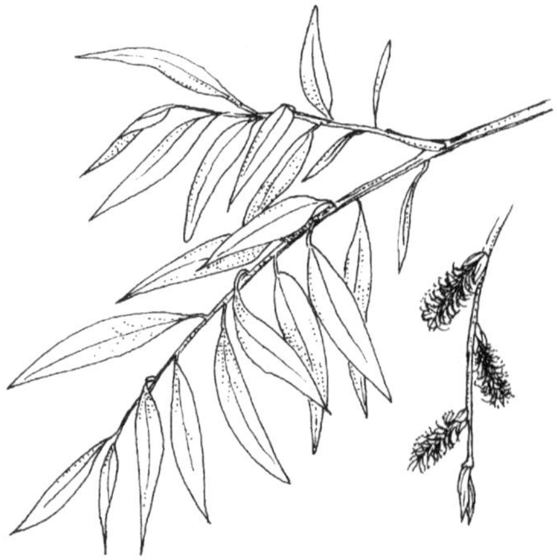

Description: The willows are a large group of shrubs or trees from the northern hemisphere, often found in wet places, with flowers in spikes called catkins that grow on separate plants. The seeds are attached to a bit of cottony fluff that is often released into the air when the capsules are ripe. The bark is an ancient medicine and a source for aspirin. You can find willow bark in the bulk herb section of many herb shops. The tincture is available, but isn't very strong.

Uses: Willow bark contains the mild aspirin-like compound called salicin. Use willow bark tea if you have a headache, fever, pain, or an inflammatory condition like carpal tunnel syndrome, rheumatism, or arthritis.

Dosage: Make a decoction by simmering 1 tablespoon of the cut and sifted bark for every cup of water for 10 minutes, then let the brew steep for another ten minutes. Drink 1 cup, 2 or 3 times daily.

Wild Oats

Latin name: *Avena fatua* L.

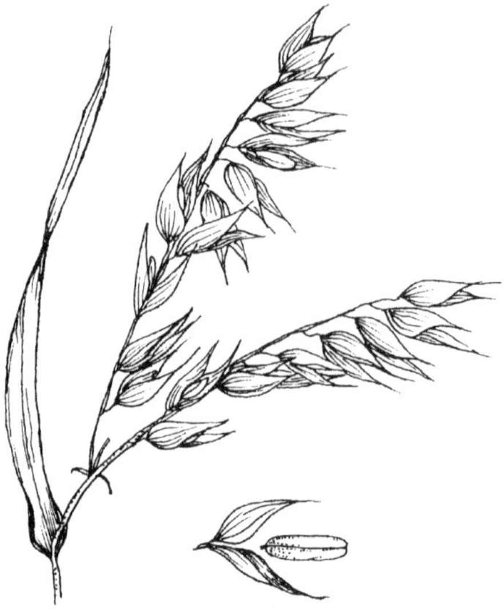

Description: Wild oats are common grasses throughout the northern hemisphere. Observing how rapidly they spread to form vast and dense fields, you can easily understand the old saying, "sow your wild oats." The small fruiting parts, known as *spikelets,* are collected when the starch of the grain is still liquid white. You can buy wild oats as a bulk herb to make tea and as a tincture of the fresh spikelets, harvested in the milky stage. Other preparations aren't effective, in my experience.

Uses: Consider taking wild oats if you have trouble with depression, nerve weakness from too much mental work, depression, or an addiction (like smoking) that you're trying to eliminate from your life. Science hasn't caught up with the traditional use of wild oats yet, but herbalists regularly recommend the herb.

Dosage: Make a tea by simmering 1/4 cup of the spikelets for every cup of water for 20 minutes. Drink 1 cup of the tea or take 1/2 to 1 teaspoon of the tincture in a little water, 3 or 4 times daily as needed. Best results come after taking wild oats for a few months, and you can take the herb up to a year or more.

Wild Yam

Latin name: *Dioscorea villosa* L.

Description: Wild yam is a vine-like perennial plant of the eastern United States with slender, stiff stems, heart-shaped leaves, and small greenish flowers. The rhizomes are harvested for medicine. The Mexican wild yam has large tubers, up to fifteen or twenty pounds. You can find wild yam in bulk for making teas, but be careful not to try grinding it in your blender — it's so tough that it can break the blades! Buy the herb already cut and sifted. Wild yam is also available in tinctures and in extract and powder form in capsules and tablets.

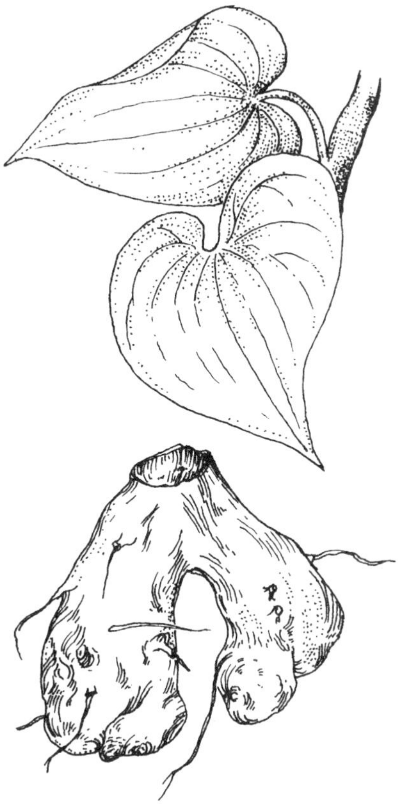

Uses: Wild yam has a history of medical use for easing the cramping of colic, intestinal and uterine spasms, and gallbladder pain. You may find that the herb is an effective addition to herbal formulas for nausea, morning sickness, and chronic rheumatism. Wild yam doesn't have progesterone-like activity, but rather a weak estrogenic effect. Many wild yam creams actually contain human progesterone created in the laboratory, often synthetically derived from a compound that naturally occurs in wild yam called *diosgenin.* In this case, they are really progesterone creams with a little inert wild yam extract added to make it seem more natural. Birth control pills are also derived from diosgenin from wild yam or other sources like fenugreek seed.

Dosage: Make a tea by boiling 1 teaspoon of the herb for every cup of water for forty minutes. Drink 1 cup, or take 2 to 4 droppersful of the tincture in a little water, 2 to 3 times daily.

Witch Hazel

Latin name: *Hamamelis virginiana* L.

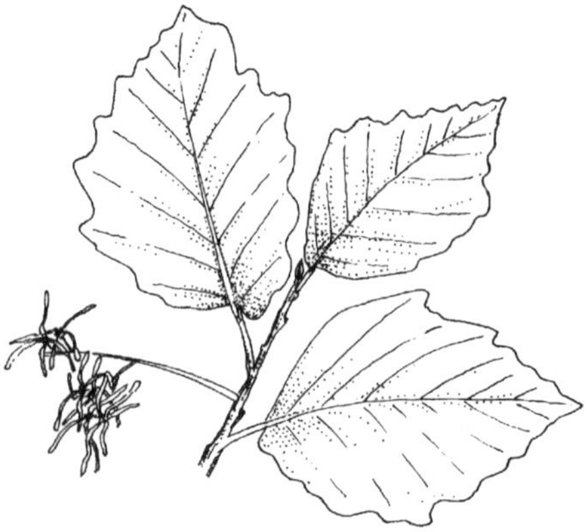

Description: Witch hazel is a shrub or small tree of hardwood forests of the eastern United States, but also a favorite garden shrub for its bright-yellow flowers that bloom in the winter. Buy witch hazel in bulk to make teas or as a tincture. You can also find it in lotions, washes, and liniments.

Uses: Consider taking witch hazel internally if you have hemorrhoids, varicose veins, or diarrhea. Externally, witch hazel is a favorite remedy for stopping the bleeding of cuts, for removing spots and blemishes, and for toning the skin.

Dosage: Use 1/4 to 1/2 cup of the bark or dried leaves to make a light decoction by simmering for 20 minutes. Take 1/2 to 1 cup of the tea, 2 or 3 times daily, or apply the lotion externally as needed.

Caution: Use of witch hazel tea or tincture for more than a few days can worsen constipation in some cases.

Wormwood

Latin name: *Artemisia absinthium* L.

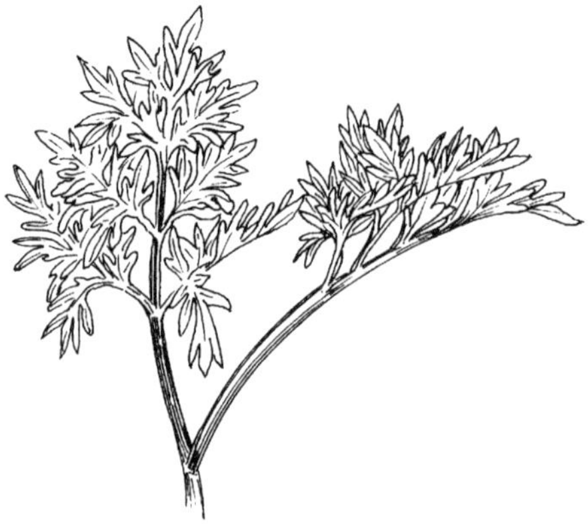

Description: Wormwood is a large woody garden plant from Europe with profuse gray-green, feathery leaves and tiny, yellowish flowers. The whole plant is pleasantly aromatic, but quite bitter. The herb is harvested to make teas and extracts. Wormwood is available as a bulk herb for making teas and as a tincture. Other forms of the herb aren't very effective.

Uses: Wormwood is a classic herb of Western herbal medicine. Try using it if you have a poor appetite, sweet cravings, stomach weakness, painful digestion, or worms. Herbalists often recommend taking a course of wormwood for helping you gain back your strength after a prolonged or serious illness or operation. Wormwood tea is a popular healing drink in Europe for easing the symptoms of stomach irritation and gastritis or for strengthening and lifting sagging digestive organs.

Dosage: Make an infusion of wormwood by steeping 1 teaspoon to 1 tablespoon of the dried herb for every cup of water for 20 minutes. Drink 1/2 to 1 cup of the tea or 20 to 30 drops of the tincture in a little water, several times daily, before meals.

Caution: Avoid use of this herb during pregnancy or nursing. Don't exceed recommended dose. Don't use the tincture for more than a few weeks at a time without first consulting an herbalist.

Yarrow

Latin name: *Achillea millefolium* L.

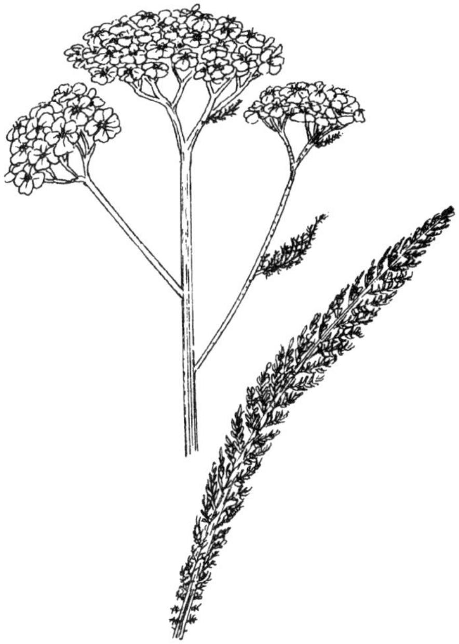

Description: Yarrow is an upright aromatic plant with finely dissected leaves and flat-topped, umbrella-shaped, white, flowering parts. The upper parts of the plant are harvested for making medicines. Yarrow is available as a bulk tea and in healing tea blends, in tinctures, and as a concentrate in some herb formulas. Avoid the ground-up herb in capsules or tablets because many of the active constituents break down over time. The best form of yarrow is the fresh herb right from a wild place or garden, but a good quality dry herb works fine.

Uses: Try taking yarrow for easing mucus congestion, inflammation, and fever of colds, flu, and other upper respiratory infections. Yarrow helps regulate blood flow throughout the body, aiding pain relief from arthritis and rheumatism. You can also use yarrow for sluggish or painful menses. fever, delayed menstruation, poor appetite, and convalescence. Yarrow helps relieve spasms and inflammation, and you may find it helpful for irritable bowel complaints, colic, and intestinal and uterine cramps. The herb acts as a bitter tonic and is highly recommended with other digestive herbs like gentian or centaury to help relax the bowels and improve digestion, as well as help prevent and treat gallstones and gallbladder inflammation.

Dosage: Make an infusion by steeping 1/4 cup of the bulk herb for every two cups of water for 20 or 30 minutes. Drink 1 cup of the tea, or 1 to 3 droppersful of the tincture in a little water, 2 or 3 times daily. Take yarrow for several weeks or months to experience the best results.

Caution: Avoid use of this herb during pregnancy.

Yellow Dock

Latin name: *Rumex crispus* L.

Description: Yellow dock has long, lance-shaped leaves and a tall spike of greenish flowers turning to masses of rust-colored seeds. The root is harvested for medicine. Besides your back yard or local field, look for yellow dock in tincture form and as a powder or extract in capsules.

Uses: Yellow dock is a common weed, but don't underestimate its powers — the root is a magnificent bowel balancer and blood tonic. You can benefit from the herb if you have either constipation or sluggish bowels, or loose stools. Midwives often recommend yellow dock to pregnant women to keep their bowels regular and to help keep their red blood cell count up. I prescribe the root for damp heat conditions of the bowel accompanied by vaginal yeast infections, bladder infections (cystitis), diarrhea, or gallbladder problems. Consider adding yellow dock to formulas to help cleanse parasites and worms from the intestines and to perk up the appetite.

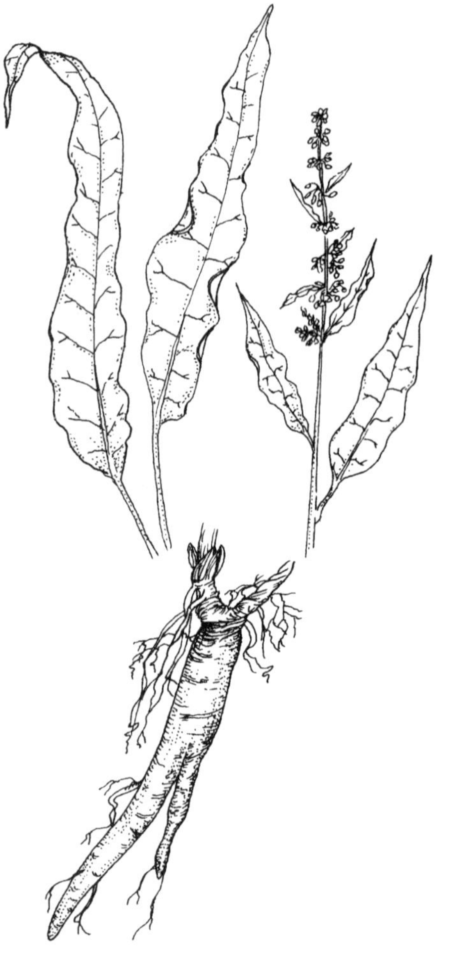

Dosage: To make a tea, simmer 1 teaspoon of the cut and sifted herb for every cup of water for 20 minutes. Drink 1 cup of the tea, or 3 to 5 droppersful of the tincture in a little water, 2 or 3 times daily.

Caution: Avoid use of this herb if you have kidney stones.

Yerba Santa

Latin name: *Eriodictyon californicum* [Hook. Et Arn.] Torr.

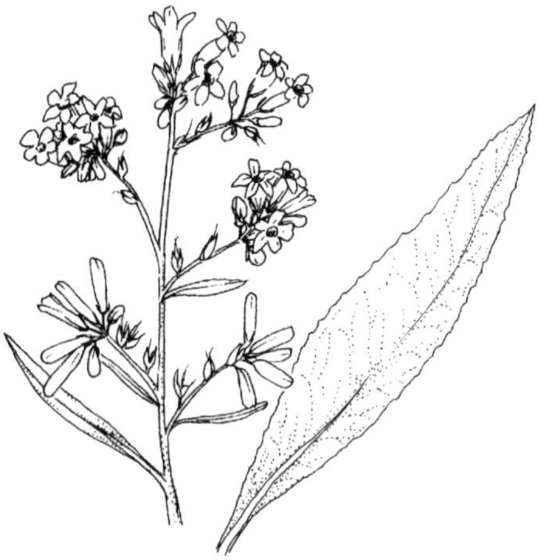

Description: Yerba santa is a sticky herb with graceful sprays of lavender flowers. Yerba santa is available as a bulk herb (for making teas) and as a tincture.

Uses: Consider yerba santa if you have respiratory congestion, a cold, asthma, or moist cough. Yerba santa is a warming expectorant that helps remove excess damp cold mucus and help you breathe. The herb is especially useful during the cold damp months of the year.

Dosage: Make an infusion by steeping 1/4 cup of dry herb for every 2 cups of water for 30 minutes. Drink 1 cup of the tea, or take 10 to 30 drops of the tincture, 3 times daily.

Appendix A

Herb Talk Glossary

abortifacient: An herb that causes a fetus to abort.

active constituent: A chemical molecule that can alter some biochemical process in the body. Most plants or herbs contain dozens, sometimes hundreds, of active chemicals that work together to alter functioning processes of the body, usually in a subtle way.

adaptogen: A safe and mild herb that helps the body adapt to any kind of stress or change. An adaptogen works to balance the activity of the nervous, hormonal, and immune systems.

alterative: An herb that slowly alters the activity of tissues or organs by enhancing nutrition, energy, and vitality.

amendment: An addition to the soil that helps make up nutrients in which the soil is deficient — rock phosphate, kelp, compost, and manure.

annual: A plant that goes through a complete life cycle in one year.

anodyne: A pain-relieving herb.

antiemetic: Counteracts or relieves nausea or vomiting.

antihydrotic: Slows the production of sweat.

anti-microbial: An herb used to fight infections.

antioxidant: A substance that inhibits oxidation and subsequent damage of important chemicals, enzymes, membranes, cells, and tissues in the body. Damage caused by oxidation is brought about by potentially dangerous chemicals called *free-radicals.* Free radicals are created in your body, by your immune system, in the process of killing disease-causing agents (like bacteria) and during the everyday process of living. Herbal antioxidants include milk thistle for the liver, ginkgo for the circulatory system, and hawthorn for the cardiovascular system. Other well-known antioxidants include vitamin E, vitamin C, and grapeseed extract. See also ***free radicals.***

antiparasitic: An herb that helps eliminate parasites.

antiperiodic: An herb that helps relieve cyclic fevers, especially those caused by malaria.

antitussive: An herb that reduces the urge to cough.

aperient: A gentle stimulant to the digestion and a mild laxative.

aphrodisiac: An herb that increases sexual desire.

aquaretic: A mild herbal diuretic that doesn't deplete potassium.

aromatherapy: The use of fragrant plants or plant essences (such as essential oils) by inhaling and smelling them, consuming very small amounts orally, or applying them to the skin, to alter your mood or change a physiological process of the body. See also ***essential oil.***

assimilation: The process of absorbing or incorporating substances into the body, usually nutrients or active constituents from plants. See also ***active constituents.***

atherosclerosis: Hard plaque formation in the arteries that leads to blockage.

Ayurveda: A 5,000-year-old East Indian system of healing. It is possible that Ayurveda, Traditional Chinese Medicine (TCM), and Western herbalism all had a common ancestor, because they all have some features in common.

base: A thick, sweet, or creamy substance that can carry herbal extracts into the body. For example, a sweet sugar or honey base is used in cough syrups, and an oily, waxy base is used in salves.

biennial: A plant that grows for two years before dying.

bitter tonic: An herb or blend of herbs that has a bitter taste and is used to stimulate and improve the digestion.

blood mover: An herb that moves the blood in the vessels, removing stagnation in the tissues and reducing pain. A circulatory stimulant.

calm the spirit: A traditional Chinese concept that means to relax the mind, emotions, and body, creating a peaceful, centered feeling.

calmative: An herb that reduces nervous system hyperactivity and has a gentle calming effect on the mind, body, and emotions.

cardioprotective: An herb that nourishes and protects the heart.

carminative: Herbs or essential oils that help the bowels release gas, relieving pain.

carrier: An herb, herbal blend, or plant essence that helps carry active chemicals (active constituents) into the bloodstream, where they can act on the body's tissues and organs.

cataplasm: A warm, gooey pack placed on various parts of the body to help draw out infection and speed the healing process of boils, sores, cysts, and other lesions. A flaxseed poultice is an example.

cholagogue: An herb that increases the flow of bile output from the liver and gallbladder.

choleretic: An herb that helps bile flow more smoothly.

compost: A complete fertilizer made up of decaying organic material, such as grass, leaves, and manure.

compress: A cloth soaked in herbal tea and applied to wounds, rashes, sore muscles, or sprains.

damp heat: An accumulation of dampness and heat together in your tissues and organs. These substances can block the proper flow of nutrients and increase your risk of having infections like vaginal yeast infections, bladder infections, chronic bronchitis, and acne.

dampness: An accumulation of excess water in the tissues of your body that can interfere with healthy cellular function. Dampness is often caused by a weak digestive system that cannot properly manage the water from food and drinks. Practitioners of Traditional Chinese Medicine say that excess dampness in your system can cause symptoms like swelling of your joints with pain of arthritis.

decoction: A tea preparation for roots, barks, and twigs. To make a decoction, simmer 1 ounce of herb to 10 ounces of water for 20 to 60 minutes. When you take the simmered herbs and add them to fresh water and simmer again, you make a *double-decoction.*

demulcent: A mucilaginous (thick and slimy) herb which soothes irritated or inflamed tissue or mucous membranes.

diaphoretic: An herb that promotes perspiration and facilitates the elimination of toxins through the skin.

digestant: An herb that benefits the process of digestion. A *bitter digestant* is a bitter-tasting digestant.

digestive: An herb that strengthens or supports good digestive function.

double-ought ("00") capsule: A gelatin capsule or vegetable fiber capsule that holds about a half a gram of powdered herb or herb extract.

elixir: A liquid herbal extract that contains alcohol and a sweet base to render it more pleasant to drink. The Chinese make longevity and energy elixirs from tonic herbs like ginseng and astragalus.

emollient: An herb applied externally to soften and soothe the skin.

essential oil: An extremely light and *volatile* (quickly-evaporating) concentrated oil used in aromatherapy products and obtained from the herb by distillation. Not for internal use without professional advice.

febrifuge: An herb that reduces fever.

free radicals: Oxygen and other molecules with an unpaired electron that gives the molecules the ability to strongly react with and damage cellular structures, genetic material, and the tissues of the body. Many scientists believe that free radicals are a major cause of tissue degeneration and hardening of arteries as aging occurs. Free radical scavengers or *antioxidants* can help protect you from the damaging effects of these dangerous molecules, perhaps slowing the aging process. See also ***antioxidant.***

galactogogue: An herb that increases the flow of breast milk.

glycerite: Liquid extract that contains glycerin rather than alcohol.

healing crisis: When you start taking cleansing herbs that increase the release of toxic wastes from your cells and tissues, they start circulating in your blood. As they begin to go out of your body through your urine, sweat, and bowel movements, the wastes can irritate your tissues, causing pain, a feeling of irritability, fatigue, and sometimes an upset stomach, or loose stools. This healing crisis (also called a *cleansing reaction*) usually lasts only a few days to a week or ten days, depending on how regularly you cleanse and how much toxic waste products are stored in your cells and tissues.

hepatic: An herb that affects the liver. A hepatic cleanser, such as boldo, helps your liver throw off toxic wastes. A hepatic tonic, such as milk thistle, helps strengthen the liver.

homeopathy: A system of medicine whose practitioners believe that highly diluted solutions of herbs and minerals can stimulate the healing process of the body.

hypotensive: An herb that helps lower blood pressure.

infusion: A tea preparation of leaves or flowering tops. To make an infusion, pour 1 pint of water over 1 ounce of herb, and let it stand, covered, for 20 minutes.

light decoction: Simmering herbs in water for 5 minutes, then steeping the brew in a covered pan for 15 to 30 minutes. This process extracts the active constituents from thicker leaves and other moderately dense part of herbs, like seeds.

liniment: A liquid preparation made from a liquid herbal extract, alcohol, oil, and an emulsifier (like gum arabic) that forms a smooth herbal liquid for external use.

liver cooler: An herb that reduces pathogenic heat and irritation in the liver.

macerating: Soaking or steeping herbs in alcohol, oil, or water. The actual preparation of the herbs soaking in a liquid is called a *maceration.*

marc: The waste herb material that has the liquid extract removed from it by squeezing or pressing during the tincture-making process.

menstruum: The solvent blend used to make a liquid extract, usually alcohol and water.

moxibustion: Burning a compacted stick of mugwort herb over areas on the skin to stimulate energy flow and facilitate healing. Moxibustion, also called *moxa,* is used by practitioners of Traditional Chinese Medicine to treat arthritis, pain, and diseases involving hormone and immune weakness.

naturalized: A plant that is originally from a foreign continent and escapes from cultivation, often wandering far and wide. Plantain, for example, is originally from Europe, but it is a common weed in North America and on other continents.

ointment: A semi-solid herbal preparation for external use that's made up of olive oil, beeswax, and herbs.

oleoresin: A sharply pungent, oily, resinous extract from certain herbs, such as ginger or cinnamon.

Old World: Plants from the *Old World* are originally from Iran, Iraq, Egypt, and the Middle Eastern countries — the cradle of western civilization.

palmately compound leaf: A compound leaf where the separate leaflets fan out from a central point of attachment like the fingers from your palm.

pathogenic heat: A disease-causing condition in the body that happens after extended periods of stress and the use of metabolic stimulants like caffeine-containing beverages, refined sugar, and red meat. Pathogenic, or disease-promoting, heat often underlies infections like vaginal yeast infections, bladder infections, and acne. Herbalists recommend cooling herbs like Oregon grape root to eliminate the heat and help get rid of the infections.

percolation: The process of removing the active chemicals (also called *active constituents*) from herb powders that are packed into a large funnel by allowing a *menstruum* (often an alcohol and water mixture) to slowly flow through the herbs. The menstruum flow is controlled at the bottom of the funnel stem with a valve, so that only a few drops fall each minute.

perennial: A plant that grows indefinitely. Shrubs and trees are woody perennials. Some herbaceous plants like ginseng completely die back each year, then resprout in the spring from their roots.

phytoestrogen: Natural estrogen-like compounds that occur in plants, especially in the pea family and in flax-seeds, which give a more balanced, estrogen-like activity than pure estrogen. Some scientists claim that phytoestrogens can help protect you from cancer and heart disease, as well as help women have an enjoyable menopause. Phytoestrogens (like genistein) are a major component of the traditional diets in Asia and other parts of the world.

pinnately compound leaf: A leaf that has a number of separate smaller leaves called leaflets, arranged on the central leaf rib instead of one solid leaf blade. A pinnately compound leaf (a fern leaf is a good example) has the leaflets arranged along one straight axis or midrib.

poultice: A mass of fresh, ground-up herbs applied wet to an area of the body in order to encourage healing. A fresh plantain poultice is used to help reduce the inflammation and pain of cuts, stings, bites, and burns.

pressure point: Special points on your body that activate internal organs and help balance body systems. Skilled practitioners use pressure points to determine which of your organs are imbalanced or weak.

propagation: The process of creating a new plant from a part of a *mother* plant. New plants can be rooted from stems or shoots, or by dividing root masses.

resin: A semi-solid plant substance with antibacterial properties that is soluble in alcohol, but not water. Amber and pine pitch are examples.

restorative: An herb that restores balance and strength to the body and its systems.

rhizome: An underground stem from which roots and shoots grow. The rhizomes of ginger, turmeric, and valerian are all collected for medicine.

salve: A medicinal preparation made from an herb, such as calendula or St. John's wort, soaked in vegetable oil and combined with beeswax for application to your skin.

sialogogue: An herb that increases the secretion of saliva.

single-ought capsule: A small gelatin capsule that holds about one-third of a gram (300 mg) of an herb powder or herb extract.

spike: A type of plant *inflorescence* (flowering part) where the flowers are arranged densely along a stalk. Cattails and lavender are good examples.

spikelet: The flowering structures of grasses, including the half-ripe milky grain of wild oats.

solvent: A liquid capable of dissolving and removing chemicals from plants and carrying them in a liquid solution, like dissolving salt in water to form a salty solution.

spp: A botanical term that is short for *species,* signifying any one of a number of species in a plant group called a *genus,* where the individuals cannot sexually cross and form a new plant. For instance, herbalists mostly feel that any member of the genus *Valeriana,* the valerians, are good for making relaxing and sleeping remedies. This is written as *Valeriana* spp.

standardized extract: A type of herbal extract in which a known chemical that is specific to each herb is identified and adjusted to a specified level to make a finished standardized extract. The potency of that compound (if it is known to have biological activity) or group of compounds is then listed on the label to help assure you that the extract company has done their homework and is selling the right herb at a guaranteed minimum of some of the active compounds. Herbalists feel those highly purified standardized extracts, like ginkgo 24 percent, are not as nature intended and perhaps going too much towards pharmaceutical drugs. Instead, herbalists prefer whole plant extracts, in which very little is removed from the original herb during the extraction process, except inert (non-active) cellulose and starch. This discussion between herbal pharmacy companies, scientists, and herbalists is ongoing, but both approaches have their benefits.

strobile: A fruiting structure with rows of overlapping scales, such as the mature *inflorescence* (flowering part) of hops.

thallus: The vegetative body of lichens and seaweeds.

tincture: A concentrated herbal extract made by soaking ground up herbs in solvents like alcohol and water and then pressing the liquid out. Some manufacturers add glycerin after removing the alcohol to make an alcohol-free liquid extract, called a *glycerite.*

tonic: An herbal product that strengthens various organs and systems. You can find immune tonics, liver tonics, blood tonics, heart tonics, and so on.

Traditional Chinese Medicine (TCM): An ancient system of holistic medicine and healing that developed over at least four or five thousand years in China. The system first spread to other parts of Asia, like Japan, and then to other parts of the world. Many licensed practitioners of TCM, of which acupuncture and herbal medicine are a part, are practicing in North America, Europe, and on other continents.

volatile oil: See ***essential oil.***

whorled: The leaves of this type of plant form the spokes of a wheel around one point on a stem. Cleavers is a good example.

wildcrafting: Picking uncultivated herbs from the wild. Wildcrafting is done in woods, yards, waste-lots, fields, and pastures. Most herbalists feel that wildcrafting also implies picking the herbs with reverence and ecological awareness.

woods-grown: Herbs grown in their natural habitat without excessive human intervention. Growers cultivate woods-grown herbs (like ginseng) without added fertilizer or water, but they watch over and manage the plants.

Appendix B
Herbal Dosage Guide

The following table gives you information on dosages for the herbal remedies listed throughout this book. You can purchase herbs and herb products from your local herb shop, natural food store, or pharmacy in tincture form, in bulk herb form (to make a tea), or in powder or extract form in capsules or tablets. You can also order them by mail or through the Web (see Appendix C for more information).

Read this before you begin!

The information in this reference is not intended to substitute for expert medical advice or treatment; it is designed to help you make informed choices. Because each individual is unique, a professional health care provider must diagnose conditions and supervise treatments for each individual health problem. If an individual is under a doctor's care and receives advice that is contrary to the information provided in this reference, the doctor's advice should be followed, because it is based on the unique characteristics of that individual.

Herb	***Action***	***Standard Therapeutic Dose and Preparation***
Alfalfa leaf	Tonic	1 cup infusion, 2 times daily.
Aloe leaf	Liquid gel: soothing, anti-inflammatory, bowel cleanser; resin: stimulant laxative	Drink 1/4 cup of the liquid gel, morning and evening with meals. Follow the label directions for capsules of the resin powder. Apply the leaf pulp externally.
Angelica root	Appetizer	1 cup decoction 3 times daily, or 1/2 teaspoon of the tincture in a little water, before meals.
Anise seed	Expectorant, carminative	1 cup decoction, 2 to 3 times daily.
Arnica	Reduces inflammation, helps heal injuries	Homeopathic tablets as directed; apply cream or salve as directed.

(continued)

(continued)

Herb	*Action*	*Standard Therapeutic Dose and Preparation*
Artichoke leaf	Digestive and bile stimulant	2 to 3 droppersful tincture or 1 cup infusion, 2 to 3 times daily before meals.
Balsam of Peru	Antiseptic, antifungal	External use. Follow label directions.
Black cohosh root, rhizome	Reduces spasms, and inflammation, regulates estrogen	2 to 4 droppersful tincture or 1/2 cup decoction, 2 to 3 times daily. *Eco-alert: an environmentally sensitive herb*
Black walnut hulls	Antifungal	1/2 to 1 teaspoon tincture, 3 times daily away from meals.
Blackberry root	Astringent, anti-diarrheal	1 cup decoction, 2 to 3 times daily.
Bladderwrack thallus	Helps normalize thyroid function	4 capsules powder, 2 to 3 times daily.
Boldo leaf	Liver regulator	1 cup infusion, 2 to 3 times daily.
Buckthorn bark	Laxative	1 to 2 droppersful tincture, morning and evening.
Burdock root	Alterative, tonic	1 cup decoction, 3 capsules of powdered herb, or 1/2 to 1 teaspoon of the tincture, 3 times daily.
Butcher's broom	Anti-inflammatory, vein tonic	1 to 2 capsules powdered extract, twice daily.
Cactus flowers and fresh stems	Heart tonic and regulator	1/2 to 1 dropperful tincture, 2 times daily or see your herbalist.
Calendula flowers	Vulnerary, anti-inflammatory	Externally in oils, creams, and salves; 1 cup infusion, 3 times daily.
California poppy	Calmative	2 to 4 droppersful tincture, as needed.
Caraway seed	Carminative	1 cup infusion, 2 to 3 times daily.
Cardamom seed	Stomachic	1 cup light decoction, 2 to 3 times daily.
Cascara sagrada bark	Laxative	4 capsules powder or 2 to 4 droppersful tincture, before bed.
Catnip herb	Calmative	1 cup infusion, 2 to 3 times daily.
Cayenne	Blood mover, rubefacient	2 to 4 capsules powder 1 to 2 times daily with meals or sprinkle on food.
Celery seed	Diuretic, sedative, reduces inflammation of arthritis	1 cup infusion, 2 times daily.
Centaury leaf	Bitter digestive, hepatic	1 to 3 droppersful tincture, before meals.
Chamomile flowers	Calmative, antispasmodic	1 cup infusion, 2 to 3 times daily.
Chaparral flowering tops	Liver stimulant, anti-microbial	1/2 to 1 cup or 1 to 2 droppersful tincture, 2 times daily.

Herb	Action	Standard Therapeutic Dose and Preparation
Chrysanthemum flowers	Alterative, antipyretic	1 cup infusion, 2 to 3 times daily.
Cinnamon bark	Digestant, warming herb	1 cup light decoction, 2 to 3 times daily.
Cleavers	Diuretic, lymphatic	1 cup infusion or 1/2 to 1 teaspoon tincture, 3 times daily.
Clove bud	Carminative, anodyne	1/2 to 1 cup decoction, 2 times daily, or use diluted essential oil for *external* use (1 drop only).
Comfrey leaf	Demulcent, emollient	1 cup light decoction fresh or dried leaves, 2 times daily for up to two weeks; fresh blended leaf mass *externally* as a poultice.
Corn silk stigma	Diuretic, demulcent	1 cup infusion or 1 teaspoon tincture, 2 to 3 times daily.
Cramp bark	Antispasmodic	1 cup decoction or 2 to 4 droppersful tincture, 2 to 3 times daily.
Cranberry juice (fresh or dried)	Urinary antiseptic	2 to 3 cups unsweetened juice or 1 to 2 capsules or tablets of standardized extract, daily.
Damiana leaf	Aphrodisiac	1 cup infusion or 1/2 teaspoon tincture or 3 capsules powder, 2 to 3 times daily.
Dandelion root and leaf	Cholagogue, hepatic	1 cup decoction, 2 to 3 times daily.
Dong quai root	Blood tonic, blood regulator	1 cup decoction, 2 to 3 times daily; follow label directions for other products.
Devil's claw root	Anti-inflammatory, anodyne	1 to 2 droppersful tincture, 4 times daily.
Dill seed	Digestant, appetizer	1 cup infusion, 2 to 3 times daily.
Echinacea leaf and root	Immune stimulant, antibiotic	2 to 3 droppersful tincture, 3 to 4 times daily.
Elder flower	Diaphoretic, antiviral	1 cup infusion, 2 to 3 times daily.
Eleuthero (Siberian ginseng) root	Adaptogen	1 cup decoction or 2 to 3 droppersful tincture, 2 to 3 times daily.
Evening primrose oil	Anti-inflammatory	250 to 500 mg capsules, daily.
Eyebright herb	Decongestant, anti-inflammatory	2 to 4 droppersful tincture or 1 cup infusion, 2 to 3 times daily.
Fennel seed	Carminative, galactagogue	1 cup decoction, 2 to 3 times daily after meals.
Fenugreek seed	Expectorant, galactagogue	1 cup decoction, 2 to 3 times daily.

(continued)

(continued)

Herb	*Action*	*Standard Therapeutic Dose and Preparation*
Feverfew	Febrifuge, anti-inflammatory	1 to 2 droppersful tincture or 2 capsules powder, 2 times daily.
Flaxseed	Anti-inflammatory, emollient	1 to 2 teaspoons freshly-ground seed sprinkled on food or 1 teaspoon of the oil; make a poultice by grinding 2 tablespoons of seeds, mixing with water and soaking to form a gel and apply to a boil or sore.
Garlic bulbs or oil or powder in capsules	Antibacterial, cardioprotective, anti-viral	2 to 3 cloves, daily or 1 capsule or tablet, 2 times daily.
Gentian root	Bitter digestant	$^1/_2$ cup decoction, 2 to 3 times daily or 1 dropperful tincture before meals.
Ginger rhizome or root	Digestant, anti-nauseant	1 cup decoction or 1 to 2 capsules powder or $^1/_2$ teaspoon tincture, 2 to 3 times daily.
Ginkgo leaf	Antioxidant, memory herb, and circulatory stimulant	2 to 3 droppersful tincture or 60 mg standardized extract, 2 or 3 times daily.
Ginseng root	Adaptogen, energy herb	1 cup decoction or 1 to 2 droppersful tincture, 2 to 3 times daily. *Eco-alert: an environmentally sensitive herb*
Goldenseal root	Antibacterial, anti-inflammatory	1 dropperful tincture or 1 to 2 capsules, 2 times daily. *Eco-alert: an environmentally sensitive herb*
Green tea leaf	Antibacterial	1 cup infusion or 1 to 2 capsules, 2 to 3 times daily.
Grindelia flower	Antitussive, expectorant	$^1/_2$ to 1 dropperful tincture, 2 or 3 times daily.
Guggul oleoresin	Reduces cholesterol	2 to 3 capsules, 2 to 3 times daily.
Hawthorn leaves and flowers	Heart tonic, calmative	2 to 3 droppersful tincture or 120 to 240 mg standardized extract, 2 to 3 times daily.
Heartsease pansy flower	Anti-inflammatory, anti-microbial	1 cup infusion or 1 to 2 droppersful tincture, 2 to 3 times daily.
Hops strobiles	Calmative, bitter digestive	2 to 3 droppersful tincture or 1 cup infusion, 2 to 3 times daily.
Horehound leaf	Relieves coughs	2 to 4 droppersful tincture, 2 to 3 times daily, or 1 cup infusion, 2 to 3 times daily.
Horse chestnut bark and seed	Anti-inflammatory, eases varicose veins	250 mg standardized extract every 12 hours with water.
Horseradish root	Digestive, diuretic	Use the grated fresh root sparingly or 1 dropperful tincture in water, several times daily.

Herb	Action	Standard Therapeutic Dose and Preparation
Horsetail herb	Aquaretic, mineral tonic	1 cup decoction, 2 to 3 times daily or follow label directions for tablets.
Irish moss thallus	Relieves coughs, demulcent	1 cup decoction, 2 to 3 times daily.
Jamaican dogwood bark	Relieves pain, calmative	1/2 to 1 droppersful tincture, 2 or 3 times daily.
Jewelweed leaf	Anti-inflammatory	2 to 3 droppersful, several times daily, or use tincture externally.
Kava root	Relaxant, calmative	200 to 500 mg standardized extract or 2 to 4 droppersful tincture, 2 to 4 times daily.
Lavender flower	Calmative	1 cup infusion, 2 to 3 times daily, or 30 drops tincture, 2 to 3 times daily.
Lemon balm herb	Anti-viral, calmative	1 cup infusion, 2 to 3 times daily.
Licorice root	Anti-inflammatory, demulcent	400 mg standardized extract, 2 times daily (DGL); 1/2 to 1 cup infusion, 1 to 2 times daily; follow label directions for other products.
Ligustrum berry	Immune tonic	1 cup decoction or 2 to 3 droppersful tincture, 2 to 3 times daily.
Linden flower	Calmative, hypotensive	1 cup infusion, 2 to 3 times daily.
Lobelia leaf and flower	Relaxes bronchial airways	10 to 15 drops tincture, 2 to 3 times daily or 1/4 cup infusion, 2 to 3 times daily.
Loquat leaf	Relieves coughs	1 cup decoction, 2 to 3 times daily or follow label directions for syrup.
Marshmallow root	Demulcent	1 to 2 cups decoction or 2 to 4 droppersful, 2 to 3 times daily.
Milk thistle seed	Liver tonic, protective	100 mg standardized extract or 2 to 4 droppersful tincture, 2 to 3 times daily.
Motherwort herb	Heart tonic and regulator	1 cup infusion or 2 to 4 droppersful tincture, 2 to 3 times daily.
Mugwort leaf	Bitter digestive, cholagogue	1 cup infusion, 2 to 3 times daily.
Muira puama root	Aphrodisiac	1 to 3 droppersful tincture, 2 to 3 times daily.
Mullein leaf and flower	Relieves coughs, soothes bronchial airways	1 cup light decoction, 2 to 3 times daily for leaf, or follow label directions for mullein ear oil.
Myrrh gum	Antiseptic, astringent	For external use as a mouthwash in tincture form.

(continued)

(continued)

Herb	*Action*	*Standard Therapeutic Dose and Preparation*
Nettles leaf and root	Mineral tonic, prostate tonic	Leaf: 1 cup decoction, 2 to 3 times daily. Root: 2 to 4 capsules powdered extract, 2 times daily.
Ocotillo bark	Lymphatic cleanser	1 to 4 droppersful tincture, 2 or 3 times daily.
Orange peel	Digestive	1 cup decoction, 2 or 3 times daily before meals.
Oregon grape root	Liver cooler, cholagogue, alterative	1 cup decoction or 1 to 3 droppersful tincture, 3 times daily.
Osha root	Expectorant, immune stimulant	1 dropperful tincture or 1 cup light decoction 3 or 4 times daily. *Eco-alert: an environmentally sensitive herb*
Parsley leaf and root	Diuretic	1 cup decoction, 2 to 3 times daily.
Passion flower herb	Calmative	1 dropperful tincture or 1 cup light decoction, 3 to 4 times daily.
Peach leaf	Relieves nausea of morning sickness	1 cup infusion, 2 to 3 times daily.
Peppermint leaf	Carminative, diaphoretic	1 cup infusion or 1 capsule essential oil, 2 to 3 times daily.
Perilla leaf	Relieves nausea of morning sickness; helps relieve symptoms of a cold	1 cup decoction, 2 to 3 times daily.
Periwinkle	Anti-microbial, astringent	1/2 cup infusion, 2 to 3 times daily, or 1 to 2 droppersful tincture, 2 times daily.
Peruvian bark	Bitter digestive	1/2 to 1 dropperful, 2 or 3 times daily.
Pipsissewa leaf	Urinary antiseptic and soother	1 to 3 droppersful tincture or 1 cup light decoction, 3 to 4 times daily. *Eco-alert: an environmentally sensitive herb*
Plantain leaf	Soothes and speeds healing of wounds, bites, inflammation	1 cup infusion, 2 to 3 times daily, or use external poultice.
Poria	Digestant, diuretic	1 cup decoction, 2 to 3 times daily, or follow label directions for capsules and tablets.
Prickly ash bark	Alterative, sialogogue, circulatory stimulant	1 to 3 droppersful tincture, 2 to 3 times daily.
Psyllium seed and husk	Bowel cleanser, gentle laxative	1 tablespoon ground up in a seed grinder or blender, soaked for fifteen minutes in a cup of hot water in the morning or follow label directions for commercial products.

Herb	Action	Standard Therapeutic Dose and Preparation
Pygeum bark	Reduces prostate inflammation	Follow label directions. *Eco-alert: an environmentally sensitive herb*
Quassia bark	Antiparasitic	1 to 2 droppersful 2 to 3 times daily.
Red clover flower	Blood cleanser	1 cup infusion or 1 to 3 droppersful tincture, 2 to 4 times daily; follow label directions for extracts in capsules or tablets.
Red root	Astringent, lymphatic cleanser	1 to 2 droppersful, 2 or 3 times daily.
Reishi mushroom	Immune tonic, calmative	2 or 3 capsules or tablets standardized extract or 1 cup decoction, twice daily.
Rosemary herb	Digestant, nerve tonic	1 to 2 droppersful tincture or 1 cup infusion, 2 to 3 times daily.
Sage leaf	Antihydrotic, antiseptic	1 cup infusion, 2 to 3 times daily.
Sarsaparilla root	Alterative	1 cup decoction or 2 or 3 droppersful tincture, 2 to 3 times daily.
Saw palmetto berry	Genital and urinary tract tonic	160 to 240 mg standardized extract, 2 times daily.
Senna leaf	Laxative	½ cup infusion or 1 or 2 tablets or capsules before bed as directed by manufacturer.
Shepherd's purse	Stops bleeding, reduces blood pressure	1 to 3 droppersful tincture as needed, up to 3 or 4 times daily.
Shisandra berry	Adaptogen, hormone and liver tonic	1 cup decoction or 1 to 2 droppersful, 2 to 3 times daily.
Shiitake mushroom	Immune tonic, anti-viral, cancer protective	2 to 4 capsules or tablets of the standardized extract, 2 times daily.
Skullcap	Antispasmodic	1 to 3 droppersful tincture, 2 or 3 times daily.
Slippery elm bark	Demulcent	1 cup decoction, 2 to 3 times daily.
St. John's wort leaf and flower	Antidepressant, anti-viral	2 300 mg tablets standardized extract, morning and evening, or 4 droppersful tincture, morning and 3 evening.
Stone root or rhizome	Astringent, vein tonic	1 to 2 droppersful tincture, 2 to 3 times daily.
Sweet annie whole plant	Antiparasitic	½ to 1 cup infusion or 1 to 2 droppersful tincture, 2 times daily.
Tea tree oil	Antiseptic	For external use in oil form; apply several drops, 1 to 2 times daily.

(continued)

(continued)

Herb	Action	Standard Therapeutic Dose and Preparation
Teasel root	Adaptogen, circulatory stimulant, strengthens bones	1 cup decoction, 2 to 3 times daily.
Turmeric rhizome	Liver protector, anti-inflammatory	400 to 600 mg standardized extract or 1 to 4 droppersful, 2 to 3 times daily in water.
Usnea	Antibiotic	1 to 3 droppersful tincture, 2 to 3 times daily.
Uva ursi leaf	Astringent, antiseptic	2 to 3 droppersful, 3 times daily, or 1 cup infusion, 3 times daily.
Valerian root	Calmative	2 to 4 droppersful tincture or 1 cup light decoction, 2 to 3 times daily.
Vitex berry	Hormone regulator, promotes mother's milk	1 to 2 droppersful tincture or 4 to 6 capsules powder, first thing in the morning.
White willow bark	Analgesic, febrifuge	1 cup decoction or 2 capsules standardized extract, 2 to 3 times daily.
Wild cherry bark	Antitussive, expectorant	1 cup infusion, 2 to 3 times daily; for cough syrup follow manufacturer's label instructions.
Wild indigo root	Anti-viral	1 cup infusion or 2 to 3 droppersful tincture, 2 to 3 times daily.
Wild oats spikelets	Nerve tonic	3 to 4 droppersful or 1 cup light decoction, 3 to 4 times daily.
Wild yam root	Relieves intestinal and uterine spasms, relieves nausea	2 to 4 droppersful tincture or 1 cup decoction, 2 to 3 times daily.
Wintergreen leaf	Analgesic	1 cup infusion, 2 to 3 times daily, or in creams for external use in essential oil form.
Witch hazel leaf	Astringent, vein tonic	1 cup decoction or 2 to 3 droppersful tincture, 2 to 3 times daily, or use the tea or lotion externally.
Yarrow flower	Diaphoretic, regulates menstrual flow	2 to 3 droppersful tincture or 1 cup infusion, 2 to 3 times daily.
Yellow dock root	Liver cleanser, relieves damp heat from intestines	3 to 4 droppersful tincture or 1 cup decoction, before meals, morning and evening.
Yerba mansa root	Anti-viral	2 to 3 droppersful tincture or 1 cup decoction, 2 to 3 times daily.
Yerba santa leaf	Antitussive, expectorant	1 cup infusion or 1 dropperful tincture, 2 to 3 times daily.
Yucca root	Anti-inflammatory	2 to 4 capsules powder, 2 times daily, or follow manufacturer's label instructions.

Appendix C
Resources

I consider myself fortunate to live near a town that perhaps holds the record for per capita herb stores, natural foods stores, herbalists, and acupuncturists. The herb store closest to my house is open from 9 a.m. to midnight, 365 days a year!

If you don't live in an area that's as herbally well-endowed as mine is, I include some helpful resources, such as how to find alternative practitioners in your area, how to subscribe to newsletters and magazines written by herbalists, and where to find out about herb classes and correspondence courses. You also discover some great places to order herb plants and seeds, herb products, and herbal essential oils, as well as places to order supplies that you'll need to make your own products. Where available, I list Web sites so that you can order online.

Ready-Made Herbal Products

While I encourage you to support your local herbalists and herb suppliers whenever possible, you may not always have access to quality herbs in your area. The following online and mail order herb companies carry most of the herbs mentioned in this book and ship high-quality herbs and herb products right to your door.

Avena Botanicals

209 Mill St.
Rockport, ME 04856
207-594-0694
Tinctures, oils, salves

Green Terrestrial

328 Lake Ave.
Greenwich, CT 06830
203-862-8690
Tinctures and other herbal products

Herb Pharm

Box 116
Williams, OR 97544
800-348-4372
Tinctures and salves

Herbalist and Alchemist

51 S. Wandling Ave.
Washington, NJ 07882
908-689-9020
Tinctures, Western and Chinese herbs

Jean's Greens

119 Sulfur Springs Rd.
Newport, NY 13416
888-845-8327
Herbs, oils, and containers

Mayway Corporation

1338 Mandela Pkwy.
Oakland, CA 94607
800-262-9929
Chinese herbs and ready-made products

Moonrise Herbs

826 G St.
Arcata, CA 95521
800-603-8364
Web site: www.moonrise.botanical.com
Herbs, body products, aromatherapy products, and containers

Mountain Rose Herbs

20818 High St. North
North San Juan, CA 95960
800-879-3337
Bulk herbs, medicinal tea blends, tins

Rainbow Light

P.O. Box 600
Santa Cruz, CA 95060
800-635-1233
Tinctures, caplets, and nutritional systems

Sage Mountain Herb Products

P.O. Box 420
E. Barre, VT 05649
802-479-9825
Tinctures and other herbal products

Way of Life

1210 41st Ave.
Capitola, CA 95010
831-464-4113
Web site: www.wayoflifeca.com
Herbal products, body products, clay, castor oil, dried herbs, jars, and oils

www.allherb.com

Web site: www.allherb.com
Herbal information and products online.

Pet Information and Herbal Products

The following sources help you help your pets naturally.

American Holistic Veterinary Medicine Association

2214 Old Emmorton Rd.
Bel Air, MD 21015
410-569-0795
Publishes a journal about alternative healing for animals

Animals Apawthecary

P.O. Box 212
Conner, MT 59827
406-821-4090
Extracts and books for pet care

Herb Plants and Seeds for Gardening

If your local nursery can't supply all your herbal needs, contact these herb companies for plants and/or seeds.

Forest Farm

990 Tetherow Rd.
Williams, OR 97544
541-846-7269
Herb plants

Elixir Farm Botanicals

General Delivery
Brixey, MO 65618
417-261-2393
Chinese and indigenous medicinal herb seeds and plants

Gardens of the Blue Ridge

P.O. Box 10
US 221 North
Pineola, NC 28662
704-733-2417
Herb plants and seeds

Glasshouse Works

P.O. Box 97
Stewart, OH 45778
614-662-2142
Herb plants

Horizon Herbs

P.O. Box 69
Williams, OR 97544
541-846-6704
Seeds for medicinal herb plants

Peaceful Valley Farm Supply

P.O. Box 2209
Grass Valley, CA 95945
888-784-1722
Medicinal seeds, live plants, and cover crop seeds

Richters

357 Highway 47 Goodwood
Ontario, Canada L0C 1A0
905-640-6677
Herb plants (including scented geraniums) and books

Seeds of Change

P.O. Box 15700
Santa Fe, NM 87506-5700
800-957-3337 (catalog requests)
888-762-7333 (customer service)
Organic herb seeds

Shepherd's Garden Seeds

30 Irene St.
Torrington, CT 06790-6658
860-482-3638
Herb seeds

Well-Sweep Herb Farm

205 Mt. Bethel Rd.
Port Murray, NJ 07865
908-852-5390
Herb plants (catalog $2)

Bulk Herbs

You can order dried herbs, such as echinacea, ginger, or valerian root, in bulk from the following companies.

Frontier Herb Co-op

P.O. Box 299
Norway, IA 52318
800-669-3275
Bulk herbs and products

Pacific Botanicals

4350 Fish Hatchery Rd.
Grants Pass, OR 97527
541-479-7777
Fresh and dried herbs by the pound

Trinity Herbs

P.O. Box 1001
Graton, CA 95444
707-824-2040
Bulk herbs and herb books

Essential Oils

Most natural food stores and herb shops carry essential oils. However, if you don't have one in your area, the following companies mail-order high-quality essential oils and essential oil-containing products.

Oak Valley Herb Farm

P.O. Box 2482
Nevada City, CA 95959
Essential oils and body products (catalog $1)

Original Swiss Aromatics

P.O. Box 6723
San Rafael, CA 94903
415-479-3979
Essential oils

Simpler's Botanicals

P.O. Box 2534
Sebastapol, CA 95473
800-652-7646
Essential oils, facial products, and carrier oils

Alcohol for Solvents

If you decide to make your own tinctures, you'll probably choose to use alcohol as a solvent. You can use vodka to make your tinctures, but pure grain alcohol acts as a stronger solvent and is available from the following companies.

Aaper Alcohol Company

P.O. Box 339
Shelbyville, KY 40065
502-633-0650

McCormick Distilling

1 McCormick Lane
Westin, MO 64098
816-640-2276

Home-Product Equipment

These tools for processing herbs are often available from your local natural foods store or can be ordered by mail from the following companies.

Mountain Home Basics

P.O. Box 1834
Gaylord, MI 49734
800-572-9549
Food dryers

Miracle Exclusives

P.O. Box 8
Port Washington, NY 11050
800-645-6360
Grinders

Sweetwater Spring

1950 N. 21st St.
Grand Junction, CO 81501
Juicers

Online Herb Information

You can access the following Web sites for the latest health and medical news.

www.allherb.com

Web site: www.allherb.com
Herbal information and products online

Infobeat

Web site: www.Infobeat.com
Health news sent daily as an e-mail message

Intelihealth

www.intelihealth.com
E-mail and Web-based health information service

Napralert

Call 312-996-2246 for access
Subscription-based herbal on-line database

National Library of Medicine

Search site: igm.nlm.nih.gov/
World's largest medical database — free to search anytime

Dr. Duke's Phytochemical and Ethnobotanical Databases

Web site: www.ars-grin.gov/duke/index.html
Jim Duke's information database for finding the uses of numerous herbs

Associations

Contact the following excellent organizations for information on finding alternative practitioners, schools and correspondence courses for herbal studies, the latest research on your favorite herbs, and ideas for saving endangered medicinal plants in the United States.

American Association of Naturopathic Physicians

601 Valley St., Suite 105
Seattle, WA 98109
206-298-0125
Provides a referral directory of naturopaths

American Botanical Council

P.O. Box 201660
Austin, TX 78720
800-373-7105
Web site: www.herbalgram.org
Herb books and peer-reviewed herb journal

American Herb Association

P.O. Box 1673
Nevada City, CA 95959
530-265-9552
Offers quarterly newsletter and directories of herbal education and mail-order sources

American Herb Products Association

8484 Georgia Ave., Suite 370
Silver Springs, MD 20910
301-588-1171
The only national trade organization for herbal product manufacturers in the United States

American Herbalist Guild

P.O. Box 70
Roosevelt, UT 84066
435-722-8434
Web site: www.healthy.net/herbalists
E-mail: ahgoffice@earthlink.net
Publishes directory of herbal education for $8

Herb Research Foundation

1007 Pearl St., Suite 200
Boulder, CO 80302
303-449-2265
Provides online database searching, scientific articles, and access to herbal experts and consultants

National Association for Holistic Aromatherapy

836 Hanley Industrial Court
St. Louis, MO 63144
800-566-6735
Publishes a list of aromatherapy sources, schools, and practitioners

National Association of Holistic Dentists

P.O. Box 5007
Durango, CO 81301
Web site: www.holisticdental.org
Offers a list of holistic dentists in the United States

National Center for Homeopathy

801 N. Fairfax St., Suite 306
Alexandria, VA 22314-1757
703-548-7790
$7 for a directory of practitioners, pharmacies, bookstores, and study groups

United Plant Savers

P.O. Box 420
E. Barre, VT 05649
802-479-9825
Web site: www.plantsavers.org
E-mail: info@plantsavers.org
Working to save endangered medicinal plants; publish a newsletter

Herb Periodicals

The following herb magazines and journals provide you with information on what's hot in herbalism, the latest tips to keep you healthy, herb gardening tips, and much more.

American Herb Association Quarterly Newsletter

P.O. Box 1673
Nevada City, CA 95959
530-265-9552

Herbalgram

P.O. Box 201660
Austin, TX 78723
800-373-7105
E-mail:
custserv@herbalgram.org

Herbs for Health

741 Corporate Circle, Suite A
P.O. Box 4101
Golden, CO 80401
800-272-2193
Web site: www.interweave.com

Medical Herbalism Newsletter

PO Box 20512
Boulder, CO 80308
303-541-9552

The Herb Companion

741 Corporate Circle, Suite A
P.O. Box 4101
Golden, CO 80401
800-272-2193
Web site: www.interweave.com

Index

• B •

• D •

• E •

• F •

• H •

(continued)

• I •

• M •

• N •

• O •

• P •

• T •

• U •

• V •

• W •

• Y •

• Z •

Save Money on These Fine Quantum Products!

Limit 1 coupon per household

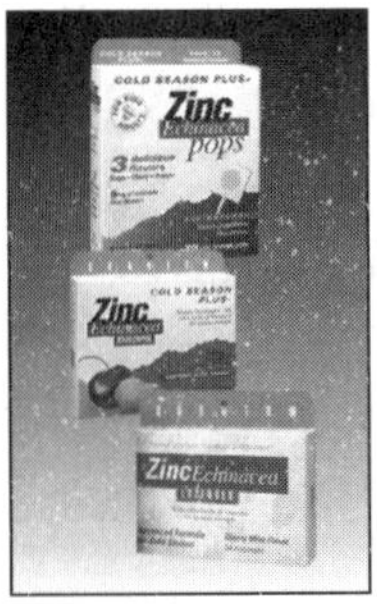

ZincEchinacea Lozenges, Pops & Drops

$1 Cash Back

Buy one or more of our Cold Season Plus+ ZincEchinacea products and receive $1.00 back on each. All items must be purchased at the same time and be listed on a single receipt. Just send this coupon (no photocopies) with your proof of purchase receipt to:

Quantum Mail In Rebate

PO Box 2791, Eugene, OR 97402

No expiration date on this cash back rebate.

For Store Information Call: 1-800-448-1448 www.quantumhealth.com

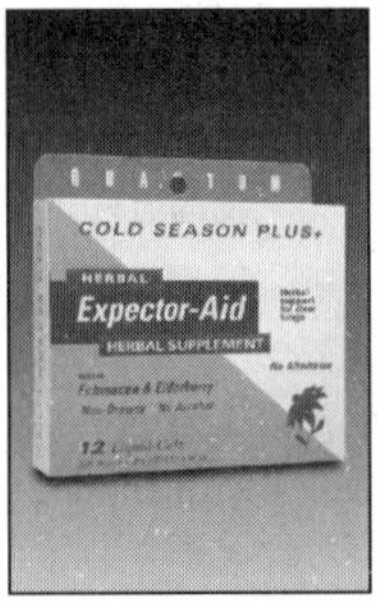

Expector-Aid

$1 Cash Back

Buy Cold Season Plus+ Expector-Aid and receive $1.00 back on each. All items must be purchased at the same time and be listed on a single receipt. Just send this coupon (no photocopies) with your proof of purchase receipt to:

Quantum Mail In Rebate

PO Box 2791, Eugene, OR 97402

No expiration date on this cash back rebate.

For Store Information Call: 1-800-448-1448 www.quantumhealth.com

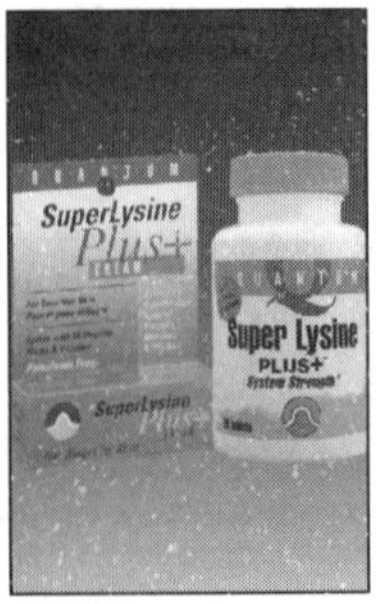

Super Lysine Plus

$1 Cash Back

Buy one or more of our Super Lysine Plus + products and receive $1.00 back on each. All items must be purchased at the same time and be listed on a single receipt. Just send this coupon (no photocopies) with your proof of purchase receipt to:

Quantum Mail In Rebate

PO Box 2791, Eugene, OR 97402

No expiration date on this cash back rebate.

For Store Information Call: 1-800-448-1448 www.quantumhealth.com

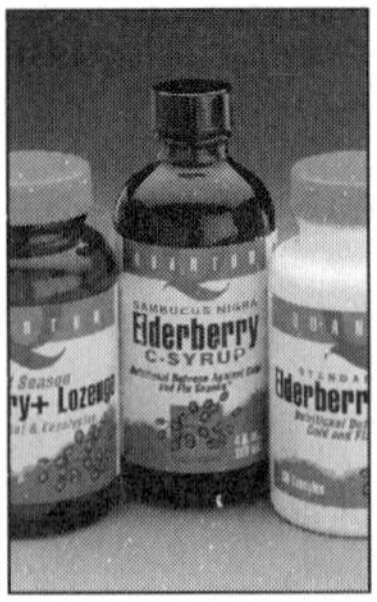

Elderberry

$1 Cash Back

Capsules, Liquid, Lozenges, C-Syrup

Buy one or more of our elderberry products and receive $1.00 back on each. All items must be purchased at the same time and be listed on a single receipt. Just send this coupon (no photocopies) with your proof of purchase receipt to:

Quantum Mail In Rebate

PO Box 2791, Eugene, OR 97402

No expiration date on this cash back rebate.

For Store Information Call: 1-800-448-1448 www.quantumhealth.com

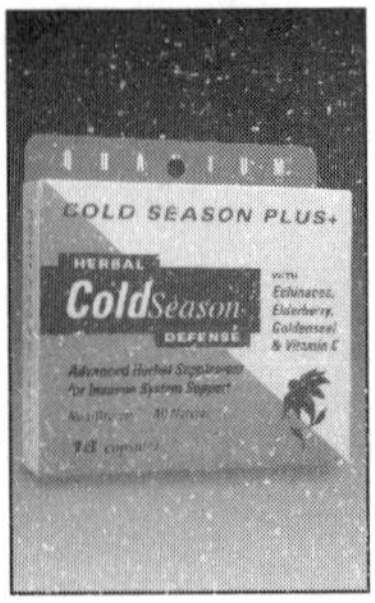

Cold Season Defense

$1 Cash Back

Buy one or more Cold Season Plus+ Cold Season Defense and receive $1.00 back on each. All items must be purchased at the same time and be listed on a single receipt. Just send this coupon (no photocopies) with your proof of purchase receipt to:

Quantum Mail In Rebate

PO Box 2791, Eugene, OR 97402

No expiration date on this cash back rebate.

For Store Information Call: 1-800-448-1448 www.quantumhealth.com

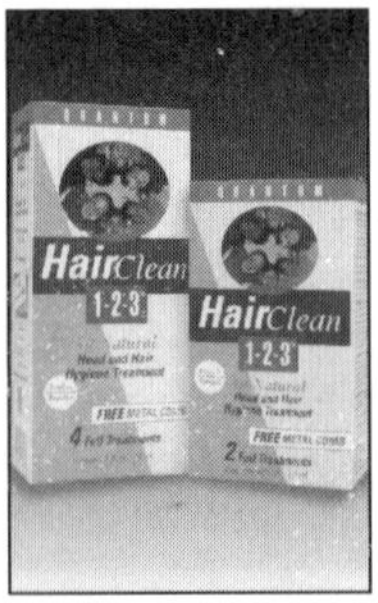

HairClean 1-2-3

$2 Cash Back

Buy any of our HairClean 1-2-3 products and receive $2.00 back. All items must be purchased at the same time and be listed on a single receipt. Just send this coupon (no photocopies) with your proof of purchase receipt to:

Quantum Mail In Rebate

PO Box 2791, Eugene, OR 97402

No expiration date on this cash back rebate.

For Store Information Call: 1-800-448-1448 www.quantumhealth.com

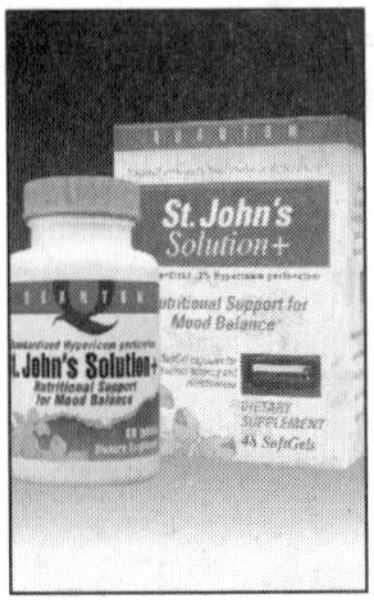

St. John's Solution

$1 Cash Back

Buy one or more of our St. John's products and receive $1.00 back on each. All items must be purchased at the same time and be listed on a single receipt. Just send this coupon (no photocopies) with your proof of purchase receipt to:

Quantum Mail In Rebate

PO Box 2791, Eugene, OR 97402

No expiration date on this cash back rebate.

For Store Information Call: 1-800-448-1448 www.quantumhealth.com

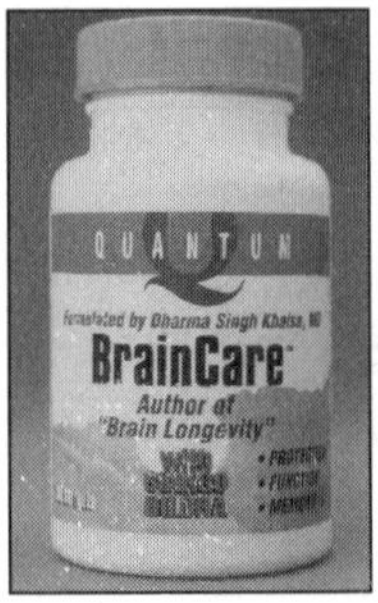

BrainCare

$2 Cash Back

Buy one or more of our BrainCare and receive $2.00 back on each. All items must be purchased at the same time and be listed on a single receipt. Just send this coupon (no photocopies) with your proof of purchase receipt to:

Quantum Mail In Rebate

PO Box 2791, Eugene, OR 97402

No expiration date on this cash back rebate.

For Store Information Call: 1-800-448-1448 www.quantumhealth.com

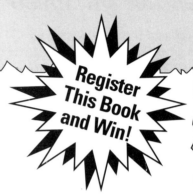

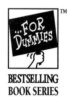